The Nutrilite Story:
Past, Present, Future

With a Dream, Anything is Possible

By Sam Rehnborg, Ph.D.

ENVIRONMENTAL STATEMENT: The Nutrilite Story is printed on Rolland Enviro 100 Print, which contains 100 percent post-consumer waste (PCW) & is manufactured 100% with Renewable Energy. The paper is FSC certified by the Forest Stewardship Council, which promotes environmentally appropriate, socially beneficial & economically viable management of the world's forests.

This issue used 55,000 lbs of 100 percent PCW paper. The environmental savings from using this paper in lieu of virgin paper is equivalent to:

- 468 Trees saved.
- 1,274,680 Liters of wastewater flow saved.
- 29,590 Kilograms of green house gases prevented.
- 13,475 Kilograms of solid waste prevented.

Estimates were made using the Environmental Defense Paper Calculator.

This entire book was printed with vegetable-oil based inks on recycled paper that contains 100 percent post-consumer waste.

Editor: Lorna Williams
Designer: Marie deVera Seiden
Cover design: William Young
Imaging and Production: Amway Paper Products

©2009 Amway Corp. All rights reserved.
Printed in U.S.A.

TO MY FATHER, C. F. REHNBORG, 1887–1973,

and to the millions of distributors past and present who have carried his message of good nutrition and optimal health to the people of the world.

Table of Contents

Introduction		7
Prologue		9
Part I: Between Heaven and Earth		15
Chapter 1	My Father	17
Chapter 2	A Place of Golden Opportunities	35
Chapter 3	Soul Searching	51
Chapter 4	Milk from Contented Cows	59
Chapter 5	Food for Thought	67
Chapter 6	The Entrepreneur	83
Chapter 7	A Pearl from the Orient	93
Part II: Building a Dream		103
Chapter 8	Desert Interlude	105
Chapter 9	From Stovetop to Storefront	113
Chapter 10	Burning the Midnight Oil	125
Chapter 11	Vita-Man	133
Chapter 12	The Birth of NUTRILITE	143
Chapter 13	The Salesman and the Educator	165
Chapter 14	Jackpot!	175
Chapter 15	The Potentates	187
Chapter 16	DOUBLE X and Double Jeopardy	203
Chapter 17	BEST OF NATURE, BEST OF SCIENCE	217

Chapter 18	Global Citizen	227
Chapter 19	South Seas Adventure	241
Chapter 20	The Clash over Cosmetics	253
Chapter 21	Amway	261
Chapter 22	Weathering the Storm	267
Chapter 23	Passing the Torch	279
Chapter 24	The Golden Years	291

Part III: Making a Difference — **303**

Chapter 25	Reunion	305
Chapter 26	My Sabbatical	315
Chapter 27	Coming Full Circle	323
Chapter 28	The Perfect Balance	333
Chapter 29	A Look at Today and a Glimpse into the Future	349

Acknowledgements — **362**

Appendix — **366**

	Appendix 1. What's In a Name?	366
	Appendix 2. Nutrition and Nutrilite Timeline	369
	Appendix 3. The Nutrilite Opportunity	392
	Appendix 4. Best of Science (Publications List)	394

Reference Materials — **402**

Index — **416**

"With a dream, anything is possible."

– Sam Rehnborg

Introduction

Sam Rehnborg, at 73, could easily be mistaken for a man 20 years his junior. At least that's the conclusion anyone would draw from an objective assessment of his energy, fitness, intellectual capacity, alertness, and overall disposition. There is something else. It's in the voice: a certain familiarity and a youthful tenor. It's also in his actions: a determined amiability and unflagging optimism that reclassifies problems as "challenges." It must be DNA. The longevity of a Scandinavian burnished by Southern California sunshine. Or, passionate diet and exercise. Or is it, could it be, the products he takes daily, the products he has taken for as long as there has been a NUTRILITE™ brand?* The regimen he, in a literal sense, embodies. No, it couldn't be the products. Or could it?

In this long-awaited book, Dr. Sam Rehnborg, the youngest son of Carl Rehnborg, shares the story of his father's journey as he developed what is believed to be the first multivitamin/multimineral supplement in North America. It's a classic "rags to riches" story—sparsely but vividly told that demonstrates what it takes to follow your dreams. It's an incredible journey. You're in for a great ride!

Steve Van Andel
Chairman, Amway

Doug DeVos
President, Amway

*NUTRILITE is a trademark of Alticor Inc., Ada, Michigan.

"Genius consists
in looking at
what others look at,
and seeing what others
do not see."

— Albert Szent-Györgyi

Prologue

NUTRILITE is in my blood. My father, Carl F. Rehnborg, often referred to me as the first Nutrilite guinea pig. After seven decades, it's a moniker that I continue to treasure with pride and have proudly repeated thousands of times to millions of people around the world.

While I've eaten NUTRILITE™ food supplements every day since childhood, it's more than just a trusted brand and a thriving business. Nutrilite is the realized vision of my father's lifelong passion to see human nutrition brought back into natural balance. More than that, Nutrilite is a network of millions of people around the globe—scientists, business owners, employees, and consumers—whose lives have been touched by the enduring idea of "THE BEST OF NATURE - THE BEST OF SCIENCE™."[†] I came to Nutrilite by birth, but I have embraced it as my own lifelong passion because I believe that my father was right, and the world is finally catching up to his ideas.

The story of Nutrilite is inextricably linked to the story of my father. By the time he passed away in 1973 at the age of 85, my father had achieved success by any measure. He had created what is believed to be the first multivitamin/multimineral dietary supplement sold in North America. He was instrumental in the development of an often misunderstood, but fundamentally brilliant, marketing plan known today as multilevel marketing. He even made significant contributions to the world in such diverse fields as eco-tourism, organic farming, religion, and profit sharing. Still, the quality I most admired in him was his insatiable curiosity about the world. He taught me to do what I'm good at, and keep at it.

At its core, the story of Nutrilite and of my father is the quintessential American dream. For those with no previous knowledge of Nutrilite, this book describes the story

[†] THE BEST OF NATURE – THE BEST OF SCIENCE is a trademark of Alticor Inc., Ada, Michigan.

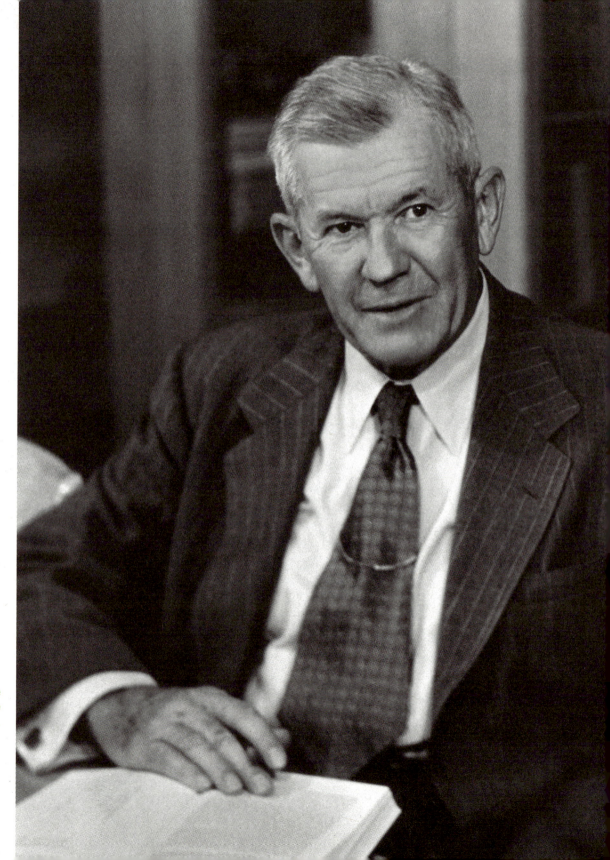

Carl F. Rehnborg at the age of 66, 1953. Books were never far from his sight.

PROLOGUE

of a man with an enduring entrepreneurial idea who survived World War I, the Great Depression, World War II, legal battles with the U.S. Food and Drug Administration, unscrupulous characters, and many false turns to launch what would become the world's leading brand of vitamin, mineral, and dietary supplements.[‡] For those who are familiar with Nutrilite and know the basics, this book will fill in the details and provide never before published information and insights behind one of the men responsible for spawning the worldwide dietary supplement industry that today exceeds $50 billion annually.

People have described my father as a man of powerful contradictions. He was an unfocused youth who became a man of singularly obsessive direction, a college dropout who made himself a scholar in many disciplines. He fell victim to con artists, yet possessed a genius IQ. He eventually achieved financial success, but probably was happiest in his laboratory making the products he loved. He was stubborn and obstinate, yet passionate and tenderhearted. He was an entrepreneur long before it was either a common term or an accepted career path. Above all, he was his own man who had courage and commitment to blaze his own trail.

My father's lifelong path began in China where his inspiration for a plant-based nutritional supplement first emerged. In China he became deeply impressed with the holistic wisdom of traditional Chinese culture and medicine. He was interested in balance—in the Chinese philosophy of yin and yang. This can be seen in his philosophy of bringing the diet back into balance with the use of food supplements and also in his keen awareness of the balance between man and the universe that he wrote about extensively in his later life.

When he returned to the United States, he worked almost obsessively to create, manufacture, and market the products he envisioned. It wasn't easy—food supplements were a novel concept, and the American medical establishment and federal regulatory agencies were vigorously opposed to the idea. Depression-era timing and the field of nutritional sciences still in its infancy didn't help matters. He persevered through it all because he believed that he had a product that people needed, and he was determined to get it to them.

While trying to market his food supplements, he pioneered a new method of selling based on his belief that the most effective way to sell a product was word of mouth. He

---

[‡] Based on 2008 sales as supported by research conducted by Euromonitor International.

reasoned that people trust their friends, so money that would otherwise be spent on advertising should instead be used as an incentive for individuals to share products they already used and trusted with their friends. In effect, to encourage people to be a "product of the product," and thereby inspiring others to want to use the same product. It's an idea that is as relevant today as it was then. This is the foundation of multilevel marketing, now in use by more than 30 million people worldwide. One of the biggest multilevel marketing businesses, Amway, grew indirectly out of my father's idea for selling NUTRILITE food supplements.

During his lifetime my father was fortunate to have had the opportunity to meet many people, dignitaries and world leaders alike. Charles S. Rhyne was one of those people. Charlie was a famous attorney with a prestigious law career that included among other things arguing several cases before the U.S. Supreme Court. During his long and influential life, Charlie met with Supreme Court Justices, every president from Franklin Roosevelt to Bill Clinton, and world leaders including Winston Churchill and Nehru. He was featured on the cover of *Time* magazine for his work creating what would become World Law Day. When asked who, of all the impressive people he had met in his lifetime, had in fact impressed him the most, Charlie hesitated a few seconds to ponder before answering: "Carl Rehnborg."

Throughout history, Nutrilite has been at the vortex of two industries that have had their fair share of controversy: food supplements and multilevel marketing. Yet, when you read this book and come to understand the history and foundation upon which they are based, I expect that many of the common misconceptions about both will be cleared up and you will gain a new appreciation for the origins of two very important fields.

In the end, I hope my father's life and enduring vision for Nutrilite inspires you: Do what you're good at and keep at it. Along the way, maintain a healthy curiosity about the world, seek truth, and pay attention to the details.

Prologue

Part I:
Between Heaven and Earth

"Man cannot discover new oceans unless he has the courage to lose sight of the shore."

— Andre Gide

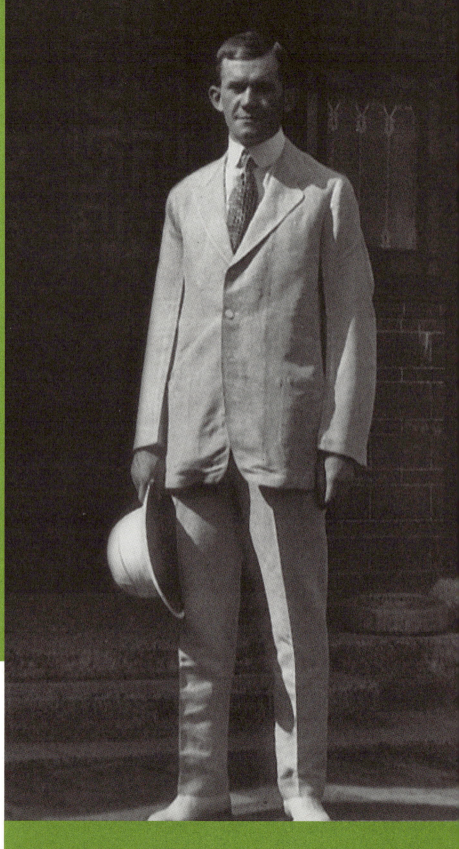

Carl F. Rehnborg In Tsinanfu, China, July 1916. The negative of this photograph, along with 55 others, was discovered in September 1997 tucked inside old, fragile film envelopes.

Chapter 1 | My Father

I look at the photograph and smile. Serendipity has stepped in, bringing it to life. It's a photograph of my father, Carl F. Rehnborg. He's standing bathed in a light so bright that the khaki of his linen suit looks almost white. Wearing a sporty tie, crisp collar on his white shirt, pith helmet in his right hand, his bearing is confident and casual. It's standard-issue summer attire for a representative of the Standard Oil Company of New York, his employer. Behind him, cast in shadow, is what looks like a temple. It's the summer of 1916 and my father is in China.

In the photograph, there's no hint of the heat and humidity that pervades coastal China during that time of year, not even a drop of sweat on my father's face. Even in the early morning hours, the temperature is pushing into the 80s, yet the creases of his trousers are as crisp as the part of his hair. He looks the epitome of the successful American businessman.

The photograph was printed from a negative discovered by one of my daughters among others lost in the garage of my father's widow. The image is of a man with his career and life ahead of him. On my father's face, there's no trace of the false starts he left behind in the United States. Poised and assured, his future awaits him.

My dad is in China because of what must have been an inherited sense of adventure. Over three decades earlier, his father, Carl Johan Paulus Rehnborg, emigrated from his home in Sweden to a new life in the United States. Paul, as he was known in the States, settled in the fledgling resort community of St. Augustine, Florida. It was a land of opportunity; a town where wealthy East Coasters flocked during the winter months.

The Nutrilite Story

With his gift for conversation, keen mind for business, and more than his fair share of entrepreneurial prowess, Paul parlayed his training as a silversmith into a thriving jewelry business and quickly became a well-respected member of the community. Things were so good, he encouraged his brother, sister, and widowed father to come to America and set up shop in St. Augustine.

As Paul's business grew, he was pleased to have his family with him. He soon began to think of starting a family of his own when a local painter by the name of Alice Maria Upton caught his eye. Alice would often stroll from her father's photography shop on Hypolita Street into Paul's jewelry store on Treasury Street. While visiting, she probably couldn't help but notice the designer. Always dressed impeccably with short, well-groomed hair, Paul had Swedish good looks that made him stand out from the crowd. With his gregarious good nature, Paul enjoyed the give-and-take of conversation with his customers. Not only would he discuss his artisan-crafted jewelry, but he would find out more about his visitors. He discovered, for example, that many of them could afford to winter in Florida and summer in New England where their kids could play in the fresh air and open countryside. Many of his customers had three homes or would make hotels their homes in the resort areas. There was definitely an opportunity to expand his business if he chose. At the same time, as he saw more and more of Alice, he was becoming increasingly enchanted with her ways.

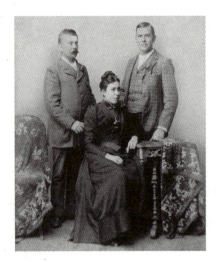

Formal portrait of Paul Rehnborg (far right) with brother Gustav Emanuel "Manny" Rehnborg and sister Lydia "Lillie" Rehnborg, circa 1879. This photograph was taken prior to Paul's emigration from Sweden to America.

Paul soon began to adjust his inventory to make souvenirs that his visitors could take home with them. He introduced "Florida curiosities," such as alligator jewelry, as well as colorful seashells. Paul also started selling Alice's artwork, which consisted of painted scenes of Florida.

Paul and Alice began to see more of each other. Sometimes, they would sit quietly listening to the scratchy cylinders playing classical music on the phonograph or reading one of the many books in Paul's growing library. Other times they might be found roaming the few blocks to the Alameda, also known as Lover's Lane, to linger under the shady live oaks past the cathedral. In the evening, they would often take a stroll under the stars with Paul expertly pointing out the constellations. When the weather was bad, they could watch the storms brewing off the Atlantic Ocean.

Chapter One: My Father

Paul also got to know Alice's father, Benjamin Franklin Upton. Mr. Upton was a pioneering photographer in Maine and Minnesota before he and his family relocated to Florida for his wife's health. Ben Upton enjoyed the outdoors and would go camping in the wilderness of Central Florida with the Rehnborg brothers to photograph the landscape. Even in his 80s, Mr. Upton was known to pack his glass plates and box cameras onto his bicycle and ride off into the woods to take photos.

The relationship between Paul and Alice blossomed into an engagement and, on May 5, 1885, the 26-year-old Paul and his nearly 30-year-old fiancée piled onto a train with their families and headed for a 25-mile trip to the city of Jacksonville (St. John's County) where they tied the knot in a Methodist service. Mr. Upton recorded the event in his well-used family Bible. The newlyweds settled in Paul's home above the jewelry shop in St. Augustine.

It was a happy time, but it was also a time tinged with sadness. Alice lost her mother due to respiratory complications. The town also suffered a crippling blow. On April 12, 1887, Paul and Alice woke up in middle of the night to the scream of sirens and the smell of smoke. They rushed outside and saw firefighters dragging their fire wagons to the St. Augustine Hotel. A fire had started in the boiler room of the wooden hotel and had swiftly swept to the rafters. Leaping from the building, the flames ripped through the old Spanish structures lining the Alameda until they began licking at the 200-year-old cathedral. While priests and parishioners hurried to save the chalice and altar pieces, sparks flew across the tree-lined street to the public market, igniting the roof. The whole town, it seemed, was on fire. Paul and his brother rushed to their shops to save what they could, while Alice helped her father move his equipment to safety. When the cathedral clock chimed at 5:30 in the morning, the fire had burned itself out.

It was a somber scene. Where row after row of shops and houses had once lined the road, only coquina pillars remained, standing like sentries amid the smoldering wreckage of the buildings they had once supported. Paul and Alice were lucky, and so was Mr. Upton—their stores had been out of the path of destruction. The family banded together to help Paul's brother, whose watch shop was left in rubble.

Despite the disaster, two months after the fire, on June 15, 1887, Paul and Alice had something to celebrate. My father, Carl Franklin Rehnborg, was born. He was named after his two grandfathers, Carl Gustaf Rehnborg and Benjamin Franklin Upton.

The birth of my father coincided with the rebirth of St. Augustine. However, it would take some time before the little resort town could get back on its feet and again flourish with tourism. Until then, the southern end of the tourist trail had shifted back north to Savannah, Georgia. With a family to support, that's where Paul and Alice realized they needed to be. They packed their belongings and journeyed up the coast to their new home to begin a new chapter in their life.

When Paul and Alice arrived in Savannah, they found the residential area to be charming. The city had a European feel, a kind of stateliness and elegance that the more rough-hewn towns in Florida lacked. It may even have reminded Paul a bit of Stockholm, with its neat rows of brick houses lined up along each street, except of course for the lush, semi-tropical gardens planted in Savannah's many squares.

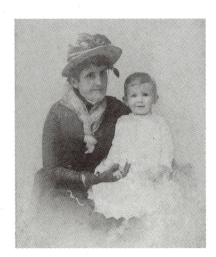

My father at age 2, with his mother Alice Rehnborg, circa 1889.

Paul's new shop, the Florida Bazaar, was walking distance from home and located on bustling Broughton Street. Here at his shop, he would dust off his display cases filled with colorful seashells and pieces of coral and straighten Alice's paintings. Between customers, he would sit at his little workbench surrounded by the tiny tools of his trade, shaping pieces of silver into pins, brooches, and lockets.

It was here by the sea that my father spent his idyllic early childhood years. And here, on March 3, 1889, when he was just learning to speak, his baby sister was born. Paul and Alice named her Pauline, in the family tradition of reusing the tried and true family names. But my father couldn't pronounce her name yet, so she became known as "Pump."

In 1891, when my dad was about four years old, the Rehnborgs moved a little further from Paul's shop to a quieter residential neighborhood of Savannah. The narrow row house at 150 Taylor Street had a deep backyard where my father and Pump could play, surrounded by high brick walls that separated their world from their neighbors. Just outside their front doorway was Chatham Square, an acre of flowers, grass, and stately trees. A few blocks away was the even grander Forsyth Park where

Chapter One: My Father

the children could see the flower gardens, a Confederate memorial, and a giant fountain whose waterspouts shot a dozen feet into the air. It was a wonderful place to grow up.

It wasn't long before they had company. Their brother Kay Porter Rehnborg entered the world in November 1892. The family was growing and needed more space, so in 1894, they moved again to a larger home on Whitaker Street near the Savannah River.

About this time, when my father was seven years old, he contracted a mild bout of polio, which affected his feet. During those days, many people were affected. The practice of medicine had only just become more reliable than folk remedies for the treatment of many illnesses. Alice was like most mothers of the era. She no longer believed in many of the old tales she had been told by her own mother, but wanted to help her family and so would try those remedies she found worthwhile. She gave my father sulfur and molasses every spring, telling him it would "thin the blood." She didn't explain why his blood had gotten thicker during the winter, or how sulfur and molasses would effectively make it thinner, or what the value of thin blood was in the first place. Instinctively, Alice used recipes that called for boiling herbs for teas or adding them to soup to cure colds, but she had no idea of the science behind it, as vitamins had yet to be discovered.

My father found it uncomfortable to run long distances or participate in typical childhood games like tag because of the polio, so he turned to swimming, which became his favorite sport. He also took to riding a unicycle. It was just like him to find a solution when a challenge arose; the first of many.

In Savannah, Dad's love of adventure took root. He could hear the shrill sound of whistles blowing as trains from the nearby train station departed for distant metropolises like New York and New Orleans. He could walk with his parents to the docks just a few blocks from their home and watch the sleek clipper ships sailing into port with heaps of silk from China, or observe steamers bound for Europe with loads of cotton. Even at home, tucked into bed as the gentle river breezes rustled the curtains of the open windows, he could listen to a symphony played by the deep bass steamship horns as they passed in the night to faraway places. In his dreams, he could imagine himself sailing to a distant land, just like his father had done before him.

Life in Savannah was full and busier than it had been in St. Augustine. Paul had essentially tripled his market. Not only could he sell his goods to tourists vacationing in the

THE NUTRILITE STORY

city, but also to those traveling further south who might have left some jewelry behind and needed a replacement, as well as to those traveling north who had forgotten to buy souvenirs to give to friends.

Paul's business was prospering, so much so that he moved his shop from Broughton Street into the De Soto Hotel, the "leading tourist hotel of the South," according to its brochure. Although Broughton, the main business street, had undoubtedly been a good location for local traffic, Paul couldn't have asked for a higher profile spot than the De Soto. When passenger liners arrived at the lively city, waiting carriages whisked the travelers straight to the nearby hotel, where they visited Paul's new shop, buying his latest creations.

As an astute businessman, Paul was always looking for new opportunities. One thing that he began to notice was the cyclical nature of his business, which dropped significantly during the hot summer months when few tourists visited. For a while, Paul watched as the business trade disappeared north with the coming of the warm weather, but in the summer of 1896, he took the leap and moved his family north to the tiny town of Huntington, Connecticut, just up the hill from Shelton and a short trolley and then train ride to New York City.

Meanwhile, the family continued to grow. Franklin Huntington Rehnborg was born on June 26, 1896, and three years later on June 6, 1899, Sara Alice Rehnborg, known as Sallie, arrived. She was born a twin; however, the other baby didn't survive. It was Sallie who my father was perhaps closest to in the family. As a protective and older brother by 12 years, he doted on his sweet baby sister. All in all, there were now five children in the Rehnborg clan—three boys (Carl, Kay, and Frank) and two girls (Pump and Sallie).

The move to Huntington proved to be a good one. Paul was soon able to afford a summer farm in Bethlehem, New Hampshire, a newly popular summer destination for East Coasters to beat the heat and humidity of the big cities.

From early on in life, my dad grew accustomed to moving and taking family trips to follow the seasonal migrations of the wealthy East Coasters. The family would stop at county fairs and resorts along the way, traveling up and down the East Coast from New York to Florida to sell his father's jewelry and mother's artwork. Accompanying them on their travels were several animals,

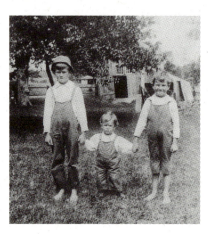

Dad, about age 11, with younger brothers Frank and Kay (from left to right), circa 1899. The Rehnborg children spent quite a bit of time enjoying the outdoors.

Chapter One: My Father

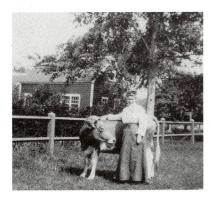

The homestead in Huntington, Connecticut and Bossie the cow (with unknown woman), circa 1896. Bossie supplied the Rehnborg family with fresh milk.

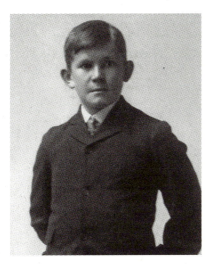

My father at age 12, posing for a studio portrait, 1899.

including Bossie the cow who supplied the family with milk. During these trips, my father was exposed to a wide variety of environments and people, which kindled his interest in the histories and cultures of the world. These trips were also a welcome chance for him to read. He loved to absorb the *National Geographic Magazine*. As the new century dawned, nearly every issue was filled with articles about a mysterious country called China on the other side of the world. Even at a young age, my father devoured everything he could find on what was called the Orient. Everything about it seemed so different—the art, the culture, even the unusual way of writing.

In a way, my father already lived between different worlds, both geographically and culturally as well. While the Rehnborgs weren't poor, the family depended on income from the wealthy who could afford Paul's jewelry, so their worlds overlapped. My father attended Shelton High School in Connecticut with children whose parents worked for the stair factory and the woolen mills. Yet, Paul made sure his family was well-dressed and, most importantly, that they were well-educated. Thanks to Paul's library, my dad was surrounded by books. They jammed the shelves at home, which fueled his respect and love for knowledge. My father figured he had the best of both worlds—he was able to socialize with kids from well-to-do families if he wanted, while attending school with the most ambitious of the working-class students who would have to work hard if they were to achieve success.

It was assumed that my dad would follow in his father's footsteps, entering the family business. And so, after graduating from Shelton High School around 1904, he set out on the road to work as a sales representative for Paul's jewelry business, traveling in a circuit around New England. However, it soon became apparent that my father's personality and upbringing weren't going to coalesce into the usual track. There was something a little too unsettled, a little too stubborn, a little too curious and philosophical about him that yearned for a vocation quite different from the family business.

Perhaps that was the contribution of his mother's side. Alice was from a cultured family, herself an accomplished artist. My father took to painting at a young age and had an especially keen eye for detail as was evident in a scene he painted during a family outing of

The Nutrilite Story

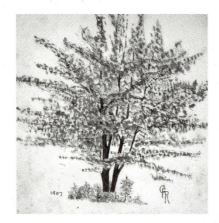

A watercolor painting of an arbutus tree created by Carl Rehnborg, 1907. Painting was one of the many activities my father enjoyed.

a blooming arbutus, capturing the tree at its peak, alive with pinkish flowers and red, strawberry-like fruit. His grandfather, Ben Upton, who had become well known for his photographs of the Chippewa, Winnebago, and Crow tribes in Minnesota, also played a role in his artistic upbringing, guiding my young father and instilling in him a love for photography and for the wilderness, where they would go camping on photographic expeditions.

During his late teen years, my father's little sister Sallie gave him a present that led to another lifelong habit: a composition book decorated with stickers that he turned into his first journal. He peppered it with quotes from writers and thinkers, including Cicero and Confucius, Byron and Sallust. Stuffed in the back were scraps of paper—tracing paper, graph paper, and artist's vellum covered with illustrations of things that captured his attention: a woman's hairstyle, an elaborate wrought-iron railing, designs for jewelry. You could also find some of his first attempts at poetry:

> *'That young Fibbs comes round too much,'*
> *said Sally's parents grim.*
> *'Now the very next time he comes round here,*
> *You want to sit on him.'*
> *Now Sally was an obedient girl,*
> *And obeyed parental powers,*
> *So the very next time young Fibbs came round*
> *She sat on him—two hours.*

He also practiced his puns:

> *I always thought that fleas were black,*
> *But now I know 'taint so;*
> *For Mary had a little lamb*
> *With fleece as white as snow.*

At times he would let weeks or months pass without a single entry. He used his journal to discuss his thoughts and what he had learned, rather than recounting what happened every day. Occasionally, after a long period without a single entry, he would

Chapter One: My Father

return with a new style of penmanship, ranging from an early imitation of typewriter script to a large and loopy middle style, to a tighter hand that seemed aimed more at efficiency than his earlier florid styles. By the end of the journal, he began crossing his T's with a strong, upward slash that would mark his handwriting for the rest of his life. It was about this time that his personal image began to change as well from a shy, childlike 19-year-old to a sophisticated man-about-town.

An unusual interlude, small in its own right, but huge in the impression it left on my father, came during the winter of 1906 when his family moved to Pinehurst, North Carolina, where the world's first golf resort, designed expressly to please the rich and famous could be found.

During this time, my dad worked for his father, seriously learning the jeweler's trade. He also continued painting, setting down his observations, and reading anything he could find. However, here in Pinehurst, he was also able to hobnob with some of the brightest and best. While in the past my father may have looked for role models in books, now he could also find them all around at Pinehurst. He didn't have to look far. He was surrounded by duPonts and Morgans and Mellons. According to the *Pinehurst Outlook*, John D. Rockefeller was back for his second season in 1905, and enjoyed it so much that he intended to return for a third season. My father also would have encountered renowned writers and performers as well. The Village Chapel's first pastor, Edward Everett Hale, wrote the best-seller, *A Man Without a Country*. Poet Edgar A. Guest, a frequent visitor to Pinehurst, may have inspired some of the doggerel in my father's journal. The world famous composer of *The Stars and Stripes Forever*, John Phillip Sousa, would go trapshooting near Pinehurst, and former cowboy Will Rogers, later a successful vaudeville and movie star, rode a pony in the polo matches in town.

The proximity to such extraordinarily successful people at Pinehurst must have had an impact on my father. Many people in his position, from a family of what were sometimes referred to at the time as "tradesmen," might have felt insecure in such a

A page from my father's 1906 diary. From a small start with diaries, he continued journaling throughout his life—keeping scores of journals and voluminous notes on his observations and correspondences.

surrounding, but these folks gave my father a self-confidence that continued to grow throughout his life. He seemed never to doubt himself. He felt as good as anyone he talked to, and conversely, that they were as worthwhile as he was. He held the quintessential American attitude—the same attitude that drove those who would have been pointed to as his role models growing up, like Thomas Edison or George Westinghouse: it took tenacity, intelligence, and hard work to make things happen rather than mere wealth.

Back at Pinehurst, it probably didn't hurt that my father was actively nurturing a dashing persona. In almost every photograph from his youth and young adulthood, he was sharply dressed—just like his father—in crisply pressed suits complete with a stiff, clean collar and well-polished shoes.

21-year-old Carl (left) and his father Paul Rehnborg, circa 1908.

Interestingly, at the back of his journal, next to a comical clipping about Lydia Pinkham's Vegetable Compound, he tucked a long list of "Rules" he invented for himself about self-conduct and successful accomplishment of what seemed to be his real passion in those younger years: attracting the attention of women. Not only was he dashing, but in conversation he made women feel special—as if they were alone in the room. In fact, most people who knew him later in life—men as well as women—felt that way. Coupled with his wide knowledge base groomed from avid reading and the gift of easy conversation, he was able to carry on a conversation with just about anyone about almost anything. In his journal, he copied and listed his 26 rules in all, numbering them one by one with Roman numerals, like this:

Rule II [2]: Even if you were voted the handsomest man in your class, don't presume that a lady is 'pinning roses on herself' simply because you are monopolizing all her calling hours.

Rule XVII [17]: Make up to the little sisters and all small girls. You may be able to lord over them when they are ten and you are twenty, but someday when they are twenty and you are thirty, the tables will be turned—and they don't forget!

Rule XXII [22]: Carry yourself with confidence but not over-assurance, remembering at the same time that everything is your fault.

CHAPTER ONE: MY FATHER

The rules seemed to work. He had gone dancing at the fancy Hotel Carolina and according to his journal:

> *I had a fine time! One dance I was standing in the door of the ballroom because I didn't care to dance and Miss Harris came up to me as I stood there. Miss Harris is one of the guests, a young woman of probably twenty-five. There were perhaps eight young men standing there, too. Well, she came up to me and said, 'Do you want to dance with me? I want to dance with someone who can.' Whew! Two or three for me and just a few for them. I could hear them gasp. And they were most awfully jealous. I recovered quickly and as we started off, I said, 'If I had only known you wanted to dance with me, I would have asked you long ago. I just didn't dare.' About the best thing I could have said for a starter, wasn't it?*

He was applying Rules 3 and 14, being sure to flatter and making sure she knew that he was impressed. As they danced, he also practiced Rule 5: "Dance a few extra steps and seem loath to let her go." This experience may have led him to come up with Rule 25: "Don't be timid about 'butting-in' at a ball. No girl in this world was ever annoyed because a man made her look popular."

My father was having a wonderful time; however, as a sales representative trying to establish distribution outlets for his father's jewelry business, his performance lacked focus. He worked hard by his own account, but it seemed to take second place to his passions for socializing, dancing, and making sales rounds riding his unicycle. After traveling down south to the Carolinas and Georgia to step up distribution outlets for the family business in Lakewood, Asheville, Camden, Augusta, Savannah, and Aiken, he returned home owing more money than he had earned. As he put it in his journal:

> *Business has been so poor for two years, and I have been so little of a man, that Dad and I amicably concluded that I would reap benefit from working for someone else.*

And that's exactly what he did, finding himself a job as a supervisor at R.U. Bassett Company, a garter and corset manufacturer. He lasted only a few weeks. His boss reluctantly let him go because his amiable style failed to motivate the crew. Being friends with the men and getting them to work were two entirely different things, my father found. He summed up the experience in his journal:

Now make all possible excuses for me, old book, for I have been fired! Of course, Mr. Northrup, the Super, assured me that the only reason was my inability to make my men work. Reasons are bald—the fact remains. He also told me that he would be glad to recommend me to anyone I named, and that he would make a point of seeing Dad, and of explaining it all to him in the most favorable light. Then he said that he regretted my going, that he had confidence in me, etc. A bean in the lion's mouth.

Mr. Northrup was true to his word and put the best spin on the situation, but my dad was now back working for his father. "Dad and I are now one, and I do earn my pay," my father wrote in his journal. My dad was happy that his father took him back into the business and, in typical fashion for him, celebrated with an adventure. He bought a new pair of shoes. In his journal he wrote:

They were nice high shoes that included my trousers when they folded about my young bovines (fearfully witty).

I put on the shoes and started on a walk. The first day I walked to Southington, 32 miles, and the next day to Hartford through Farmington, 17 miles, where I arrived at 2 PM. Then I felt tired of walking and went back home by train.

Even all that walking couldn't keep my father from getting restless. No matter how much he tried to stick to the jewelry business, things kept pulling him in another direction. At the age of 22, he had written in his journal:

I want to go on the stage and to that end I shall go to New York and try for a position there, in some store or office, to the end that I may seek to find an opening into the theatrical profession.

However, by the fall of 1909, it looked like things were settling down on a track. My father was accepted to the Pratt Institute in Brooklyn, New York, to begin serious study in the jewelry design program. Pratt was (and is) a marvelous institution offering the highest quality of art education to those accepted to the program.

At Pratt, my father met a fellow student named Hester Hawkes, a young heiress whose family had an estate called Wingaersheek, up in Gloucester, Massachusetts. They became friends as they found themselves consistently attending the same classes. They shared their big dreams in some lively conversations, discovering a common love for adventure and travel, including a mutual interest in China, a mysterious place that was suddenly

CHAPTER ONE: MY FATHER

in the news because of huge shifts in its political situation. To an adventurous young man or woman, China at that time was like the Soviet Union after the fall of the Berlin Wall, full of danger and opportunity. Hester put together a scrapbook that contained cutouts of photographs and printed drawings of exotic places like the Forbidden City and the Cloud Rock Temple and the Great Wall of China, along with her own drawings. Dad included similar drawings in his journal.

My father's relationship with Hester might have blossomed further, but within a year he was no longer attending Pratt. Why did he leave? There isn't a clue in his journal. A likely possibility is that he decided once and for all that he just wasn't cut out for the jewelry business. It may have been a great occupation for his father, grandfather, and uncle, but it wasn't for him—his heart wasn't in it. However, his days at Pratt weren't entirely a waste. Deciding "not" to go into the jewelry business is still a certainty of sorts.

So what did he do? My father, always the optimist, knew something would turn up, his brown eyes sparkled with ideas. For my father, it was a time of infinite possibilities. He could become an artist like his mother, or maybe a poet or writer. He could be a photographer like his grandfather, Ben Upton, or maybe go into the sciences. He had many interests—which made it tough to choose one. Every opportunity was filled with potential.

And, something did turn up. What my father chose to do at this time was break new ground. Sometime after dropping out of Pratt, my father went on to develop a revolutionary flooring material made out of melted rubber, sawdust, and other special ingredients. It was fireproof. It was waterproof. People told him it was good, a surefire success. He and his partner envisioned it covering the floors of the world. They took samples to various warehouses to sell their idea. Finally, one company consented to let them put down a sample floor as a test of the product. He and his partner worked feverishly installing the flooring. Unfortunately, according to Hester, "…it cracked! Was most unsatisfactory." My father just didn't have the money to do further research or experimental tests, so he gave it up.

To make matters worse, his mother, Alice, became ill. She may have inherited a susceptibility to her own mother's bronchial condition, which had originally brought her family to St. Augustine. She contracted pneumonia and died in August 1911 at the age of 56. Less than one year earlier, Grandpa Upton had also died after a good, long life of 92 years.

For my dad, it was a very difficult loss. It was also tough for his father, Paul, who was now a widower with five children, three still in their teens. Business also appeared to be slow, as Paul was forced to sell some of the Bethlehem farm at a tax sale in 1912. But for a man like Paul, who was used to assessing a situation and reacting accordingly, he took matters into his own hands and moved his business south for the winter to Camden, South Carolina. There, he set up shop in a house that he called Flower Cottage, where he made his "absolutely safe safety pins," which he was quite proud of for their usefulness. From Camden, he also corresponded with Lillian Glynn, a young widow who lived about 650 miles away in Derby, Connecticut, down the hill from Huntington. Her husband had died of typhoid fever after seven years of marriage. In his letter, Paul described their meeting at a party and promised to return to New Haven in the spring. "You know I am a lonely fellow and while I love the ladies in a general way, like some others, I love some in a more particular way." About a year after Alice's death, Paul and Lillian were married.

My dad was also living in Camden, but he and Paul were no longer "as one," as they were just before he left for Pratt. Perhaps it was due to Paul's high hopes for his bright, yet restless son. During this time, my father found work as a street car conductor in Columbia, South Carolina. He was now 26 years old and beginning to feel pressure to accomplish something with his life.

With newfound motivation in the fall of 1914, my father made his second attempt at college, this time at the University of South Carolina. He passed the entrance exam and enrolled in September. He chose a more general course of study this time with classes in math and science, but also medieval and modern European history, German, and composition and rhetoric. It was here that my dad may have written an essay called *Is Conformity Desirable?* that provides a glimpse into his state of mind at the time. He wrote:

> *We conform to the rules of society, the rules of a household, the rules of the classroom, or the rules of a game, because these are the mechanics of convenience in living. So we may witness, or take part in, pranks and parades and picnics, and enjoy ourselves highly doing it, without changing the fact that we should not imitate a senior classman because he sets a campus profile, or acquire a phony accent to be like a self-appointed superior class, or even agree completely at all times with the professors…Instead we have to be concerned consciously and for all our lives with creating, from the materials of the universe which*

CHAPTER ONE: MY FATHER

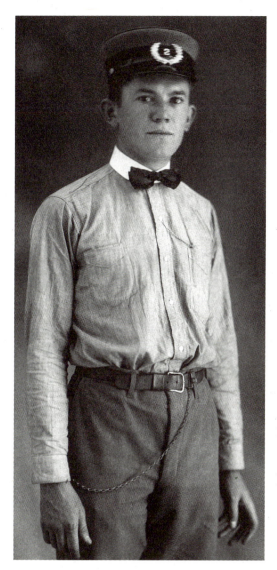

Carl Rehnborg in his streetcar conductor uniform in Columbia, South Carolina, circa 1913. One of many jobs my father held.

came into our possession, the thoughts and things only we can create because we happen to be our individual selves, unlike any other self anywhere. And we have to do it with pride and with humility—humility in realizing that other men may do as well or better, and pride in doing our best with the tools and the materials the Boss made available to us.

He did well in most of his classes, especially chemistry and physics, but despite a strong beginning with all A's and B's, by spring he had dropped out. He had begun missing more and more of his classes while supporting himself in a full-time job as a copy editor at one of the city's three newspapers—the *Columbia Record*.

As a copy editor, he would have had difficulty getting up for an early class after a late night in the newsroom, putting the paper to bed instead of himself. And he had to be on his toes: he needed his full wits for copy editing. He would have to read column after column of typeset text upside down and backwards before it was made into printing plates, checking for errors and jokes that the typesetters or crusty reporters deliberately included just to trip up greenhorn copy editors. It was tough, but the experience taught him how to swiftly read a book—two pages at a time! I remember conducting a test on him while I was a young boy, hoping to prove he really wasn't reading. I gave him a book I knew he hadn't seen and asked him to read a few pages. After he zipped through the pages, I promptly gave him a pop quiz. He not only knew the facts, he knew the context. Not only did he become an adept speed reader thanks to that job at *Columbia Record*, his appetite for books became even more voracious—regularly reading a book a day for the rest of his life.

The University of South Carolina was Dad's last stab at formal education, with the exception of a three-month training course. In many ways, this was the beginning of what would be a non-traditional, but highly effective lifelong education for him. He took it upon himself to follow his natural curiosity—studying and absorbing the world and people around him, drinking in knowledge and taking in all that he could from books. To those who knew him and had experienced his brightness and energy, his zest for life and unforced geniality, it seemed just a matter of time and circumstances until the directed, focused part of his personality would awaken.

But what now? Even for my dad, it was hard to escape that sense of time running out, the frustration at all the dead ends. Although his early experiences and insights would contribute to the man he would become, it was a small consolation. He was 27 years old and had nothing much to show for his life but a series of dead ends. He had already run through more jobs than many people see in a lifetime: salesman in his father's jewelry business, supervisor at a corset and garter plant, aspiring actor, jeweler, inventor of a seamless flooring material, street car conductor, and copy editor. About the only common thread in all these jobs was his restlessness and natural curiosity.

He was interested in the world around him and wanted to see more of it. He loved to wander and explore new places. He was the kind of young man who would celebrate rejoining his father's business by buying a new pair of boots and walking for 49 miles in a couple of days or riding his unicycle for 52 miles through the mountains just for the fun of it. However, at this time, the phrase, "Go west, young man," may have been reverberating in his ears. Inspired by the tales of Jack London, he was drawn to Seattle with a dream of joining the Alaska gold rush, but once arriving discovered it was too late. There weren't any more prospectors striking it rich, just placer miners working like slaves for mere ounces of the precious mineral.

Seattle, however, opened the doors to a new adventure that would prove to be the right one for my father: China. China was the new Yukon, the place where young men of adventure discovered their future. People were making fortunes there. And the biggest fortunes were being made by the oil companies, the largest of which was Standard Oil Company of New York. My father returned home immediately to look into pursuing employment in China. The time was definitely right. He was ready for the adventure, to set sail for distant shores, and to discover his future.

CHAPTER ONE: MY FATHER

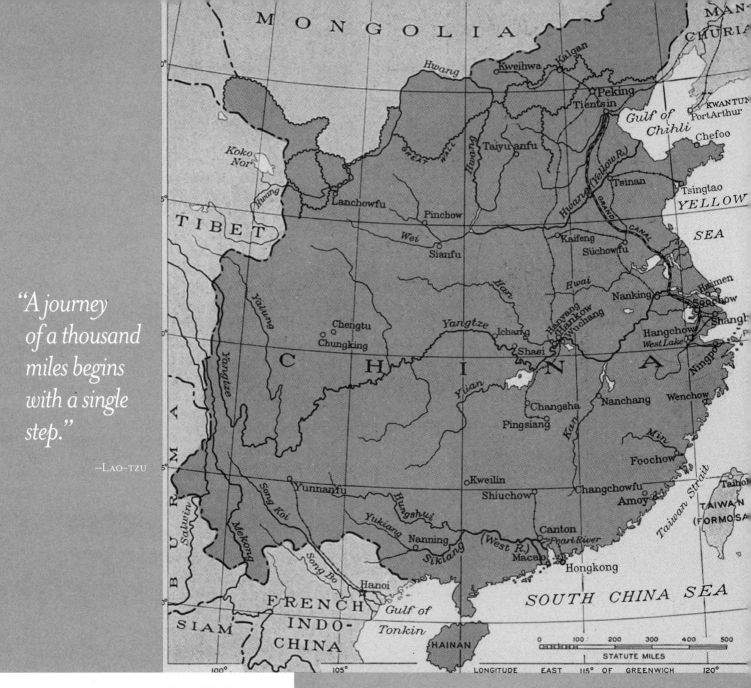

"A journey of a thousand miles begins with a single step."

—Lao-tzu

Map of China, 1927. The names of many cities have changed since this map was created. For example today Tientsin is known as Tianjin; Peking is known as Beijing; and Nanking as Nanjing. [A.H. Bumstead, National Geographic Stock]

Chapter 2 A Place of Golden Opportunities

When your destiny is to blaze new trails, it can make you feel like a square peg in a round hole. But when you find the right fit, magic can happen. So it was for my 28-year-old father during the fall of 1915 when he packed all his goods into a steamer trunk, stepped onto a train in Grand Central Station, and embarked on a journey that would take him halfway around the world. He would begin a new career in China as an accountant for Standard Oil Company of New York, which everyone called Socony for short. Beyond the obvious adventure of it all, the Socony job offered him the means to fulfill a deeper pull: something that had been tugging him powerfully since his days at Pratt Institute, or possibly before, toward that mysterious, inscrutable faraway land.

Before my father could leave, he had to pass a rigorous training program in New York, a program that would prepare him for his new life. During this time, he learned all about the oil business—about oil, solvents, fractionation, and vacuum distillations. He studied Chinese culture, history, and philosophy. He also learned about life as a foreigner in China—how visitors could live in foreign concessions that had the look and feel of their home country. The course was fascinating, but the competition was brutal and the pressure was intense. The class was whittled down from 100 to 20 students in three months. My father not only survived the cut, he thrived in the competitive environment, graduating with honors. His final 200-page project was so good that Socony accepted it as a model for assignments to other men, even putting some of his recommendations into effect. At graduation, the names of the students and their stations were read out. My father's home for the next two years would be Tientsin (today known as Tianjin), the "City of the Heavenly Ford," a large port city not far from Peking.

It must have been humbling for my father to stand under the canopy of golden stars in the expansive ceiling of Grand Central Station, his pith helmet and pongee suit carefully tucked away in his trunk, and try to imagine the adventure that lay ahead. Would it be like anything he and Hester imagined as they had pored over the news, events, and culture of China during their days at Pratt? His long journey began with a train ride from New York through the Midwest to catch a steamship from Vancouver, British Columbia, bound for China, after stops in equally exotic Honolulu and Yokohama.

At first, it seemed as if the train would never leave the endless city that surrounded New York, but it soon caught its rhythm and sped through the low mountains on its way to the Midwest. Looking out on the landscape as the train churned on, my father could see the rolling hills of Ohio where John D. Rockefeller had started Standard Oil. He changed trains in Detroit, the city where Henry Ford's amazing assembly line was cranking out Model T's so fast that almost anyone could own one. It was hard to imagine that just a few years before gasoline had been a waste product of the oil refining process, while kerosene for lamps and paraffin for candles were the primary products. In China that was still the case, but when all 400 million Chinese could afford motor cars, well, the future was almost unimaginable. It was a new century and a new world in which technology fueled by oil would make everyone's life better, and my father was now to play a part in this business, a business of almost limitless potential.

At night, my father drifted off to sleep to the soft heartbeat of the rails, padum-padum, padum-padum. He could look out at a sky with stars so thick that the Milky Way looked good enough to drink. Soon the artificial sky he had seen in Grand Central Station became only a memory. That was just a big building with a fancy ceiling. This was the universe. During the days, he could sit for hours reading and thinking in the light of the window as the Great Plains passed by outside. At night, he could read under the tulip lamps. He was fascinated with astronomy and the world around him. By this time, he had read books by Copernicus, Tycho Brahe, and Galileo, as well as books from other great thinkers such as Bacon, Descartes, Hegel, Kant, Spinoza, Schopenhauer, and Voltaire. He would tell people that "on a rich diet one sometimes gets mental indigestion." So he would spice it up with novels, popular histories, books about agriculture, religion, science, and nature. To him, it didn't really make any difference what you read, as long as you learn. It will all help you in the end.

When my father's train reached Calgary, more steam engines were added. Even with their massive horsepower, they still strained to pull the train over the Canadian Rockies. Every time my father thought they must have reached the Continental Divide, they began to climb again, the engines puffing with effort sending a cloud of smoke that carried a scent of the city back over the cars, while streams below ran with whitewater from pure mountain runoff. Waterfalls plunged through breaks in an almost continuous forest of Douglas fir, cedar, and pine. High trestles carried the train over rivers so clear my father could see salmon swimming upstream between the rocks that lined the bottom.

The regions past the Rockies reminded my father of the forests near Bethlehem, where he had spent so many happy summers growing up. Only here, in places, lumberjacks had been busy at work; where majestic pine trees once stood, now only an eerie wilderness of stumps remained. It seemed a shame to my father to see such wanton destruction. In the distance, he could see giant buildings shaped like saltshakers with glowing tops that burned sawdust from the lumber mills. Leech pits in phantasmagoric colors held the residue of the mining process, some of it seeping off in orange or purple streams.

Farther down in the Okanagan Valley, the streams cleared again, cattle grazed on lush alfalfa, and the fall harvest was beginning on some farms, with farmhands harvesting their crops or preparing them for shipment on rail. Then the mountains began again; the Cascades, just as high, but far greener than the Rockies. Occasionally the train would pass a line of flatcars loaded with massive logs taken from the apparently endless supply of timber in the mountains. A surprisingly short time after reaching the crest of the Cascades, the train descended into Vancouver where my father transferred to the steamship that would take him toward China.

That first evening on the steamship, the water glowed like soft fire. Ever curious, my father found out that the glow was caused by blooming phytoplankton that floated near the surface of the water. The trip was filled with wonders: whales on the horizon spouting and then diving to feed on the plankton, dolphins racing the ship like silver messengers, and schools of fish swimming in shiny streaks as they rushed to get out of the way of the steamer.

During the long voyage, my father spent much time with a Mr. Rich, General Manager of Socony operations in India. They struck up quite a good friendship. Mr. Rich saw something unusual in my conversant father who spent such a large part of his day reading. He was so impressed he tried to steal him away from Socony's Chinese division. "Come to India instead. I'll send you to Karachi," Mr. Rich said. "It's a very beautiful city." But my father was not tempted.

The steamer stopped briefly in Hawaii and then made its way to busy Yokohama, Japan.

After a brief stop in Yokohama, the steamer set sail again. On the way out of the city, my father could see massive battleships in the harbor. Whereas steel had once been restricted for use in making samurai swords, it was now being used to build rifles, mobile cannons, and ships. A day out of Yokohama, passengers on the deck were surprised to see what looked like a giant mud bank in the middle of the East China Sea. It was the water of the Yangtze River, carrying runoff from the deforested mountains of China. With nothing to hold the soil, enough silt was carried to the sea to extend the Yangtze's mouth eastward by several inches each day. The river's cream refused to mix with the sea's coffee. The dividing line between the two was visible for miles. The steamer waited for high tide, then continued up the Yangtze a short distance before branching into the Huangpu River where busy farmers with their harvest could be seen on the flatlands along the riverbank. Every inch of ground appeared to be cultivated—except where canals cut through the land. But even in the canals, my father could see people scooping rich silt from the bottom into their boats to spread on their fields.

The ship steamed slowly up the Huangpu. It seemed like a lifetime since my father had boarded the train in New York. At last, he was now standing at the railing watching a collection of enormous black oil tanks lining the riverbank like squat sentries welcoming him to China, painted in Chinese characters that he knew spelled the name Socony used in China: MEI FOO YANG HONG. "Mei Foo" meant "beautiful country," while "Yang Hong" meant "foreign business."

And so he entered China. His first stop was the bustling city of Shanghai. From the steamer, he could see the city itself as he looked across the river and upstream from the oil tanks. Even from the middle of the river where the steamer dropped anchor, my father

Chapter Two: A Place of Golden Opportunities

could feel the energy vibrating from the city. It was a city where fortunes were made and just as quickly lost. Countless river steamers, freighters, junks, and sampans made their way up and downstream. Sailors and marines drilled on gunboats anchored nearby. On the shore, construction cranes lifted bricks and steel to the tops of unfinished buildings, while derricks on freighters transferred everything from shiny new automobiles to cages of squealing hogs onto the docks. Car horns honked as frustrated drivers pounded on their rubber bulbs trying to get balky rickshaw pullers and wheelbarrows out of their way. Dozens of sampans and launches descended on my father's ship to unload the cargo and transport the passengers to the docks along the shoreline or *bund* where foreign businesses flourished.

In Shanghai, my father quickly learned that China was a land of contrast, like the waters of the Yangtze, coexisting but refusing to mix with the sea. Modern office buildings rose next to dilapidated tenements; affluent Chinese in elegant silk gowns being pulled in rickshaws by men whose sole possessions were a loincloth and a ragged shirt. All of these contrasting elements added to the richness of his experience and the challenges he would face in understanding the place he would call home.

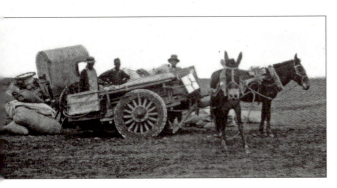

My father took hundreds of photos while living and working in China. On the back of this photograph he wrote: "Traveling cross country- stuck in mud ... there are no roads in inland China only paths and an occasional cart track," circa 1915-1917.

After the brief stopover in Shanghai to meet the general manager and review operations, my father headed north for the last leg of his journey by train. The study in contrasts continued. The train that carried him to Tientsin was even newer than the one in which he had crossed North America. His American-style breakfast was served on white linen with fresh flowers in a little vase that rivaled the most advanced of western luxury, yet he was looking out on a landscape reminiscent of the 15th century: a boatman on a canal sculling his sampan with a long oar called a *yuloh*; a pair of peasants using foot power to run a small waterwheel made of bamboo and scraps of wood; and farm families stacking rice stalks to dry for fuel. He also observed a small boy leading a mule that powered a stone grinding wheel and a fisherman waiting patiently while his cormorant, a bird with a long neck, dove to catch a fish, unable to swallow it because of the ring the fisherman had placed around its throat.

My father's train finally pulled into Tientsin's east station past what looked like a slice of Vienna, followed by a slice of Rome. It was as if he left China and entered a miniature Europe. He was met at the station by a representative of Socony. Together, the men journeyed by rickshaw to Socony's offices at Number 8, Quai de France. My father may have preferred to walk, but was told it was best and more honorable to ride. According to the representative, "It's his rice bowl." If you could afford the service, but chose not to ride, it was tantamount to stealing someone's bread—and it was clear there was no shortage of men whose primary job was to ferry people and their goods through the crowded streets.

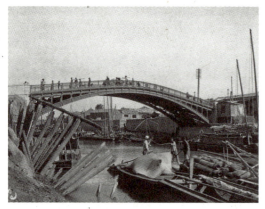

My father wrote on the back of this photograph, "A bridge on the Grand Canal as it enters Tientsin. Looks grand, doesn't it?," circa 1915-1917.

On his way in the rickshaw, my father passed through what looked like a bit of St. Petersburg, Russia, and while he crossed the river he noticed what appeared to be French carriages along the Seine. Just as his cart was making its way around the next river bend, he could make out some buildings in the distance that appeared to be from a Prussian industrial suburb or maybe even from Yokohama.

Finally, after having to struggle through the press of carters, wheelbarrows, and people balancing bundles on their shoulders, the rickshaw puller deposited my father at the office along with his steamer trunk, carried in a second rickshaw. The Socony representative paid the pullers, but was careful to watch out for being "fobbed off" as they said, with brass coins in place of silver for change.

"Welcome to Tientsin!"

My father had made an oral agreement to stay in China for the standard three-year term that Socony offered. After three years, he would receive a free passage home and a six-month furlough at full salary. Not only was he working for one of the largest and most efficient selling organizations in the world, he had also entered a whole new realm of self-worth, at least in Chinese terms. By entering China, my father had crossed the "Dragon's Gate." The Chinese considered their land to be exalted, far removed from the mundane world of their neighbors. Not that China was heaven of course—that kind of overbearing pride would be sure to invite punishment from the gods. But neither was China of the earth. China was the Middle Kingdom, between heaven and earth. Little had my father known it at the time, but by coming to China, in a real way he had come home.

CHAPTER TWO: A PLACE OF GOLDEN OPPORTUNITIES

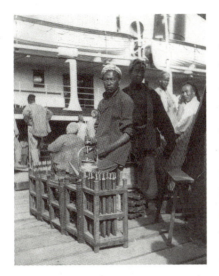

On the back of this photo my dad wrote: "The Tallyman and his Teakettle," circa 1915-1917.

But which China? There was a choice to be made; two very different experiences of China lay ahead of him, and the decision was his. It was possible to live in China within the thin, but seductive safety net of a veneer of European civilization—or to cut the umbilical cord and enter China. He had arrived in China, to be sure. But which China would he decide to encounter? During the previous 75 years, China had gradually and begrudgingly opened its gates to European trade: gates that had swung shut firmly in the 15th century. After the conclusion of what had been known as the Opium Wars in 1842, the British had wrested from the Chinese the right to build concessions. These were rather like cities within a city, with a familiar architecture and their own legal systems. The British and French concessions were the earliest to be created in Tientsin and were joined by Japan, Germany, Russia, and by countries without concessions elsewhere in China including Austria-Hungary, Italy, and Belgium.

In these compounds, it was possible to live a completely insulated Western lifestyle of wealth and privilege—walled off from the poverty, disease, and the danger of the world outside. In this bubble-like existence, a foreigner could speak his native tongue, eat his favorite national dishes, and read newspapers in his home language. He could live here in these foreign concessions for decades and never truly enter China—literally, because the foreign concessions were foreign territory governed by the laws of the home country.

For the time being, the westernized safety zone was the world my father would inhabit. He moved into a house by a canal shared by other young agents of Socony. One of the terms of the deal was Socony's strong preference that their young agents, known as *griffins*, remain single for at least two years. The frequent field trips would require arduous travel, and Socony felt that family responsibilities softened a man and divided his loyalties. The compensation was a college fraternity-type arrangement known as a bachelor mess. But, unlike most fraternities, it was amply staffed with servants whose wages were measured in pennies per day. My father had his own personal servant, or houseboy, Hua, who attended to his every need. At first, he was a bit uncomfortable about the idea, especially the part in which tradition suggested he call Hua by the name of "Boy." However, he was able to rationalize his dilemma by saying:

…the French call servants 'garcon,' which means boy, and so people who live in foreign lands have got in the habit of always calling their native servants 'boys.' The servants don't mind at all; in fact, my boy called me 'Master.'

My father learned that there was a classification applied to all those who helped around the bachelor mess. So the cook was known simply as "Cook," and if there were more than one cook, the boss would be "Number One Cook," and the assistant "Number Two Cook," and so on. And so my father and his friends lived in a kind of luxury that was almost unheard of back home. Each day, before my father woke, he'd find his bath ready and his clothes laid out neatly for the day. At night, he'd find Hua's handiwork again, his bed covers turned down and his pajamas set beside the edge of the bed.

It must have been hard for my father to concentrate on work the first few days after his arrival. It was a whole new world in so many ways. He had never been to Europe, yet he found himself living in a company house in the French concession that would have been right at home in Paris. On his way to work, it would have been easy to mistake his new home for some place in southern France. Plane trees lined the avenue, their trunks whitewashed to eye-level and their leafy canopies providing much needed summer shade. Behind the trees, he could see the elaborate doorways and French-style windows of the apartment blocks and the art-nouveau scroll work on the grilles and the signs announcing the local patisseries and boulangeries.

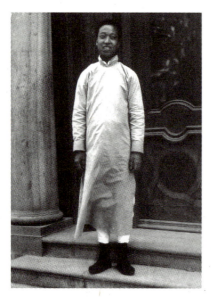

My father's personal assistant, Hua, June 4, 1916. Dad wrote on the back of this photo, "This is Hua (means flower) or Hughie standing on the steps of the hotel."

He had a wonderful time exploring this exciting city, and all the while he kept in contact with Hester—sending letters and photographs so she could enjoy, albeit vicariously, this strange and exotic world. He roamed the streets and temples taking photographs with his trusty Brownie and sent them to her by the score. In most ways, it was completely different from home, but there were some surprising similarities. After all, China had been a nation long before Europe had its first emperors and kings. It had been the scientific leader of the world up to the 15th century, developing the compass, paper, the first printing press, the first moveable type, and gun powder, and making tremendous contributions to anatomy, astronomy, and mathematics.

Chapter Two: A Place of Golden Opportunities

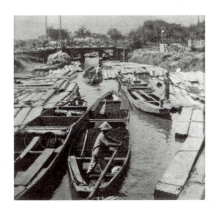

Tientsin, China, circa 1915-1917. My father wrote on the back of this photo, "This is the canal in front of the house on a busy day."

At his office, my father could look out the windows and see flat-bottomed riverboats and sampans moving upstream toward Peking or downstream toward the ocean or the Grand Canal. A few feet down the slippery canal bank floated a raft-like wharf made of rough-hewn timbers, where Chinese laborers unloaded fresh fish and other goods to be delivered to the nearby houses. My father could also see a boatman standing on the back of his sampan, shouting and cursing at the other boats that were blocking his path, as he pushed and pulled on the yuloh to guide his boat carefully between the close-set pilings of the low bridge just up the street.

My father knew Socony, too, had its own launches tied up outside the building. Much of the company's business was conducted via the waterways. The road system was still primitive outside the cities in China, so the fastest way to move people and goods was frequently via the network of canals and rivers. The railroads were also an efficient alternative, but they only connected the major cities.

My father worked at the Tientsin headquarters at first, training with Mr. Burns, the local manager. Socony had its own offices in all the treaty ports like Shanghai, Nanking, and Tientsin, which were run by Americans, but they also had agencies throughout the country owned and operated by the Chinese who had been carefully selected from an enormous pool of applicants, eager to cash in on the growth of the oil-fueled light business. My father, as an inspector, would travel out to these agencies and check the books and stock.

This was an auspicious beginning, but as soon as possible, my father vowed he was going to break out of the safety net and encounter China face to face. Neither his own curious nature nor his hunger for life and experience would allow him to remain sheltered in the foreign concessions. China stirred his interest, as well as elevated his passion for intense intellectual activity. Somewhere in that welter of early impressions and the magnetic tug of China still drawing him, my father resolved to become a *keeper of custom*, as it was known—not just an expatriate living the western life, but one who could move beyond the safety net and open himself fully to China.

What would be required? First, of course, was to learn the language. A rudimentary familiarity with the language was required in the basic training so that he would be able to

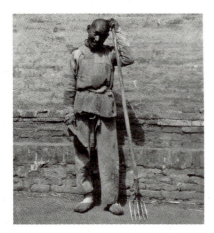

"Silly Billy," circa 1915-1917. Dad wrote, "Silly Billy—he watches the public latrine, so nobody will steal the odiferous contents—useful for fertilizer. His is a self-appointed job. He's cracked and funny as a crutch."

understand the agents and his own interpreter who would travel with him on his inspection trips, but my father wanted to learn more. He set out to learn to speak fluently, with a goal to learn at least 3,000 Chinese characters—enough to read the newspaper or get the meaning of a business letter.

More complicated was learning the system of Chinese tones. A single syllable could mean four different things depending on inflection. Even knowing the vocabulary and characters, it was easy to disgrace oneself in business. The usual compromise was to conduct business dealings in pidgin—basically modified English and other foreign words with Chinese grammar. The word "pidgin" meant "business." It was a way for people to communicate without fully learning each other's language, and for the Chinese to communicate with any foreigner in one common language. For example, the word "savvy" is based on a Spanish word and means "understand." The word "chop" was borrowed from India and denotes the official stamp used to seal a deal. And "chop-chop" means "quickly." So if my father wanted his seal quickly, he would say, "Bring chop chop-chop, you savvy?" It may have sounded a bit clumsy, but at least in pidgin, everyone sounded funny. However, my father wished to do better—to assimilate as fully as possible.

The language was possible to master with some hard work, but fully understanding and integrating into Chinese culture was much more challenging. Still, Dad was game to try. In America, he had learned and valued directness. "Say what you mean and mean what you say." In China, business was a complicated dance of gestures and saving face. It was an art to be learned—with long periods of silences and puffs on the water pipe. During these negotiations, one had to be very wary of missteps. My father's job was to make sure that the amount of oil alleged to arrive at each agent's office was the amount that actually arrived. The oil was shipped in five-gallon tins that were made in a factory in Tientsin's Russian concession. From there, the tins would be piled high onto carts drawn by a team of mules or oxen. It was not unusual for a thin trickle of oil to leak from the tins, leaving a trail behind. Some agents were known to claim some oil had been lost and to sell the missing oil on the gray market. Others would water down the oil, which caused the lamps it fueled to flicker and hiss, rather than burn with a steady flame. The merchant might regard shorting the

Chapter Two: A Place of Golden Opportunities

customer or inspector as proof of his own shrewdness as a trader, while Socony, with its own reputation to maintain, insisted on delivering a quality product.

Even when my father thought the negotiations had ended, when the agent called for his chop, the negotiations would begin all over again. Every agent seemed to do his best to wear down his honorable opponent, representative of the oil kings, trying to get the best deal. It made Dad's earlier days as a traveling representative for his father back home in the States seem so straightforward. Sometimes the only thing preventing the inspectors from melting down completely in the face of such dogged persistence were the limits that Socony set on what they could concede. Nevertheless, the experience was extremely valuable and my father adapted and became adept at the process.

Meanwhile, my father continued taking pictures of what he saw and sent them along with letters back to Hester. The relationship grew despite the distance and the weeks it took for a letter to arrive. My father asked a friend to take a picture of him posed in front of a Chinese house like a movie star in a white suit with a pith helmet at his side. It is the photo at the beginning of Chapter 1. He sent the photo to Hester and in the letter wrote:

> *Doesn't this pongee suit look fierce? I've been holding this by the side of the snap-shot of you, and saying—'just look who gets who.' You're not getting value received—but I hope you don't think so, because I love you, dear.*

Within a few months, my father had developed a basic proficiency at his job. He had finished the formal training required by Socony, but was also well along on the personal training he had undertaken for himself to leave the security of the expatriate life and enter into the heart of China.

In his travels from village to village, practicing his Chinese with local people, my father picked up local lore that may not have seemed very important to him at the time, but stuck with him. He could see children with bowed legs and old women hunched over like question marks, their bones as brittle as dried twigs. Drawing from his own childhood and the emphasis his family placed on drinking milk, he wondered if their conditions could be alleviated by drinking milk, which was known to contain calcium, an important mineral

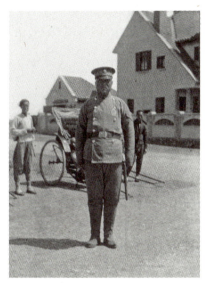

Chinese police officer, circa 1915-1917. Dad wrote, "My friend the cop. Just a second before he was laughing and talking with me, standing at ease. But the second he saw I was taking his picture he must—Chinese fashion—draw himself up straight and look as if he was being shot."

for strong bones. Were they getting enough calcium in their diet? He learned that pregnant women often lost their teeth. However, those who drank a soup containing vinegar and chicken bones managed to keep their teeth. Thinking back to his days at the University of South Carolina, my father figured that the acid in the vinegar helped leach, or make available, calcium from the animal bones.

In other places, people used local plants, like crabapple or spiraea, to make teas that would help with some ailment or another—very much like his mother did during his childhood days. Willow bark tea, he learned was good for headaches. This was something my father could understand since he knew that willow bark was used in the United States to make the newest headache remedy at the time: aspirin.

Dad was curious and had an amazing ability to make connections. He had questions though. One disease seemed to affect the wealthier more than the poor peasants in the field. It was a disease called beriberi, which literally means "I can't, I can't." My father had seen the victims of the disease. They were so weak that they would lie around all day, unable to move, uninterested in food, as their legs and arms went numb. The strange thing was that the disease seemed to affect the wealthy more than the poor peasants. During those days, it was believed to be caused by germs. My dad began to wonder if it might instead be caused by something missing from their diets. The affluent could afford white polished rice, whereas the poor sustained themselves on brown rice. My father had many questions, but few answers.

As he traveled, my father saw other kinds of diseases that he had never seen back home. In one gruesome case, the victim's hair appeared to bleed, mysterious bruises appeared almost spontaneously, and his teeth fell out of his bleeding gums. Although the disease had a name, scurvy, its cause was still unknown. My father had seen this disease in areas where people were scavenging for anything to eat—rats, spare bits of rice, bugs. However, in other areas, where villagers had managed to grow bean sprouts, there appeared to be no scurvy at all. Just as calcium from milk might help strengthen people's bones, could these diseases be a result of a poor diet? My father filed these questions away in his mind, hoping some day to discover the answers.

During his travels, he noticed how intricately all phases of the natural cycle were linked. He noticed how fertile the fields were in China, even after three millennia of

Did You Know

… in 1884, Kanehiro Takaki, the Director General of the Japanese Navy cured sailors of beriberi by giving them more meat, barley, and fruit during their long ocean voyages? He concluded (incorrectly) it was the higher protein content of the diet that was responsible for the cure.

… in 1897, Christiaan Eijkman, a Dutch physician, proved that feeding polished white rice to chickens caused a disease very similar to beriberi? When the birds were fed the rice husks or unpolished brown rice, they recovered. Eijkman thought there was something in the white rice that caused beriberi—a kind of poison—and the antidote was in the polishing. Although this was erroneous, this discovery revolutionized the thinking of the day—giving birth to the field of nutrition and leading to an intense period of investigation during the early 1900s.

constant use. One reason, as he had witnessed on his arrival, was that farmers would scoop silt from the bottom of the canals and then spread it across their fields. The silt functioned as a natural fertilizer, a kind of compost that had washed off the mountains and fields. It was rich in calcium from mussels and snail shells and brimming with organic matter from the fields, along with decaying fish, and water plants. Often the silt was combined with leavings from the fields, eggshells, food waste, and animal dung in large piles. The piles were then watered and turned until all the components had broken down into sweet-smelling compost. Even "night soil"—human waste—was collected daily from the chamber pots and placed into the mix.

Steam launches, which moved people and goods easily up and down the rivers, were a leap of efficiency for China, but some people complained that they destroyed the effectiveness of silt as a fertilizer by churning up the muck. They also felt that these launches possibly affected the purity of the water by killing the shellfish that filtered the water for food. This idea was scoffed at by some of the progressive Westerners, but to my father, the idea of protecting nature was beginning to show some merit. Here in China, he was beginning to see the intricate links that tied together everything in nature. The Chinese were still close to the land. There were few factories to pollute the waters, and their careful systems ensured that even the sewage was too valuable to dump in the canals. Until water reached the larger cities, it was relatively clean, considering the vast population it served.

In the course of his travels, my father met many different kinds of people, including missionaries. While he respected their commitment, he disagreed heartily with their approach. My dad believed that each man had his own direct, personal relationship to God. In his mind, churches weren't necessary to nurture that

Did You Know

… the Frenchman, Jacques Cartier, back in 1500s discovered a tree that cured his men from a disease that was later known as scurvy? He brought seedlings of the tree back to France. The king dubbed it arbor vitae, or tree of life. The leaves, like oranges, contained what became known to scientists centuries later as the anti-scurvy (antiscorbutic) factor.

… a couple centuries later, in 1753, the chief doctor for the British Navy, Dr. James Lind, proved that an unknown nutrient (vitamin C) in citrus foods prevented scurvy? It was a common and deadly disease—with more British sailors being lost to it than to war. After that, British sailors were given rations of lime—which led to their nickname, "Limey."

connection. As he saw it, Jesus taught that religion was not merely rituals or observances, but rather a mental attitude. To my father, Jesus stood above it all. My dad believed that love is at the center of it—not only the love of the Golden Rule, but the love of men and women, family love, the love of friends, and even love of enemies. Under this logic, it made no sense that God would punish a poor, but good-hearted, Chinese man simply because he had never heard of Jesus.

My father would get into some ardent debates with the missionaries on whether it was morally correct to impose their religion on the Chinese. He himself felt that this is too wonderful a universe to spark from nothing, and there had to be a creator to set down the universal laws. However, it made more sense to him to study the Chinese faiths. Maybe there was something the Westerners could learn from the Chinese. Centuries before Jesus lived, Lao-tzu had advocated in the *Tao Te Chiang* the same kind of virtues as the Sermon on the Mount: meekness, simplicity, temperance, charity, sincerity, and kindness.

However, in other ways, my father and the missionaries were similar. Most of the missionaries chose to live among the Chinese to learn the language and the culture so that they would be better able to teach. My father was doing the same as he traveled out to towns and villages for his work, spending hours memorizing the tone tables, and immersing himself in the environment.

The paradoxes in China amazed him, raising questions in his mind that he couldn't yet answer. As a Swede who grew up drinking milk, he wondered why the Chinese never seemed to keep a cow, never drank milk. And yet in some ways the poor peasants in the field seemed healthier than the milk-drinking Europeans who kept themselves locked up in the foreign concessions, eating only polished rice and importing their fruits and vegetables to avoid contamination from the notorious Chinese night soil. And yet, was this as crude as the Europeans assumed? There seemed to be relatively few outbreaks of cholera and other diseases. While he would see the inevitable results of deforestation and soil erosion, there was also a care for the soil, putting things back into the soil that allowed even this huge population to live off and remain close to the land. The questions sharpened as my father observed how Chinese peasants lived and as he soaked up impressions from the amazing world around him. These vivid and powerful sights opened his mind and elevated his consciousness.

At this point, my father was not only a valued employee in a thriving, expanding business representing an essential product in what would seem to be an unlimited market, but he was also well on his way to becoming a "keeper of custom." But his entrepreneurial spirit was emerging again, and he began to think about the next move. He also found himself increasingly thinking of Hester and wishing she were by his side.

As my father's devotion to Hester grew, his position at Socony became shakier. For one thing, he had trouble accepting the two-year rule—expecting to work in China for at least two years before getting married. He was in love with Hester and wanted to marry her. But beyond the marriage issue, he found his interests diverging from the company's corporate culture. Socony needed followers—not yes-men, but men who would carry out the wishes of the company with little questioning—not men with their own ideas on how things should be accomplished. My father, with his willingness to question authority, began to wonder if he still fit in at Socony.

Here in China, my father was learning much about himself and acquiring internal riches that would continue to grow and upon which he would draw for the rest of his life. Here, he was beginning to realize he was different from many other men, and those differences were not weaknesses, but rather strengths. He had ideas of his own, and he had come to value them. This was China, where Thomas Lipton, who had started as a greengrocer in London, went on to become a multimillionaire tea merchant, a man could be whatever he wanted. And it was here in China that my father chose to be himself.

*"A discovery is said to
be an accident meeting
a prepared mind."*

— Albert Szent-Györgyi

Chapter 3 | Soul Searching

Well, call it Dad's adventurous spirit, but within a year of his arrival in China, my father had a new job. He had left behind the "blue chip" security of Socony to begin a more "seat of the pants" life as an importer-exporter for the China American Trading Company. According to Hester, my father "found himself in disagreement with [Socony's] policies or their way of conducting business. He criticized freely. He tried to tell top management what they should do—and they resented it, and let him go, perhaps regretfully, but with finality."

He had been fired before, but this time was different. He had gained his freedom and could marry the woman he loved. He had a new job that allowed him to shape more of his own destiny and indulge his sense of adventure, exploring the length and breadth of China on purchasing and sales trips. What more could he have asked for?

In his new line of business, profits were made only if a deal went through—sink or swim. The traders were risk takers; if you bought cargo and delivered it successfully, you made money; if not, you lost. Dad's new position called him to trade in cotton, wool, leather, furs, and other commodities, and his travels took him far and wide in China, including at least one trip into Manchuria.

As soon as he settled into his new position, my father and Hester got married. Dad sailed to Yokohama to meet Hester, who arrived by steamer in the company of her mother, Amanda. My father had everything ready: he had picked out a wedding ring, arranged for a minister, and reserved a time for the wedding at the American Consulate. On a sunny, warm day, on April 30, 1917, Hester and my father were married.

The two entered their new life as a couple during a turbulent time. Earlier that month, on April 6, the United States had entered World War I on the Allied side joining, among other nations, Japan, whose own increasing military involvement in the world was to have severe repercussions in the country where my father and his bride would make their home: China.

For a while it was a great adventure, as only adventurous newlyweds can have. My father settled Hester into their brand-new home on the outskirts of Tientsin's French concession, where she was able to live like royalty among the expatriates, in a manner well befitting her New England blueblood upbringing.

Their neighborhood was as new as their home. That they could afford to live here was a happy surprise for Hester. Dad seemed to be doing better financially than she had imagined. Perhaps even more surprising was the retinue of servants that Hua had lined up, five in total—and that didn't even count the *amah* Hua hired as Hester's own personal attendant.

Hester's job in the eyes of the Chinese was simply to enjoy the luxuries of her station and not interfere in the household accounts. It was Hua's job, as the Number One Boy, to operate the Rehnborg household. He would hire and fire the help and make sure the family's possessions were safe. Meanwhile, Hester could spend her time reading, listening to music, visiting gardens, chatting with the other wives at lunch, or *tiffin* as it was called, play bridge in the afternoon, go dancing after dinner—and show off her gifted dancer husband to the other ladies.

Hester soon began to adjust to the gilded-cage existence of the expatriate elite. She rarely carried money. To pay for anything, she needed only to sign a chit, a piece of paper that stated how much she owed. On the first of each month, hundreds of *shroffs*, or money changers, from the clubs and shops would go out to collect on the chits. My father would be given a tally sheet showing what the bills were and how much was paid. Hester would never see any money other than the coppers she carried to pay the rickshaw coolies. Even if she wanted to get involved in the running of the household, the servants would discourage her. It wasn't her place. A wife could sign chits, but she shouldn't concern herself about the finances. It was custom.

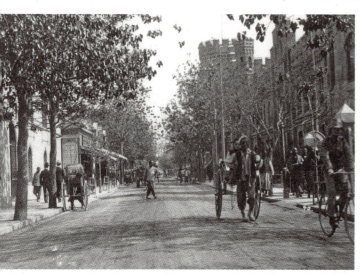

Tientsin, China, circa 1915-1917. Dad wrote for his bride-to-be, "Victoria Road. In the German Concession this is the Wilhelmstrasse, in the British, Victoria Road, in the French, Rue de France. It is Tientsin's main street. There are no white ways here. You'll miss that. The shops look more like residences than anthing else. The turrets are on Gordon Hall."

Chapter Three: Soul Searching

Although Hester was living in the lap of luxury, the enforced idleness was at times difficult to accept, particularly since she was adventurous and college-educated and wanted to see more. She was finally in the land about which she had dreamed, yet in an environment strangely insulated from it. This was not an ideal atmosphere for a young, energetic person who preferred to be active and not merely settle down.

Hester met some of my father's friends. One in particular was a colleague from Dad's Socony days—a nice young man incongruously named Fuzzy, who had already started to lose his hair. Fuzzy Vaughn was a man with a future at Socony, if he wanted it, although he was talking about enlisting in the Army to join the doughboys in Europe. As a newlywed, my father was not expected to volunteer, although there was rumor of a draft.

The shock waves from World War I, in full swing in Europe, had filtered down into Chinese politics, which had already been destabilized by the death of the dowager empress in 1908. Within the foreign concessions, it was possible to live an insulated life, but out in the field, in what had become the era of warlords, the uncertainty was right there in your face.

The treaty ports, like Tientsin, carried out business as usual. The warlords left them alone, still in awe of the gunboats and occasional destroyers and marines that came to visit. The warlords also needed the taxes generated by the foreign trade so expatriates could live a life that was relatively unimpaired. It wasn't exactly the safest place to live, even if you were a foreigner protected by extraterritoriality. However, the illusion of safety in Tientsin was easy to maintain. All your needs were taken care of by your servants. No Chinese troops would dare enter the foreign concessions.

For my father, though, whose new line of business would take him far from the security of the concessions, it was a different story. Occasionally, the rail line from Tientsin was cut by a local warlord or by bandits, and my father would have to travel cross-country by car. Northern Manchuria, with its icy wilds, was bandit country, and travel by car demanded extraordinary measures. At night, the oil had to be drained out of the engine and transmission, the water drained out of the radiator, and kerosene, unlikely to freeze, was applied to the brake mechanisms. The oil was kept warm in special containers in the kitchens of overnight inns, while the radiator and the hood were protected by a felt-lined cover or boot. In the morning, the traveling men had the innkeeper boil five or

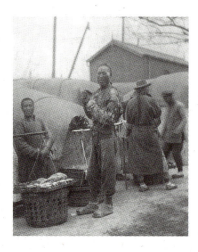

Road side market, circa 1917. Dad wrote, "Gambling for his chow. If he draws combination of numbers on the little sticks, he gets threefold. If not, nothing."

10 gallons of water and heat the oil until it was close to the flash point, then take the oil out and pour it in the engine as they started cranking it. They lifted the front flap of the boot and filled the radiator with hot water. "When you did all that," recalled my father's buddy Fuzzy, "you turn the switch on and the engine would go right off. Of course it took a little time, but it was worth it."

While in Manchuria, Dad took a photo of a roadside market. There were actually two different markets in the same place. Street vendors would set up trays on top of the large baskets they had carried to the market. On the trays were the dry goods they sold, things that wouldn't freeze in the frigid air. Behind them were structures that resembled Mongolian yurts, but were actually piles of grain, furs, and other bulk goods covered with felt mats. These were the wholesale goods that my father's boss, McGowan, would have my father buy.

McGowan's more tolerant management style allowed Hester to accompany my father on some of his trading trips. In October 1917, they traveled south to Nanking, on the Yangtze River. Only a year earlier, American Marines had been called in to quell a riot on American property in the city, but the trouble had calmed by now.

Though Nanking was peaceful and subdued, events in the outside world were impinging upon the isolation of the Middle Kingdom. In August, China had entered the War on the Allied side, freeing the Chinese to reclaim Germany's concessions, and adding an element of vulnerability to life in all the foreign concessions. In October, the Bolsheviks had risen to power in Russia, ousting the Kerensky government and guaranteeing that there would be trouble along the Siberian border. China's entry into the modern world was bringing with it involvement in worldwide conflicts.

Winter set in, bringing discomforts beyond the cold. The strong winds that swept down the loess plains of Mongolia sometimes brought clouds of dust with them, which forced their way through the tiniest of cracks, coating everything in the Rehnborg household and adding a gritty flavor to the food. Hua and the staff did what they could, stuffing cotton into the window frames and gluing strips of rice paper over the frames to seal out the dust. At night, the wind was so strong that they could hear the tiles rattling on the roof.

However, early in 1918 my father and Hester had some good news—they would soon be having a baby. Now the reasoning behind Socony's policy of having griffins wait

Chapter Three: Soul Searching

two years before marrying became apparent: it interfered with business. Many Western women wanted to go home for the birth of their child, and Hester was no exception. With huge support from her wealthy mother on Boston's North Shore, Hester encouraged my father to return to the States.

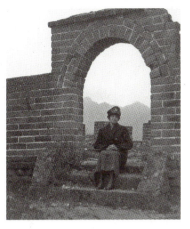

Hester Rehnborg visiting the Great Wall, circa 1918.

It wasn't easy. My father had yet to be with China American Trading Company for the standard three-year term required before a foreign employee and his family are granted free passage home. My father had to wrangle a bit, but was successful. McGowan found him a job with the Boston office, but his first "stateside" assignment took him well afield to Guadalajara, Mexico.

My father realized that this might be the last chance for them to see China, and Hester had yet to visit the two most famous attractions—the Great Wall and the Ming Tombs. So, the two had some fun doing a little sight-seeing. Hester's excitement at finally getting a chance to see the most famous construction in the world—the Great Wall—showed in her happy grin as my father snapped a picture of her, sitting crossed-legged on a spread of newspapers, on the rear platform of their train. In her left hand dangles a cigarette, and on her face is a sweet, relaxed, and unaffected smile. A mist floats over the hills in the background. She was happier than she had been for a long time.

In April 1918, my father and Hester, three months pregnant, left China and headed back to the States. My father accompanied Hester to her mother's home and then took off to fulfill his obligations in Guadalajara.

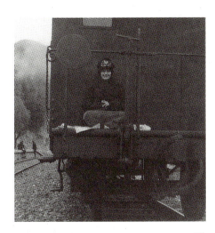

Hester on back platform of train, circa 1918.

Dad's job in Guadalajara was to buy leather, so that it could be exported to China where it would be turned into shoes. Mexico had huge herds of cattle, and China had essentially no domestic leather available, yet could churn out shoes very cheaply. The shoes would in turn be exported to America at a profit. My father, experienced now at negotiating in a foreign, primarily rural culture, was at home in Mexico, fulfilling his obligation to McGowan, inspecting the stacks of cured leather and hides, meeting new people, and learning about their lives and culture.

On his way home from the mission, Dad made a stopover in Beaumont, Texas. His entrepreneurial instinct may have smelled an opportunity. World War I continued overseas, and there was a great demand for ships. Even after the war was over, demand in the area for oil tankers would continue to grow. He knew that there was a huge opportunity in the oil business, and the Gulf Coast of Texas was its epicenter. He interviewed and was offered an executive position for the Lone Star Shipbuilding Company.

This created a marital crisis—perhaps not the first, but certainly the worst. My father wanted to live in Beaumont, while Hester preferred Boston and felt that he should take the job that McGowan had offered him there. A quarrel ensued, but Hester finally capitulated.

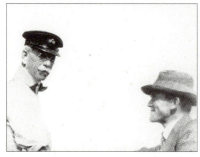

My father (right) with H.A. Wisewood in Beaumont, Texas, spring 1919. My father and Hester resided in Beaumont for about 18 months during 1918 to 1919.

It turned out to be an unmitigated disaster. Hester wrote to her mother that "Carlos was titled 'comptroller,' but found the company like a wayward child, most difficult to control." The Lone Star Shipbuilding Company seemed likely to go under, and my father almost did as well. He was felled by the vicious outbreak of influenza that gripped the United States in the winter of 1918-19, killing more Americans than had been lost on the battlefields of Europe. He was hospitalized.

For my father, it was a time of enforced isolation. Except for seeing the nurses on their rounds or the chance to speak with Hester through the closed window, my father was alone with his thoughts. He suffered through the cold sweats and the hot flashes and the delirium brought by severe flu, but in the moments of remission, he could think about what he was doing in Beaumont, what he was doing with his life, and it became clear to him once again that he really hadn't accomplished anything. There were things to be proud of—his report on the opening of a branch office for Socony, his high grades at school, the coming birth of his first child. But he was already over 30 years old and had yet to feel he brought anything new to the world. He had already dropped out of two different colleges. He had failed at his plan to develop a new type of rubber flooring, and he had been let go from Socony. Now, he was the comptroller of Lone Star Shipbuilding Company, which appeared to be beyond his or anyone's help, and he would likely soon be without a job.

What could he do that would take advantage of his skills? Even the people who had let him go had done so with regret. He saw problems in a company and wanted to address them. His employers didn't see things the same way. Maybe he just wasn't cut out for those kinds of jobs. Maybe things would be better if he were the boss. It was too late in the game to try to work his way up at another company like Socony or China American Trading.

Chapter Three: Soul Searching

Alice Tisdale Hobart, whose husband worked at Socony at the same time as my father, summed up his dilemma succinctly: companies were loath to take a risk on a man over 30 when they could train young men right out of high school.

My father had faith in himself and knew he would be good at whatever he set his mind to. The difficulty was to find something worth doing. Exporting furs and importing leather just weren't going to help the world. The oil business was a place for company men, and it was becoming more and more clear that he was too much his own man to fit in there—not the way he had back in the training classes in New York or in those exciting months after his arrival in China three years before.

But China was key. There were so many opportunities there. He wanted to do something that would make a difference—and what could make a bigger difference than helping improve the health of those people he saw? Perhaps he could do something to help the Chinese people get a more balanced diet. He had been thinking about how odd it was that they never drank milk. Brittle bone disease was very common in China. Maybe milk could help with that. There were few cows in China because they took up so much land for grazing. In a country with little available land, the best thing to do would be to import canned milk from America, a land with an apparently infinite amount of land ... and an infinite number of cows. Since canned milk could be stored almost forever without refrigeration, it could easily withstand a month-long trip on the back of a camel to a remote village and could sit on a merchant's shelf for another month before a customer bought it. And customers could use it whenever they wanted milk—whether for drinking or cooking. Like fresh milk, canned milk was a rich source of calcium. One company, Carnation, now had its products on shelves throughout America, but nobody had the agency for them in China.

What a perfect job for my father! He knew about exporting and importing from McGowan. He knew about distribution and working with Chinese agents from Socony. He knew about sales from his work with his father's jewelry business. He could put it all together and build a business his way. And it would succeed. All the elements were coming together.

It was time for my father to start focusing on what was really important to him. In 1918, catching the flu was a brush with death, and he had survived. He had been given a second chance, and he was going to take it!

"This is as complicated
as the universe."

CARNATION LABORATORY SCIENTIST
DESCRIBING ALFALFA

The Story of Carnation Milk
produced by Pacific Coast
Condensed Milk Company, 1915.

The STORY of CARNATION MILK

Chapter 4 | Milk from Contented Cows

Once the idea hit, it hit like wildfire. Dad immediately dedicated himself to bringing milk to the people of China. First on the list was to get the job. He headed out to New York in September 1919 to meet with the managing director of American Milk Products Company, C.S. Stevens.

The company had only recently formed, bringing two competitors, Carnation Company and Pet Milk Company, together to advertise and sell milk overseas. They had already established agencies in France, Germany, and England.

My father was determined to convince Stevens to hire him to build their business in China. He realized that over the past four years his track record showed that he had already been through three career changes. Although each new job was arguably better than the last, it was possible that Stevens could perceive him as a failure who couldn't hold a job.

However, Stevens found himself face-to-face with a man of action who knew when to move on to a better opportunity. Here he found a man who not only had export-import experience combined with a growing fluency in the Chinese language and years of residency in China, but a passion for improving the health of people—and improving it with the use of milk.

The combination my father brought to the interview just proved to be irresistible. According to Hester, "Carl sold himself easily and brilliantly." He had the job. He was hired on as the company's principal representative for China. He would be the first to establish agencies in China to sell Carnation Evaporated Milk. His responsibilities were to include both China and Japan, and he would have business dealings with various British, American, and Chinese firms in both countries.

The Nutrilite Story

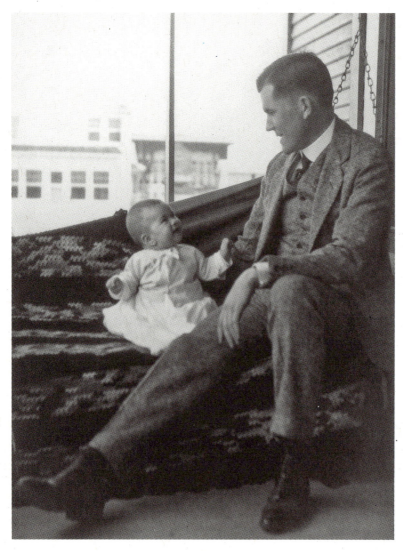

Ned at 4 ½-months and Carl Rehnborg, March 1919.

It would be two months before the family would depart to China. By this time their son, Edward Hawks "Ned" Rehnborg, was born.

While in the United States, Dad learned all he could about milk, milk production, and nutrition. Meeting with New York wholesale brokers, he found out about retail sales and distribution of canned milk in the States. He read what he could about milk—its nutritional properties and the science behind its production.

The field of nutrition was just in its infancy. At the turn of the 20th century, most people felt that a diet was adequate if it contained sufficient amounts of protein, carbohydrates, fats, minerals, and water.

My father's instinct was that there was a positive correlation between milk and health. He vigorously reviewed the scientific literature and was very pleased to see that his instinct was correct. In 1906, one of the most advanced researchers in nutrition, Sir Fredrick Gowland Hopkins, of Cambridge University in England, had reported that rats given an artificial mixture of protein (casein), carbohydrate (starch), and fat (lard) with mineral salts and water became sick and died. However, when given small amounts of milk or dried vegetables, they did fine. Hopkins concluded that there are unrecognized substances in milk and certain dried vegetables that, even in small quantities, are essential. He called these essential unknowns "accessory food factors."

Chapter Four: Milk from Contented Cows

In 1913 another pioneer in nutritional biochemistry, Elmer McCollum, along with his research partner Marguerite Davis, isolated one of those unrecognized factors found in such foods as milk and certain fruits and vegetables. They called it "fat-soluble A," because the compound was able to dissolve in fat, and they assumed it would be the first of many such compounds to be identified. It had also become known as the "anti-infective agent," because a deficiency of it was associated with eye infections in animals.

McCollum and Davis also analyzed the crystalline substance derived from rice polishing that eliminated the beriberi-like symptoms in chickens. This substance could also be extracted from milk. They called the substance "water-soluble B," because it was soluble in water. By 1919, the name "water-soluble C" was proposed for the factor in foods such as vegetables and fruits that prevented scurvy. Although these vitamins had been labeled (fat-soluble A, water-soluble B, and water-soluble C), nobody really knew what they were composed of or exactly how they worked. My father was intrigued.

One of the best places to learn more about the nutritional aspects and science behind milk was Carnation's

Did You Know

… Elmer McCollum, an American biochemist, proposed in 1909 that the lack of "palatability" of certain diets resulted in nutritive failure? He felt that if diets could be made to taste better, the animals would be induced to eat more, which would result in an adequate diet. This hypothesis was quickly shot down.

… in 1911, a Polish-born biochemist at the Lister Institute in London, Casimir Funk, precipitated out a sixth of an ounce of crystalline substance from a ton of rice polishings, which he then fed to birds with an induced beriberi-like disease? It cured them. He called the substance a "vitamine" because he suspected it was a nitrogen-containing amine vital for life. In a paper published in 1912, he suggested that all of Hopkins' "accessory food factors" were probably vitamins, and diseases such as beriberi, scurvy, pellagra, and rickets were caused by diets lacking in these elements.

largest plant and research facility near Madison, Wisconsin. Here at the Oconomowoc Condensory, my father discovered that there was quite a bit of technology that took place behind the production of what people thought of as "just milk." He found himself surrounded by what seemed like miles of shiny silver pipes—pipes made out of "stainless steel," a brand new kind of steel that would never rust. He watched milk being homogenized—the raw milk being forced through tiny holes under high pressure in order to break up the cream into particles that would stay suspended in the milk. He watched cream being made from the milk using a kind of centrifuge that spun at thousands of revolutions per minute. The heavier nonfat milk would spin to the sides and then run off into a collector. The lighter cream would stay toward the center and rise to a cream outlet. The cream could be separated into various grades: half-and-half and light cream for coffee and tea, thicker cream for whipping and ice cream, and the thickest cream for making into butter.

My father found the most interesting aspect of the visit to be the results of an experiment to create a kind of artificial or substitute milk. This milk substitute was essentially whole milk, but instead of the valuable cream or milk fat that is normally found in whole milk, cheaper coconut oil was substituted. "This resulted in a milk substitute," my father had written, "presumably the equivalent of whole milk in cooking." He wrote further that, "Everyone concerned, including the company itself, was somewhat dubious as to whether the substitution of coconut fat for cream was a feasible procedure...."

An experiment was conducted to settle the question. The investigators fed calves and other research animals the substitute milk to see whether it provided adequate nutrition. There was no question as to the results: the animals became sick and almost died. They developed night blindness and mysterious white scars on their eyes. My father had seen similar symptoms while in China—but in people whose eyes suffered from the same white scars and whose skin became rough and scaly. What amazed my father was that when the animals were fed whole milk, they got better and perhaps more surprisingly, they also recovered if they were fed the substitute milk plus "green leafy material." There was obviously something in the whole milk and in the green leafy plants that was missing in the substitute milk that contained coconut oil. In other words, coconut fat was not the same as milk fat. Coconut oil just wasn't nutritionally equivalent to milk fat or leafy green plants.

Did You Know

... earlier in 1907, two Norwegians Axel Holst and Theodore Frölich, produced a condition in guinea pigs comparable with human scurvy by feeding them a diet of cereal and eliminating fresh animal and vegetable foods?

The addition of the restricted food to the diet cured the surviving animals.

My father also had the opportunity to study Carnation's research showing that cows consuming nothing more than alfalfa and water produced the most milk and gained the most weight. They were healthy and their coats were shiny. One chemist at the condensory held up an alfalfa plant and said, "This is as complicated as the universe," because the plant contains tiny bits of all the elements found in nature. The statement deeply resonated within my father, because it confirmed what he had believed instinctively.

After Dad's visit to the condensory, the family planned to take the train to Seattle, Washington, to meet the man behind the Carnation name, Elbridge Stuart. It was Stuart, in combination with a partner, who improved the processing technology of evaporated milk to eliminate the carmelized or "cooked" flavor previously associated with it—a process my father could understand because it was similar to the vacuum distillation he had studied in Socony's training classes, which separated grades of oil from raw petroleum. Stuart also had a knack for marketing and came up with the brand name, "Carnation," which was lifted from a line of cigars. It seemed a more appropriate name for milk than cigars— a name suggesting freshness and purity. It went along nicely with their catchy slogan: Milk "From Contented Cows™."†

On the train ride toward Seattle, my father had several days to reflect on one of his hunches. As he put it, "For the animals in the experiment...some of the things provided by the leafy material had been subtracted from their diet. It was presumable (and correct) that these were the things that had been in the cream."

But those same nutrients were in the leafy material fed to the calves in the experiment and in the alfalfa eaten by the cows that produced the whole milk. "This was a key point," my father wrote years later, "although not at that moment, when it was not even the beginning of an idea."

During the train ride, as the vast emptiness of the Great Plains turned into the rugged peaks of the Rockies, my father thought about animals and plants in relation to the earth. The vitamins that had been identified as *available* in plants were, in essence, *created* by plants. Animals needed the vitamins to thrive, and they needed to eat the plants directly or indirectly to get the vitamins.

As the train pulled into the King Street Station in Seattle, my father's anticipation must have been growing. He was now able to meet Carnation's founder, Elbridge Stuart, in person, at the company's headquarters across Fourth Avenue from the elegant Olympic Hotel in the new Metropolitan Center development that Stuart and his partners had built with the money they had made selling canned milk.

Although no records can be found that document what took place during the meeting, it would have been interesting to be a fly on the wall and hear the conversation and ideas that these two impressive men—one younger and one older—might have shared. Stuart was a man who was as concerned with the ingredients that went into his milk products as he was with the process of making it. He believed that a steady supply of good quality milk could

Did You Know

… …more recent evidence has found organic milk provides more health benefits? By analyzing produce from 25 farms, researchers found that organic milk contained 67 percent more antioxidants and vitamins than ordinary milk. Scientists also found organic milk contained 60 percent more of a healthy fatty acid called conjugated linoleic acid.

CHAPTER FOUR: MILK FROM CONTENTED COWS

only be maintained by obtaining it from healthy cows. Perhaps this is something that the two men with ideas discussed?

After the meeting, Dad took Hester and Ned to Carnation's experimental farm in the Snoqualmie Valley, just 30 miles east of Seattle. The farms were a testament to Carnation's dedication to quality—here, they were breeding prize Holsteins and testing different kinds of feed, including alfalfa. Dad could show one-year-old Ned the cows, and see for himself how contented they really were.

After their visit, the family headed to Vancouver where they boarded the *Empress of Japan*—taking them toward their new home in Shanghai, China, where at last my father would be his own man. He would still report back to the export company's headquarters in New York, but in China he would be given the opportunity to run the show.

"From Contented Cows" is a trademark of Societe des Produits Nestle S.A., Switzerland.

> "A moment's insight is sometimes worth a life's experience."
>
> —Oliver Wendell Holmes

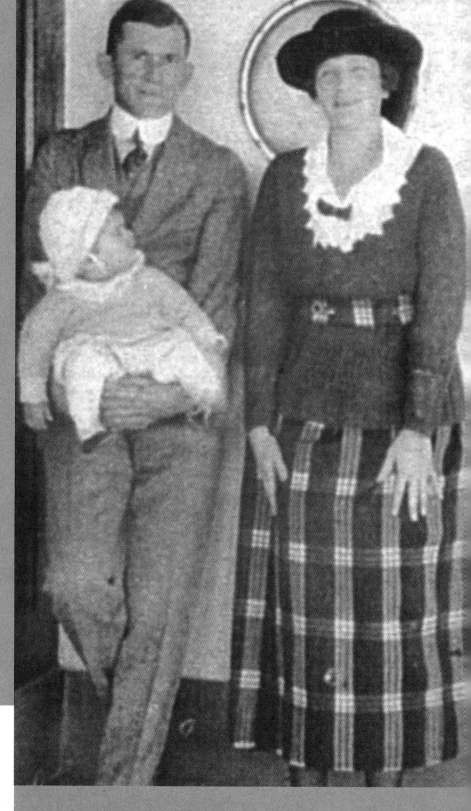

Carl, Hester, and little Ned Rehnborg aboard the *Empress of Japan* en route to Shanghai, December 1919.

Chapter 5 | Food for Thought

It was a chilly day in December of 1919 when the family arrived in Shanghai. Hester had bundled Ned in a warm coat and hat. They had crossed the Dragon's gate and had entered the Middle Kingdom, where according to the old Chinese proverb their status was elevated 10 times.

After setting up a temporary household at the Burlington Hotel and finding an *amah* to help look after Ned, my father enthusiastically set out to sell canned milk. He opened an office in an elegant building with a grand arched entranceway at 7 Soochow Road, which was just off Soochow Creek. Across the street was the Rowing Club that he often visited and, almost next door, were the broad lawns of the British Consulate. Only a few blocks to the west were shops that rivaled those found in New York, London, and Paris.

By contrast, an area called "Thieves' Market" was equally close by. Here, families were so poor they slept in shifts on planks in cramped, rented spaces under staircases, sharing their body heat. A half-man, a beggar whose body appeared to be growing out of a roof tile, could be found rocking his way down the street. Others reached out their hands as my father passed, some exaggerating their misery, many simply starving, calling out, "Do good works!" These people had nothing, and yet they could benefit most from the nutrients in milk. How could they afford it? This was a question my father had troubling answering.

My father felt that within one month of his arrival he could make a "first rate analysis" of the business opportunity before him. He had been away from China for about a year and a half and was looking at the country with fresh eyes, gathering much of the information he needed through the swirls of parties and dinners that occupied his and Hester's evening hours.

It was a changed China. After World War I, society was more open; the formerly strict lines dividing Chinese from foreigners had started to blur. In Shanghai, the changes were striking. Nearly every restaurant sported a cosmopolitan clientele. Even in the way people dressed, you could see the blending of cultures—Chinese men in gowns wearing top hats, English women in tight cheongsams, and Chinese women in the latest French fashions.

Chinese students who had graduated from American universities were returning home. My father enjoyed talking with these educated and sophisticated men on a variety of lighthearted topics such as baseball, jazz, cocktails, and horse racing. But on a deeper level, they helped guide him into the collective psyche of the time and into the thoughts of their contemporaries, the leaders of indigenous student intellectual movements like the *New Tide Society* and the *Citizens' Magazine Society* that had sprung up after the War.

These movements were composed of activist Chinese in their early 20s working with professors, who were just slightly older, in opposition to the middle-aged and elderly scholars and warlords who had come to dominate the Chinese Republican government.

Shanghai was, in many ways, the political epicenter of the country. On May 4, 1919, only seven months before my father and the family had arrived in Shanghai, thousands of students had gathered at Tiananmen Square, in front of the Forbidden City in Peking, to protest the signing of the Versailles Treaty, which handed over Germany's territorial rights in China to the Allied partner, Japan. Thirty-two students were arrested and one was injured and died three days later.

The movement exploded in reaction to the death. The authorities were unable to squelch it. On May 7, 20,000 people had swarmed into Shanghai's Hunan Stadium waving flags painted with patriotic slogans demanding self-determination: "Give Us Back Our Country."

During the next week, strikes swept through Shanghai along with an anti-Japanese boycott. Over 70,000 workers joined in. On May 31, 100,000 students and citizens gathered for a memorial meeting for the martyred Peking student. The crowds moved through the streets of Shanghai past white mourning flags hung in the doorways and listened to impassioned speeches. John Dewey, the American educator and reformer, wrote home: "We are witnessing the birth of a nation and birth always comes hard …."

Chapter Five: Food for Thought

Foreigners feared that the demonstrations would get out of hand, and they sometimes did. At one rice shop where the owner refused to close, the students fell to their knees to beg him to join in. An assistant tried to run them off. A bystander responded by throwing rocks at the shop front and rallying a mob. The owner finally appeared only to be attacked and yanked by his beard.

Outside of Shanghai, the warlords appeared insatiable in their demands. In Szechwan, taxes were being collected 35 years in advance. Yet the general resentment against foreigners had yet to extend to the expatriates in the concessions, where they were somewhat protected by the warlords.

This was the foundation on which my father had chosen to build his milk business. It appeared to be about as stable as the shifting channel of the Yangtze River. Fortunately, the flow of commerce seemed to be able to navigate these unstable channels the way the river pilots navigated the Yangtze.

Very soon after my father arrived in Shanghai, he took a canal trip. It was a kind of test run of the many trips he would take as he built his milk network. Hester and 14-month-old Ned accompanied him. Ned was bundled up in the warm clothes he had worn on the Pacific crossing. Hester took a photo of Ned nestled in Dad's lap as they sat atop the cabin, in front of the weather-beaten mast. In the canal, my father saw reflected the whole cycle of life, as he described later, "… we saw dead dogs, dead goats, and one dead buffalo. We also saw people bathing, people washing their faces, people drinking the water and dipping it up to take home to cook supper with."

Another photo taken around this time could, in hindsight, symbolize his struggles yet to come: my father appeared lost in thought, a tiny figure, almost invisible, at the

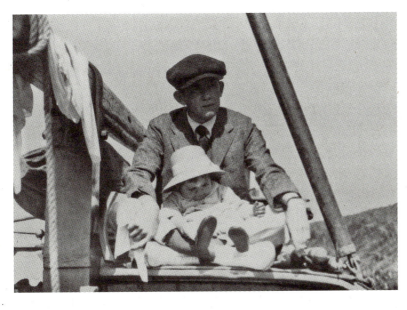

Dad and Ned, as a toddler, on a canal trip up Soochow Creek in China, circa December 1919. During such trips, my father observed the intensive farming practices that took place, which he came to believe, depletes the soil.

bottom of a massive flight of steps leading to the top of a hill in Soochow.

While he sat on those steps, he may have been pondering the best way to get canned milk to the people who needed it—in a country where most people had never seen a cow. So many in real need: little children with bellies distended from starvation, women weak and pale from pregnancy, rickshaw pullers with scaly sores of pellagra, and blind musicians with white-encrusted eyes. My father realized that the milk he was selling couldn't help all of these problems, but it could certainly help some. And, it certainly was a more worthwhile product than the ubiquitous imported British toilet paper that looked more like glazed parchment and was just as tough. He joked that they called it Bronco, because "you can't bust it." However, that didn't stop Bronco from becoming the most popular brand. My father hoped to have the same success with Carnation milk, noting that "the Chinese were very slow to pick up a new brand, but when they had, it couldn't be shaken."

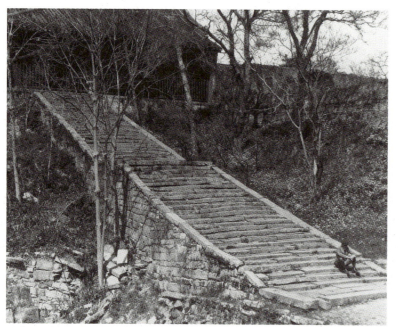

My father visiting Tiger Hill in Jiangsu Province in Soochow, China, 1920.

The nutrients in milk could be very helpful, but the difficulty would be convincing people to give it a try. Few people drank it after infancy and others associated it with the "disgusting butter smell" of foreigners. In order to market the milk and get the message through the clutter of commercial and political information, my father came up with an idea—a cross cultural strategy—involving Ned and a Chinese baby.

Deciding to photograph the two babies for a marketing shot, he posed Ned and the Chinese baby with a stack of Carnation cans. In one photograph, an amah is depicted feeding the Chinese baby milk from a porcelain cup and in another the baby holds a can of milk. In another, the amah is shown holding up a small glass bottle while Ned sits in her lap. The most striking of all looks like a parody of Michelangelo's famous painting of

CHAPTER FIVE: FOOD FOR THOUGHT

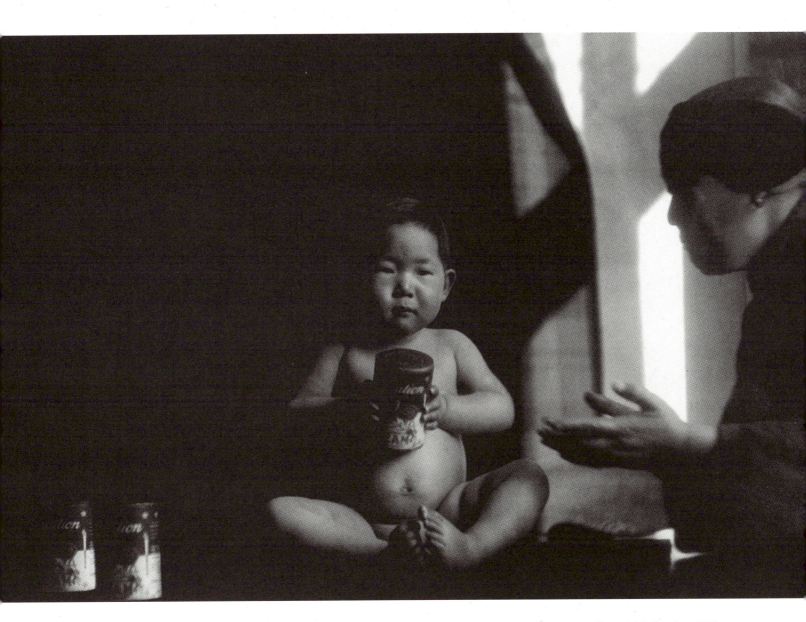

A baby holding a can of Carnation Milk, circa 1920.
One of the handful of marketing photos my
father took to sell canned milk.

Adam: Ned is stretching out his cherubic body toward a hand holding a can of milk.

My father continued to learn all that he could about milk in order to better market it. His education took place not only while reading the latest scientific journals and ancient Chinese medical texts such as the *Pen T'sao*, but also while on the streets of Shanghai talking with the people in his best Mandarin.

He visited the Chinese pharmacies where the locals went when they were ill. In the pharmacies, my father could see doctors treat patients in a manner very different from back home. The doctor would feel a patient's pulse at the wrist, trying to identify one of more than 30 different types of pulses said to represent different conditions. The doctor would also ask the patient to stick out his or her tongue in order to check its color, moisture content, and secretions or coatings. From the check-up, various symptoms could be identified: a racing pulse, high temperature, raw throat, bad teeth, infected gums, and so on.

The aromas present at the Chinese pharmacies may have reminded my father of a grocery store. It was easy to see why. Depending on the patient's condition, the doctor would prescribe a combination of natural herbs, usually to be taken as a tea or soup. The goal was to restore the harmony of the body, balancing *yin* and *yang* and aligning the flow of *chi*, or life force. To my father, these Chinese herbal remedies, like drinking an infusion of dried plants, had a kind of familiarity dating back to his childhood, when his mother implored him to drink various herbal teas to help him feel better.

Besides the pharmacies, my father also enjoyed visiting the local market in the Hongkew District. The market spread across several buildings and roads and was filled with the aromas of ginger, lichees, and sugar that seemed to mix like a nasal stir-fry with the scent of fish, raw pork, and orange duck. The sights he saw were as incredible as the variety of foods available, not always as fresh as they were purported to be. My father would smile at the vendor bent over his barrel of fish that Dad had seen floating belly-up a few moments before; now the man was gently encouraging the fish with his hands to appear a little more alive.

To the Chinese, maintaining one's health was a matter of balance. Any mildly observant individual would have noticed immediately that the blank-eyed fish in the fishmonger's hands was a little short on *chi*. But it might have been saved if its yin and yang had been brought back into balance soon enough, and the first course of action when any living

Did You Know

… recorded history on the use of plants and plant extracts for medicinal purposes in China dates as far back as 2800 BC, when the medical text *Chen Noug Pen T'sao* was published?

…yin and yang are the underlying principles of Chinese philosophy and medicine? Good health is believed to come from a balance of yin (feminine, negative, and dark) and yang (male, positive, and bright).

Yin	Yang
Female	Male
Negative	Positive
Night	Day
Dark	Light
Cold	Warm
Passive	Active

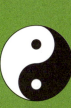

creature became ill was to examine its diet.

All around in the market, my father could see foods that, according to tradition, affected people's health. Plants were used in cooking not only for their taste, but also for their medicinal value. Ginger, served with fish, was considered an antidote to shellfish poisoning. It also was attributed with aphrodisiac properties. Fresh coriander guarded the diner from food poisoning. Squid, sparrow eggs, and abalone when mixed together and thrown into a soup were said to benefit menstrual distress; sticky rice dumplings made of Chinese yam and rice would aid low spirits. There was even a cure involving milk, mixed with honey, for weakness. Everywhere, the interest in food was linked to the interest in nutrition. In China, doctors believed they should first treat patients with food, only turning to medicine if the food was ineffective. And as my father could see by the crowd in the market at noontime, people were always searching for the freshest ingredients possible, even if that meant going to the market twice a day for perishable foods. My father was learning much as he talked with the locals and wandered through the streets. The sights percolated in the back of his mind.

While developing ways to market milk and learning more about nutrition and Chinese ways, my father was simultaneously developing a distribution network. He knew from his Socony days that the system was already in place and, once adapted, could be used to distribute milk or anything else for that matter. The rivers were key. Most of the 400 million people living in China resided in the valleys and on the deltas of three great rivers; the Yangtze, the Yellow, and the Pearl. From these giant arteries, canned milk could flow into the biggest cities and then into the tiniest villages through a dense network of canals. Freight cars, camels, or bearers carrying goods on bamboo poles were also used in places the canals couldn't reach.

My dad first established *godowns* or warehouses to hold shipments of milk as they came in from the freighters. He then set out on his distribution routes traveling by whatever means was most expedient: train where possible, riverboat, canal boat, and even those bumpy and most uncomfortable Peking carts. As my father established his distribution network for canned milk and spoke with each agent, the ritual was similar. He would arrive at a shop filled with bustling assistants and the merchant would greet him—not with a handshake, but by grasping his wrists beneath the flowing sleeves of his silk gown. And it would be business as usual with the merchant and my father going through a series of negotiations until both were satisfied with the arrangement they had hammered out. Dad was learning to negotiate as if he were Chinese—displaying patience and calmness during the discussions, unlike many foreigners who would let their turmoil show—and in the process was gaining the merchants' trust. The chop was then pulled out to seal the deal. My dad believed that "if you enforce what you can enforce and should enforce, if quite without rancor you refuse to be cheated or deceived, the Asiatic will respond nobly and will be a most satisfactory business contact."

Sealing the relationship was very important for long-term success. When it came to business, milk was distributed on consignment. An agent would take a limited quantity of the milk in exchange for a deposit. The balance would be paid off after the goods were sold. This put the bulk of the risk squarely on my father's shoulders as an employee of American Milk Products: it was up to him to enforce the contract, which meant that he or an assistant would have to come back to conduct an inventory and collect payment.

By spring 1920, my father felt that he knew his product and customers well enough to expand his distribution into what was known as the Interior. The Interior was a vast and mysterious place accessible almost exclusively by the Yangtze River, where only the most intrepid foreigner would travel. It began on the outskirts of Shanghai and continued all the way to the Himalayas and the Gobi Desert.

Dad was often the first foreigner that locals in some smaller cities had ever seen—many were probably quite surprised to see him, a man walking like a pale ghost among them. The poverty was also evident here; one street vendor sold peanuts arranged into piles of three: a quantity that even the poorest passerby could afford. It was a tough market

Chapter Five: Food for Thought

in which to be selling canned milk, a commodity so inexpensive back home that almost anyone could afford it, but one that could require a day's wage here.

Traveling by river steamer on the Yangtze, my father saw the purple heads of poppies blooming on the alluvial plain, ready to harvest to make the opium that would fund the local warlord's treasury. Around 1920, three percent of the agricultural land in China had been planted in opium. By 1929, it would reach 20 percent.

From his steamer, my father continued to observe the deforestation that was taking place along the whole length of the Yangtze and was the main cause of the devastating floods that ravaged the countryside periodically. At Chengdu, the vice-regal capital of Szechuan and Tibet, he went to see earthworks designed during the Warring Kingdoms period, around 250 B.C., to prevent flooding. The system was still in use and still effective. And, while in Szechuan, he noticed the farmers alternating rows of wheat and peas. The legumes naturally nourished the wheat by fixing nitrogen from the air.

Szechuan was a generally prosperous province of carefully maintained farms and an ancient agricultural tradition. Here were found the original plants from whose cuttings the rest of the world derived oranges, lemons, grapefruit, peaches, apricots, and European walnuts.

Around Changsha, in the province of Hunan, famine gripped the countryside. From a distance, the threadbare families staggering along the canal towpaths looked like jolly, drunken buddhas, but close up my father saw that their roly-poly bodies were not jiggling with fat, but distended from starvation. These people were described as "eaters of bark and grass." Why didn't they simply take some of the vegetables and grain that were growing in the fields lining the canals?

Changsha was actually a hotbed of educational reform, centered at its new Normal School. One of the teachers, a mop-haired young man named Mao who favored a floppy cap and padded jacket like those worn by the men he was teaching, had established the student union as an undergraduate and introduced night classes for workers.

Throughout the country, the danger of bandit and warlord activity was a continuing and growing concern. In March, a landing force was sent ashore at Kiukiang, one of the major riverboat stops on the Yangtze, following a "disturbance" that threatened American lives. At Chungking, 1,500 miles upstream from the coast, gunboats were anchored midriver to protect foreigners and their interests.

Beyond the mountains that divided the Yangtze Valley from the Yellow River was Sianfu, which had been the seat of government for 11 dynasties. Most cargo was transported here by camel caravan. Yet, even here, the Chinese were buying proprietary medicines with "secret formulas," toothbrushes, cosmetics, liqueurs, and cigarettes. The market was there if you could tap it.

Slowly and patiently educating himself further in China's geographic and political realities, Dad was assembling his distribution network for canned milk and fine-tuning it to meet the needs of China. He established agencies throughout China, including Hong Kong and other cities along the Pearl River delta.

While my father was setting up the distributor network, he would be gone from the family for weeks at a time. When he returned from these trips, he began to notice that those people who remained in the comfort of the French concession didn't look too healthy. Many of the foreigners who were preparing to go home for furlough looked ravaged—they were weak, tired, and had lost their appetite. That furlough, which seemed so generous on the part of the company, now looked like a necessity. And indeed it was. As my father observed later:

> *It had been found that the general health of the foreigner, good when he first arrived, declined very steadily after a year of service in the Orient, and very rapidly after several years of uninterrupted service.*

Whatever caused the illness, it seemed to be cured by a furlough at home. When my father asked why this happened, people told him that "the steady decline in vitality was due to the climate and the unsanitary conditions in the Orient."

The prevailing scientific wisdom was that disease was caused by germs found in food, but my father was beginning to believe that many of the diseases he saw surrounding him were due to the diet—not so much what was in the diet, but what wasn't in it. He thought about the cows he had seen at the Carnation farm—those that had a diet of only alfalfa and water produced the most milk and had shiny coats. He reflected on some of his observations during his travels—those people who lived close to the land and ate a diet rich in fruits, vegetables, and whole grains tended to enjoy better health than those living in big cities. He thought about traditional Chinese medicine—the importance of balance to health. And

Did You Know

… the germ theory of disease proposes that microorganisms are the cause of most diseases?

he was becoming increasingly convinced that a plant-based diet was key to health. He was aware through his research on milk that McCollum, the co-discoverer of fat-soluble A and water-soluble B, had been working on a concentrated cattle feed at the University of Wisconsin.

Maybe there was a way to create some kind of concentrated food for humans as well? Clearly some of the illnesses suffered by foreigners living in China could be alleviated simply by providing them with a better diet. They may have been getting adequate protein, fat, and carbohydrate; however, they appeared to be missing other important nutritional elements—other important elements that could be found in plants. If only there were some kind of supplement that provided all the vitamins, minerals, and other important but unknown compounds in plants or what he called associated food factors lacking in their daily meals. Such a supplement could help "balance the diet." The thought started to nudge at the edge of my father's mind.

He also came to a similarly intuitive conclusion about the role that soil played in the nutritional value of plants and, therefore, to the people and animals eating them. He had summed it up this way:

> *It seemed to me that the general leanness and poor health of the Chinese was not due to communicable diseases and partial starvation only, or that the foreigner failed in health because of climate or the almost universal bad smells. Instead it seemed more likely that both, eating products of the land, suffered for lack of the things that got leached out of the soil.*

Feeling that healthy soil is essential for healthy plants, which in turn is essential for good health in people, my father tested his hypothesis. He found some U.S. Department of Agriculture analyses of American-grown foods and their mineral content. He then had studies made of similar plants grown in China. These consistently revealed a deficiency in potassium, phosphorous, and iodine. There may have been other critical deficiencies, but at that time the list of "essential" elements was much shorter. This would be good information to share with his Chinese agents regarding the benefits of canned milk, since the cows that produced the milk grazed on American soils.

My father had much to think about. Meanwhile, the family was adjusting and thriving in their new environment. Ned, like most foreign children in Shanghai, was learning pidgin from the servants and proper Mandarin from Dad. The family had moved from the Hotel Burlington to an apartment in Frenchtown and would soon be moving close by to a new home on Rue Ratard.

One day, my father took the family down the street to see their new home under construction. At the site, scrap wood and slops of stucco were everywhere, but the exterior was mostly finished. It was a striking home, two stories with brick below and stucco above. The big arches framed a sitting porch that opened off the front parlor. In the backyard, a big sandbox would be built. Thinking optimistically, Dad had a garage built as well to prepare for the day he would have a car. He loved cars. It wouldn't be long. After all, this was Shanghai.

Sundays were often quiet days. Although the family rarely went to church, Hester enjoyed listening to hymns on the Victorola while my father was becoming a student of comparative religions and espousing the right of all people to think freely, whether they were Christian, Jewish, Muslim, Buddhist, or any other religion. On Sunday, or when he would get some free time, my father enjoyed going for long walks out into the country. These walks would take him miles from home. It was easy to get distracted. One day he found himself lost and far from home. He walked up to a couple of farmers and asked them in his best Mandarin, "How do I get back to Shanghai?" They shook their heads uncomprehendingly. He went up to another couple of farmers and asked again in his best Mandarin, "How do I get back to Shanghai?" They didn't understand, either. My father got frustrated. After all, he could understand what the farmers were saying. Why couldn't they understand him? Finally one of the farmers said to the other, "Isn't it funny how much English sounds like Mandarin?"

During his free time, my father much preferred exploring China rather than spending time in what he thought were some of the rather snooty country clubs that

Chapter Five: Food for Thought

many of the expatriates enjoyed visiting. Close to his home was the country club (or *The Country Club* as Fuzzy, his friend from Socony, put it). Other nationalities had their own country clubs in the area, like the Americans' Columbia Country Club and the German Country Club. My father didn't particularly care for such clubs, feeling that the attitude of some of the foreigners in the country clubs alienated the very people to whom they hoped to sell their products.

Meanwhile, Hester had some news herself: she was pregnant again. The timing was excellent: my father and Hester would be able to settle into their new home on Rue Ratard before the baby was born. It was an ideal place for the family. The American School, the school Ned would attend when he was old enough, and the French Park were just a few blocks away. Everything else was easily reached by rickshaw or tram.

Hester delivered a beautiful baby girl on February 10, 1921, whom they named Nancy Fitch Rehnborg; the middle name in honor of Hester's uncle. Nancy had trouble sleeping through the night, so my father affectionately bestowed to her the title of Little Noise, and big brother Ned was promoted to the Big Noise. Like many children, two-year-old Ned wasn't too thrilled about all the attention suddenly transferred to the little bundle of joy. To Hester, he often seemed resentful of his small sister. She explained to him much later:

> *…I just tried to ignore it and show you in every way I could possibly, how much I loved you and appreciated your fine qualities, and admired your achievements, for instance your drawings and paintings and your tiny little airplanes you made so beautifully, and such, and such. And then too, I spent an awful lot of money on giving you things to occupy your very active mind. Erector sets, airplane kits, and books and books and books. But you always had a very loving and gentle streak in your makeup, and were very tender-hearted in many ways, to animals for example or birds or when someone was injured or hurt physically. This was always a very appealing trait in your rather tempestuous character which counteracted the bad.*

My father could overlook much of the commotions going on at home. He had other very pressing issues. He was beginning to find that the Chinese weren't too accepting of the idea of adding milk to their diet—even with all his nutritional studies. He originally thought it may just be a cultural dislike, but now he was finding it might be something else.

Nevertheless, he pressed on with his own research keeping an eye on the latest nutritional developments. He also began experimenting with the family's diet.

For example, Dad decided that breakfast cereal wasn't enough to provide his family with a balanced diet, even with nutritious canned milk added. So he decided to supplement it with whatever he thought might be lacking in it. Years later, he wrote:

> *In China I fed myself, my family, and friends on things that were supposed to be healthy; for instance I bought yeast in one-pound cakes and used rice polishing and things of that sort, which were added to the diet—to the cereal we ate, for example.*

My father's growing nutritional passion, however, put him sharply at odds with Ned, who didn't welcome the substitution of yeast for sugar on his morning cereal. Ned kicked and screamed. My father and two-year-old Ned just didn't see eye-to-eye on this one. Ned, however, was no match for Dad, who was equally stubborn and didn't tolerate his rebellion.

My father continued to pursue his interest in nutrition, or what some of his friends in the expatriate colony might consider an obsession, as he looked for new things to add to the diet. He ground up bones with an old grinder for his soups. Convinced that most of the mineral value of potatoes was in the fraction of an inch nearest the skin, he used potato skins in his soups, as well as the cooking water, on the theory that it contained vitamins that had been boiled out of the potato. Among the items he urged on his friends, in addition to yeast and various selections from green leafy plants, was a beverage made from infusions of rusty nails as a rich source of iron, and a dust of powdered shells scattered over foods as a source of calcium and phosphorous. Many laughed at him. Even Dad said some of his early experiments resulted in "the most God-awful messes: concentrates of milk, kelp, fish oil, wheat germ oil, liver, alfalfa, watercress, yeast, and parsley." Needless to say, meals at the Rehnborgs were a most memorable affair!

CHAPTER FIVE: FOOD FOR THOUGHT

"You've got to go out on a limb sometimes because that's where the fruit is."

—Will Rogers

Chapter 6 | The Entrepreneur

The milk business wasn't growing as quickly as my father had envisioned. Although milk provides important nutrients to the diet, he was beginning to realize selling it would be an uphill battle. He was finding that many Chinese just didn't seem to like the taste of milk. It often made them sick, and it was expensive. It was beginning to seem like there was simply no way to create a mass market for milk in China.

My father's agents throughout the country were telling him the same thing. One agent told my father that he was "losing money" because his business wasn't growing as fast as he had hoped. He could relate. It wasn't the same as working for Socony; the Chinese could only buy so much milk, especially since they weren't very fond of the stuff. It was a lot more work than selling oil and had a lot lower return.

If he could expand his business and carry additional lines, other types of merchandise, he could get more income for himself and for his existing agents. He could use the same distribution routes he had established and include other products in his selling portfolio. Just a quick peek around and he could see the immense possibilities of representing additional products. People always needed personal care items like soap, toothpaste, shaving cream; and carrying luxuries such as perfume would also be a nice touch.

Perhaps he could step out on his own and distribute canned milk as a commissioned agent for Carnation? He had already done the major leg work of establishing a distribution network. As a commissioned agent, he could represent other products as well. It would be a bit of a financial risk; he would make money only when the products sold.

Hester wasn't very enthusiastic about the idea, preferring the guarantee of a steady paycheck. What if products didn't sell? The idea of my father owning his own business was unsettling to her, especially now with a family of four to support. In a letter, years later, Hester wrote to Ned explaining:

> *Without unlimited capital, a man with responsibilities simply cannot take the risk of going into business for himself. Even if he does make enough to scrape by on, the nervous wear and tear takes it out of him, as well as out of his wife over the <u>uncertainties</u>. Wives, mothers, need a sense of security, the knowledge that there will always be a weekly or monthly paycheck coming in. It's as vitally necessary to them as food, truly.*

My father contended that it was in the best interest of the family. He envisioned being the exclusive distributor of Carnation milk products, able to budget his own time so that he could pursue his nutritional research, and at the same time distribute other products. It seemed like a win-win proposition. He might even rival his old boss from Tientsin. Hester had to agree that she thought McGowan was very successful. Could Dad be as successful, too?

He met with the folks from American Milk Products to discuss his idea of selling Carnation milk as a commissioned agent. They weren't interested—they liked the current arrangement. My father, however, saw greater possibilities.

In the summer of 1923, he followed his instinct and took a gamble setting up his own business. He had to scramble to find companies to represent as their Chinese agent. It wasn't as easy as he might have imagined. Agencies weren't his for the taking. He realized the best course of action was to return to America and persuade companies in person.

The family headed back to the States at the end of the year. It was also a chance to show off their newest family member, three-year-old Nancy, to Paul and Lillian and to visit with Sallie who was all grown up, a 24-year-old nurse living on Madison Avenue in New York City.

The family visited Paul and Lillian out at the farm in Bethlehem. It must have hit Dad pretty hard, however, when he first saw his father. Paul was an amputee—both of his legs had been removed due to a circulatory condition. He seemed to be getting around fine in his wheel chair—and it didn't seem to slow his success at business, either. Paul had recently bought a hotel on an island in Florida where he hoped his second family could spend the season. On a happier note, it was a wonderful time for Ned and Nancy to get

Chapter Six: The Entrepreneur

acquainted with their granddad and their step-grandmother. They also were able to play with eight-year-old Aunt Betty and four-year-old Uncle Marcy—Paul and Lillian's children.

During the family's visit to the States, my father's primary objective was to visit Harry Colgate of the Colgate Company. Colgate produced a huge assortment of products—products that would do well in China—exactly the kind of line he was looking for.

Looking sharp in a new suit, my father traveled by train to Jersey City. He could see the new Colgate complex sprawled over dozens of acres. It was easy to find the headquarters with the famous 40-foot clock on top of the building and a four-story sign that said "Colgate's—Soaps—Perfumes." A lot of firsts had gone into building that massive complex over the years: the first perfumed soap in 1866; the first milled soap in 1872; the first toothpaste tubes in 1896; and the first research laboratory in 1896. By 1906, the company had several laundry soaps, 160 kinds of toilet soap, and 625 varieties of perfume! What a contrast to Carnation's handful of products, which most Chinese couldn't stomach.

With no appointment, my father stepped into the building and asked Mr. Colgate's secretary to let him see the boss. "What would you like to talk to Mr. Colgate about?" she asked. "China!" my father replied. The answer flustered her and when she went to speak to Colgate he said, "Send him in!"

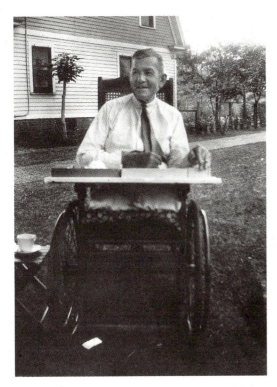

Paul Rehnborg, circa 1924-1931. Chair is outfitted with tray, on which Paul continued to make jewelry.

Selling himself as a Young China Hand, possessor of the same skills that had landed him his job with American Milk Products, my father promoted himself into the position of Colgate's independent sales representative for China. If he couldn't save Chinese teeth with Carnation Milk, maybe he could at least help keep them clean with Colgate toothpaste.

On March 19, 1924, he filed for incorporation of China Food Products Corporation in New York State—with stock valued at about $5,000 per share in 2009 dollars. The shares were issued two days later. The Colgate connection made it seem like a solid investment. One of Hester's relatives even bought six shares. They could return to Shanghai in style. But just in case, my father skipped the usual luxury liner departing from Vancouver, opting instead to book passage on the *Nile*, departing from San Francisco. On their last night in America, they stayed at the Chancellor Hotel, whose motto was *"Comfort without extravagance."*

Upon returning to Shanghai, my father had two huge "Colgate's" signs painted on his office windows and strung banners for the grand opening. Dad's office had all the latest gadgets, including a telephone about the size of a typewriter. It looked like a regular American office, except for the carpet and the wall paintings reflecting the spirit of the East. And the location of the office at 29 Szechuen Road couldn't have been better placed for excitement, between the headquarters of the Municipal Council and the sailors' dives and opium dens.

It wasn't unusual to see the gangster Big-Eared Du "sweep flamboyantly through Shanghai in his huge bullet-proof car," complete with machine-gun-toting White Russian bodyguards standing on the running boards. The city was effectively ruled by Du who, with his partner Pockmarked Huang, Frenchtown's chief of detectives, had consolidated the opium trade. Shanghai was developing a reputation for vice and corruption. However, for most expatriates, a certain amount of vice could be tolerated as long as they weren't affected and as long as there was a lid on crime. Big-Eared Du and his Green Gang had brought peace with a profit sharing scheme that allowed all factions a cut of the take. In fact, its success was enough to make businessmen like my father take note. If treating enemies like partners could bring peace among gangsters, just think what treating your employees like partners could do.

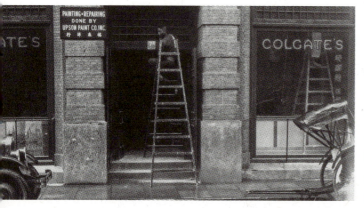

In preparation for the grand opening of China Food Products Corporation. 1924.

From the outset, my father's business was a relatively large operation. All 18 employees and a small office boy assembled in front of the building for a grand opening photograph, posed under the crossed flags of the United States and the Chinese Republic. He invited agents in for banquets, 20 at a time. While they were feasting, they could admire the posters for FAB™ detergent and Colgate™ Ribbon™ Dental Cream.**

** FAB is a trademark of Phoenix Brands LLC, Stamford, Connecticut
COLGATE and RIBBON are trademarks of Colgate-Palmolive Company, New York, New York

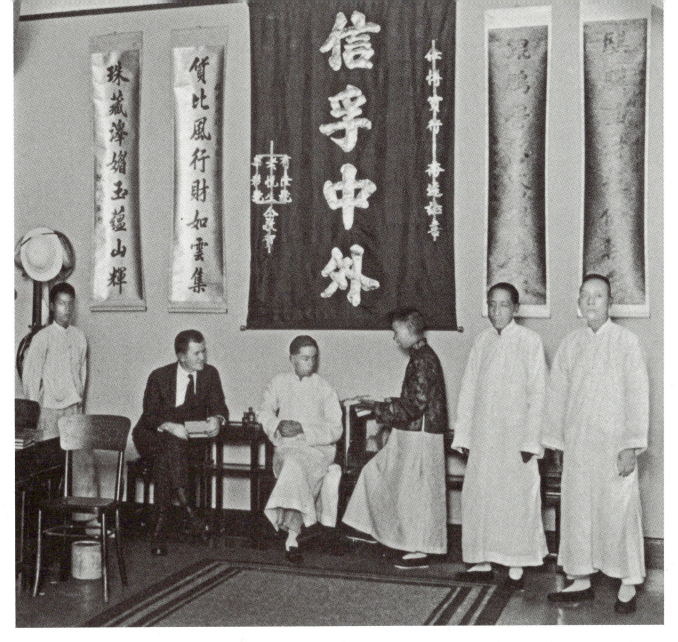

Carl Rehnborg (seated second from left) and staff at his business establishment in Shanghai, late 1920s. The four big Chinese characters on the large banner, Xin (Integrity or Reputation), Fu (Convincing), Zhong (China), Wai (Foreign Countries) means, "Well Reputed in China and All Over the World."

Did You Know

… recent science makes it clear why Dad had such a difficult time building the milk business? The problem wasn't cultural as he originally thought, it was physical. Many Chinese are lactose intolerant. They can't digest the sugar, lactose, found in milk—and without this capacity milk causes cramps, bloating, and abdominal distress.

… in 1925 Joseph Goldberger and his associates at the U.S. Public Health Services proposed a theory, which was later confirmed, that water-soluble B vitamin, identified by McCollum and Davis in 1913, actually consisted of two components? These would eventually be called vitamin B1 (thiamin) and vitamin B2 (niacin) and prevented beriberi and pellagra, respectively. Vitamin B1 was also known as vitamin F; vitamin B2 was known as vitamin G or P-P.

For other names given to vitamins and vitamin-like compounds, see Appendix 1: What's In a Name?

With no physiological intolerance to overcome, toothpaste proved popular in a way that canned milk never could. His business thrived. The combination of my father's knowledge of China, his negotiating and people skills, and the Colgate products was a winner. He could be considered a *tai-pan*, or tycoon, who could enjoy flexible hours. He now had time to do his nutritional research, read, and partake in activities he enjoyed.

One such activity was following the paleontological efforts that were happening in parts of China. Scientific expeditions had found implements used by ancient men to prepare food, as well as 1,000-year-old skeletons that revealed information about their diet. My father noted that the people were taller and their teeth had fewer dental cavities than the majority of people who currently lived in the area and wondered whether the diet somehow contributed to it. Was it out of balance? Were people getting the important associated food factors?

He continued with his interests in vitamins, preparing crude soups and gruels for his friends to try. He found that his Chinese friends liked the concoctions better than the foreigners. They were used to soups made out of alfalfa and dandelion greens. The breadth of nutritional knowledge continued to grow in the universities back home and in Europe and my father kept a vigilant eye on developments. Scientists had now broken down water-soluble B into components, including Casimir Funk's vitamin B1. Vitamin C had been isolated and identified as necessary for health in 1926.

Meanwhile, concern was growing about the sales of quack remedies in the United States, with some doctors voicing their concern that vitamins might be sold as a cure-all rather than as part of a healthy diet. The new head of the Federal Trade Commission said in 1926 that Americans "are annually robbed of hundreds of millions of dollars" through fraudulent medical advertisements.

CHAPTER SIX: THE ENTREPRENEUR

My father took it all in, and while nutrition was on his mind, so was fitness. When the weather turned warm, the family would head to the pool or the beach. Dad loved the water and loved to swim. Besides swimming, he was a member of the nearby Rowing Club. Rowing was very popular in Shanghai—and you could get a great workout strengthening your back, legs, and cardiovascular system. Dad would go rowing with his team. Fuzzy was also a member of the club, representing the Socony crowd. My father believed that exercise was every bit as important to good health as one's food choices. And at last, Dad got that long-awaited motor-car, as they called them back then. He would drive his new Rugby rag-top down Rue Ratard past nearly identical new lawns ready for mowing in front of nearly identical houses. The rapidly growing plane trees softened the new look, lending a suburban American look to the street. The neighborhood was growing more popular. Even the famous author Lu Hsun moved to Frenchtown.

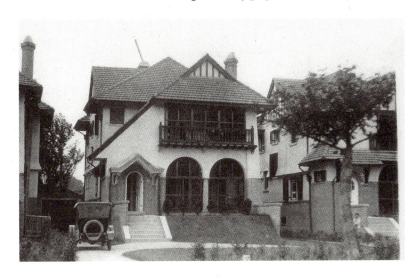

The Rehnborg home in Shanghai at 546 Rue Ratard, 1920s. In the driveway sits my father's new car.

But, the Civil War appeared to be heating up. The communists had monopolized the top posts of the Nationalist Party. Chiang Kai-shek averted a coup attempt at the Whampoa Military Academy and seized control of Canton.

Dad, along with Fuzzy who had just recently returned from the war in Europe, was recruited to join the Shanghai Volunteer Corps, a military body of some 2,000 men from all nations charged with helping maintain order in the International Settlement and protect the city from warlords.

While all this was happening, Ned wrote to his grandma, Amanda, in Boston: "Some frogs laid a lot of egges [sic] and they have turned in-to tadpoles. Your grandson." Life went on for the expatriates in Shanghai.

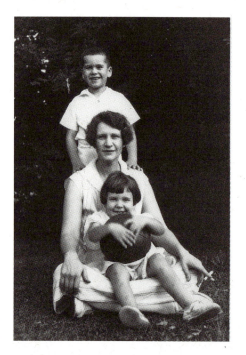

Hester, Ned, and Nancy Rehnborg, 1926

Hester wrote on the back of the photo: "Our kiddies Ned and Sister. Also Sallie Rehnborg 1926 Shanghai."

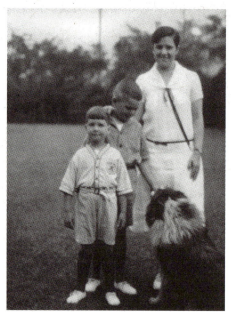

One day while my father was out and about in Shanghai supervising the unloading of some cargo, he happened to chat with the ship's captain. The captain was complaining to my father about the food on the ship—namely, the salt biscuits. Salt biscuits were a standard shipboard ration in those days and would get soggy after a few weeks at sea. My father knew the problem. The biscuits were oxidizing over time. Keep the oxygen out of the containers, and you could keep them indefinitely—just like the process used in canned milk. It was news to the captain. My father suggested that a vacuum be created in the biscuit container to remove the oxygen. The captain reportedly liked the idea so much that he became the first manufacturer of the vacuum pack.

Sallie had also moved to China, perhaps inspired by my father's adventures. She lived in a little cottage that my father had built in their backyard and worked as a surgical nurse at a well-known private hospital. Here in China, she met her future husband—a man who was a rising star in the Socony hierarchy. My father couldn't have been happier and even helped her fiancée pick out her engagement ring. It was his good friend Fuzzy Vaughn, after all!

Chapter Six: The Entrepreneur

Business was good for my father—even though the Chinese political situation was heating up. It looked like he had made a wise decision to pass over a permanent position at Carnation for the risk of being a free agent. His business flourished and he had the time to pursue his nutritional investigations and outside interests. Life was good.

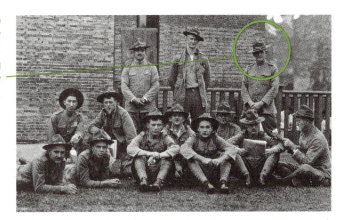

Members of the Shanghai Volunteer Corps, circa 1923-1927. My father is standing in the back row at the far right.

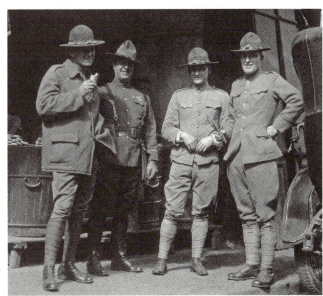

In this photo Dad is on the left.

"Out of difficulties grow miracles."

—Jean de la Bruyere

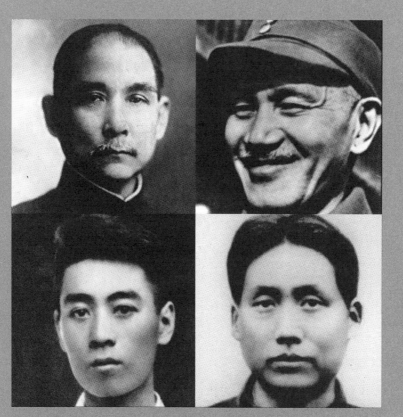

Sun Yat-sen, undated

Chiang Kai-shek, 1945

Chou En-lai, 1919

Mao Tse-tung, 1927

Chapter 7 | A Pearl from the Orient

In 1926, Chinese politics boiled over. And the boiling point was in the city where my father lived and had built his business: the Pearl of the Orient, Shanghai. One year earlier, Sun Yat-sen, who had been living in a house in Frenchtown, had died of cancer. A scramble began to fill the tremendous void he had left in the life of post-imperial China. Big-Eared Du and the Green Gang were determined to have their say, as was Big Eared Du's protégé Chiang Kai-shek, who recently returned from military training in Moscow and whose true political allegiance was unknown. The former teacher Mao Tse-tung had been working in a Shanghai laundry, while the Soviet Comintern agent Mikhail Borodin had enrolled his children in the American School. Among the Chinese Communist Party labor organizers working in the city was Chou En-lai, soon to help lead a Shanghai general strike. The political life of the wider world had come to China, and it had come with a vengeance.

Reports filtered into Shanghai on the status of warlords with colorful nicknames, as the Dogmeat General and the Christian General and their various coalitions as they dominated one area or another. The fighting had left much of the country in tatters, and the soldiers patrolling the Yangtze often appeared to be little better than pirates. In January 1925, as the failing Sun tried to unite the warlords and end the fighting, riots and demonstrations erupted in Shanghai. American Marines were landed to protect lives and property in the International Settlement. On May 30, ten protesters were shot by the Shanghai Municipal Police under British command, and a general strike and anti-British boycott were called in response. The strikes continued until September. The formerly docile Chinese were spitting on foreigners and displaying posters showing the "foreign devils" covered in blood. Foreign interests, such as those of my father, were increasingly at risk.

Life in China for the family promised to be very good indeed, if they could weather the present political difficulties. But the civil conflict seemed to be edging closer.

The accrued resentment of decades of foreign disrespect was finding voice among ordinary Chinese. At Hankow, British and American forces were landed to help suppress rioters and protect foreign businesses. In Chengtu, a warlord looted the city only to be driven out by another General, whose soldiers then looted what was left. Word came from the interior that one of my father's agencies had been wiped out. If Dad traveled to the province, it might still be possible for him to retrieve some portion of the looted goods.

Dad set off up the Yangtze. The riverboats had added steel plates along the decks to protect passengers and crew from snipers along the shore. Upriver, travelers were frequently escorted by platoons of soldiers. Dead bodies lined the trails, and foreign families were given instructions on how to reach river gunboats in an emergency. My father had to abandon this trip and return home to Shanghai.

In May of 1926, Chiang Kai-shek, an unusual combination of courtier, gunman, military officer, and politician, turned suddenly on his Communist Party allies, capturing and hanging many of the Party leaders. Awarded dictatorial powers, he formed the Northern Expedition, a military campaign to unite China, sweeping north through central China to Hankow.

In July, the British agreed to return their concessions at Hankow and Kiukiang to the Chinese over two years. Shanghai was apprehensive about the Nationalist advance. The Nationalist Party continued to enjoy the support of the Soviet Union, which was in disarray now after the death of Lenin and the subsequent power struggle between Stalin and Trotsky. Shanghai's foreign businessmen feared that the Nationalist government would implement a Russian-style communist regime.

The Northern Expedition captured Changsha, capital of Hunan Province, in August. Rumors abounded that landlords were being killed and their property seized for redistribution. Political allegiances were so confused that the Russians professed to be "aghast" at land seizures by Mao's Communists in Hunan.

Nationalist forces captured Kiukiang. In the International Settlement, small firms were beginning to go bankrupt, unable to collect payment from upcountry

A Brief Glimpse at the Political Situation in China from 1911 to 1925

1911: In October, a revolution in China begins with a bomb explosion and the discovery of revolutionary headquarters in Hankow. The revolutionary movement spreads rapidly through west and southern China, forcing the abdication of the last Ch'ing emperor, six-year-old Henry Pu-Yi. In December, the Republic of China is established. Sun Yat-sen named temporary president.

1912: Rulers of Manchu Dynasty formally abdicate. Yuan Shi-kai becomes the president of the Republic of China. The Nationalist Party is formed.

1913: The Nationalist Party stages a revolt against Yuan. The revolt fails and the Nationalist leaders flee to Japan. Yuan becomes a dictator and takes steps to establish himself as emperor.

1916: Yuan dies. Presidents continue to hold office in Beijing. The real power, however, belongs to the warlords in northern China.

1919: The May Fourth Movement begins precipitated by resentment against weak warlord governments in Beijing as well as unfair terms of the Versailles Treaty that grant territorial concessions to Japan.

1919: Sun begins to reorganize the Nationalist Party.

1921: Founding of the Communist party.

1923: The Soviet Union sends advisors to China to help Nationalists.

1923-1927: The Nationalists and Communists join forces for the purpose of wresting control of China from warlords and restoring national unity.

1925: Sun dies. Chiang Kai-shek becomes the new leader of the Nationalists.

1927: Nationalist-Communist split; Chinese Civil War.

1928: Most of China is reunited under the control of the Nationalist Party.

agents, and steamers were canceling their trips upstream. The yacht-sized gunboats that formerly kept the peace on the river were now dwarfed by destroyers and cruisers anchored in midstream.

The American Minister to China sent an urgent request for 20,000 troops to defend Shanghai's International Settlement. U.S. President Coolidge sent a Marine regiment instead. Wuhan, the Pittsburgh of China, was shut down by a general strike. Foreign refugees descended on Shanghai, turning the green waterfront bund into a lengthy refugee camp.

Hester couldn't take the children out to the public gardens any longer to look at the warships without stepping over bodies of refugees; some sleeping, some dead. The bad news from the interior continued unabated. The British concession in Kiukiang was peacefully overrun. Foreign residents were evacuated from Changsha. It was a wholesale pullback by foreigners. Nothing like this had ever happened in China before. A new self-confidence permeated the Chinese working class in the cities upstream. Even coolies began to sass the Europeans and demand unheard-of-payments to work for them.

In February 1927, the Nationalists began advancing down the Yangtze Valley toward Shanghai. Fighting around the city caused American naval and marine forces to be increased.

Nobody in Shanghai really knew what was happening in the interior. My father was cut off from his agents. A delegation was sent to Hankow and Hunan to seek information. They returned with horror stories: they had been seized by the Communists and paraded through the villages like criminals, wearing signs branding them *Imperialist Dogs*.

On behalf of the foreign business community, my father was delegated to negotiate with a warlord near Shanghai. The warlord had seized a large compound for his headquarters. The courtyard was filled with soldiers whose rifles were leaning against the tripods of covered machine guns. Some of the men were in uniforms, others in white gowns. They sat on ammunition boxes, playing mah-jongg or eating rice. My father trembled as he walked into the general's encampment, under a white flag. His previous business negotiating experience served him well enough that, even though his negotiations were fruitless, he got home alive and unharmed.

To help bring some kind of order to the country, the foreigners, who had once feared Chiang Kai-shek as another Communist leader, were now offering to raise funds in support of him as a potential savior.

The Chinese Communist Party had other ideas. They planned to remove Chiang from command of the military and strip him of his dictatorial powers. On February 19, 1927, Chou En-lai, a militant Communist labor leader, called for a general strike. Nationalist troops, meanwhile, had reached Hangchow, just a one-hour train ride from Shanghai.

Foreign troops began pouring into Shanghai, some 40,000 of them from Japan, Italy, and France, as well as from America and Britain. Their orders were to defend their countrymen, not to make war on the Chinese.

My father and Hester tried to maintain a semblance of normal life for their family, taking the kids to see the military formations and parades. Dad even wrote a poem harkening back to his own quiet childhood, where he and his brothers and sisters would swim in the old mill pond in Huntington. And in a veneer of normalcy, Fuzzy and Sallie tied the knot on December 14, 1926. They immediately departed back to the States on a six-month furlough for their honeymoon.

Chapter Seven: A Pearl from the Orient

But there was no hiding the fact that Shanghai had turned into an armed camp. For my father and Hester, the stress took both an emotional and financial toll. In fact, with all the company's stocks on consignments, my father would only be paid if and when the products sold.

Travel inland was too dangerous, assuming my father could still book passage on one of the few British steamers still making the trip. Nor could he send someone else. Mobs were snatching "running dogs of the imperialists" and abusing them.

Hearing that the Nationalist forces were less than 100 miles away, the soldiers of the local warlord guarding Shanghai became demoralized and melted away. Control of the city seemed to hang in the balance, but who would prevail? Big-Eared Du and Pockmarked Huang with their gangster-police alliance? The Communists? The Nationalists?

From his home in the French concession, Big-Eared Du released an announcement declaring that he would maintain order until the Nationalist troops arrived in the city. In response, the Communists mounted a demonstration at the capitalist heart of Shanghai, outside the Sincere and Wing On department stores. Blowing off firecrackers while leaflets rained down from the roofs of the department stores, the crowds chanted, "Down with British imperialism!" and "Down with the reactionaries!" Chinese and Indian policemen moved in, blowing whistles, clubbing demonstrators with truncheons, and tossing their bodies into paddy wagons to be taken to the city jail.

On March 20, Chou En-lai declared a general strike. The entire city shut down as 600,000 workers refused to work. There was no mail. The streetcars stopped running. The air cleared as factories stopped belching their smoke. Chou En-lai sent 5,000 armed workers to seize the police stations, the arsenal, and the old army garrison. Another 50,000 strikers were assigned to maintain order. Chou had taken City Hall, proclaiming a People's Government of Shanghai.

The following morning, the reaction set in. The Municipal Court declared a state of emergency. My father was called to assemble with his unit of the Shanghai Volunteer Corps, which was charged with setting up and manning the barricades on the Garden Bridge and at other International Settlement crossings.

At the Garden Bridge, a tram had been boxed in at the peak of the bridge. Barbed-wire barricades were drawn halfway across the bridge, leaving a narrow passage through which people and vehicles moved slowly. There was a trickle moving north, but a heavy stream heading south, into the part of the city guarded by foreign soldiers.

The refugees descended past the barricade onto the park-like bund, where there was more room. The business district buildings, once flowing with commerce, were all closed, their windows "blankly shuttered or crisscrossed with gummed paper" to protect them from the concussions of artillery, their doors blocked with barbed wire and sandbags.

More than 6,000 miles of barbed wire had been strung around the International Settlement. The Settlement was walled in with some 800,000 sandbags and guarded by 30,000 men with rifles. Entry and exit were permitted only through manned checkpoints. Concrete blockhouses had been erected on the outskirts to protect the entrances from invading troops. Artillery could be heard, firing in the distance. Shanghai's foreign enclave, the world's largest gated community, had become, in effect, a prison.

One morning, the firing dwindled. Chou's forces seemed to have captured Shanghai. Men and women wearing red armbands surrounded the International Settlement, while the telephones inside the Settlement were cut off. There was no way for my father to collect his debts or even assess the damage to his agencies.

Within the isolated Settlement, foods supplies grew short. My father noticed the signs of malnutrition among his colleagues, unable to get access to fresh fruits and vegetables, or pay the exorbitant wartime prices. His previous food experiments became crucial as he helped keep expatriates alive and strong until they could get out of China. Using whatever greens he could gather from the Settlement's parks and gardens and whatever foodstuffs he was able to persuade the Chinese guards to bring him, he prepared his soups or gruels. He added rusty nails and bones to his stew whenever he could, knowing that they would provide supplemental iron and calcium and other valuable minerals. He passed out samples to his friends and neighbors. Dad and the family ate it, and he encouraged everyone who would listen to do the same. At least one "highly successful businessman," as Dad described him, was intrigued enough to pay attention as my father collected greens from roadsides, fiddled with nails and apples, and cooked up these foul-tasting concoctions that were supposed to be of significant nutritional value. He didn't like the concoctions any better than anybody else, but he believed what my father said about their nutritional value.

Chapter Seven: A Pearl from the Orient

Meanwhile Chiang's Northern Expedition forces remained bivouacked outside the city. In a kind of truce, Chiang entered the city by gunboat on March 26. The Kuomintang Central Committee had removed him from command of the Northern Expedition, yet local generals still came aboard ship to confer with him.

Panic was spreading into the city. On April 9, the *President Taft* set sail with 300 Americans from Shanghai aboard, most of them women and children. At night, searchlights from the gunboats lit up the buildings along the bund, where women and children, sent from the interior, swelled the ranks of refugees.

For Hester, their existence in Shanghai had come to an end. A house, servants, a business, none of these was worth the risk to her family's lives. Life for her in China had changed forever. It was time for those who could to leave. At her insistence, my father made reservations for Hester and the children to return to the States. Her thoughts were clear. It was time to give up. It didn't matter if he had made a success of things several times. She had lost faith in him. On March 6, 1927, they boarded the *Empress of Russia*—the last passenger steamer to leave Shanghai during the crisis—and headed to Massachusetts to live with her mother on her estate.

For my father, it was different. The challenges didn't appear insurmountable, dire though they might appear to be. Something would turn up. It had been 12 years since he had first come to China. He loved China—the language, the friendships, his company, his continuing passion—his growing vision for the future of health and nutrition—were all here. To abandon this would be to abandon what he'd come to realize was the best part of himself. His marriage had been a mismatch—although it hadn't really become clear until the financial situation deteriorated. He and Hester were opposites. She thought he was ruined, he thought something would turn up. He was determined to stay.

Hester saw this as stubbornness, selfishness, an immature refusal to accept the reality of having to work under other men. To my father, his autonomy, pursuit of his vision, was literally a matter of life and death. If required to knuckle under, to simply survive from day-to-day like so many men, he would perish, and he knew it. He was willing to pursue a deeper challenge, a challenge that amounted to the true test of a life.

Determined to make a go of his business, Dad economized. He moved into the little backyard cottage, the same one Sallie lived in before she and Fuzzy got married. My father figured that renting out the main house would give him a little extra money while he was salvaging his business.

About one month after the family departed to America, on April 12, his application to change the name of his business from China Food Products to CF Rehnborg, Inc. was approved in New York. And on May 3, he sat in his office at 29 Szechuen Road to type a reply to a letter he received from Ned, who was nine at the time, which had been posted from a refueling stop in Hawaii. Hester, before she had left for the States, had told my father that since he was penniless, she wanted nothing more to do with him. But he kept all his worries out of the letter:

Dearest Ned,

This morning the postman was very nice to me. He brought me your letter with the picture of the two islands. I know those islands perfectly. You saw them after you left Nagasaki, on the left side of the ship. And just beyond that was a big harbor where the Japanese keep their warships. Did you see that also? It was on the right hand side of the ship.

You were lucky to see the porpoises. I have often seen them, but not always, although I always look for them. Between Japan and Vancouver I'll bet you saw some whales as well, because there are lots of them there. Then at night, near Japan and near Vancouver, there is lots of phosphorescence (bet you did not read that word) in the water, and it all looks as if it was made of soft fire. I hope you saw some of that too. The fishes in the water all swim fast to get out of the way of the steamer, and as they swim the water shines and they make long streaks in the water.

Do you remember the little house back of ours that Sallie had? That is my house now, and it is an awfully nice little place for one person. But there is one thing I notice a lot, and that is the quiet. Ned and Nancy are so far away that I can't hear them in my house at all, and I miss the Big Noise and the Little Noise. How is the Little Noise by the way? You didn't write anything about her in your letter to me, although you mentioned your watch several times.

I think it is lovely that you are Hester's time keeper. Does she have to look at the watch, or do you read it and tell her what time it says? And are you always right? And if you are, is the watch?

I love you heaps and lots. Here are some kisses (x) one for you, and (x) one for Nancy, and (xx) two for Hester. Please deliver these for me. Good loud smacks.

Please write me lots, Carlos

Chapter Seven: A Pearl from the Orient

By early May, the military emergency had eased. The foreign landing parties began returning to their ships. However, the business climate seemed to have changed irrevocably. "The plight of the Chinese merchant," reported the *New York Times*, "is pitiable." Dad found it impossible to collect from his agents or to pay for the products that had been shipped across the Pacific to him. He had been cut off from his godowns throughout the interior of China, which had been stocked to the gills with products from Colgate and other foreign manufacturers. My father had no way of knowing how many tubes of toothpaste and bars of Cashmere Bouquet soap had been looted by the warlords. The goods had all been on consignment and for all practical purposes were lost, yet their loss was his responsibility. His business was finished. He had lost it all: family, house, car, servants, office, and corporation. But the most profound loss was his wife's belief in him. There was finger-pointing, as if the convulsions of China had somehow been his fault, but no one was really to blame.

"It's been often said," Hester wrote years later to Ned, "that if a person knows his own failings and shortcomings, he can remedy them <u>if he really wants to</u>. But you have to <u>want</u> to awfully hard…We have to compromise. We have to learn to 'make do.' It's either learn this hard lesson or become a drifter, a rolling stone." My father was adrift, and he was broke. And he was alone. This was not just failure, but lost achievement, an even more discouraging form of pain. Convinced at last that nothing would turn up that would allow him to stay in his adopted home of China, he had nothing left, not even boat fare. One thing did turn up, however. His old employer, Carnation, came to the rescue and lent him the price of passage home. And so on June 24, 1927, my father picked himself out of the rubble of his marriage and his working life and embarked for the States in a third-class cabin on the *Empress of Russia*.

Although he was broke, discouraged, and disenchanted, he left China with a "pearl from the Orient" — so to speak, an idea that was better than gold. It would take awhile for the idea to flourish into reality. It wouldn't be easy. It would be a struggle. But when you have a dream, a vision, and determination … anything is possible. And my father had all three.

Part 2
Building a Dream

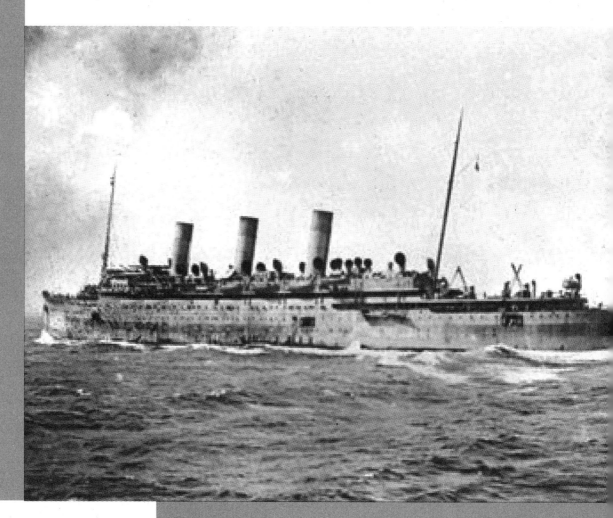

"Not until we are lost do we begin to understand ourselves."

—Henry David Thoreau

The Empress of Russia, 1914. My father boarded this ship when he returned to America in 1927.

Chapter 8 | Desert Interlude

In many of the great "vision quest" legends worldwide, the would-be warrior must undergo a season of testing in the desert. It's a time of stripping, both externally and internally, where the nonessentials are pared away and the heart is laid bare. And if he's alert, he emerges from this time of stripping having received a gift that could not have been given in any other way and that will carry him all the way.

Whether my father's vision quest can be seen as a living legend or not, the fact remains that the season in the desert was literally true. In the years immediately following his return to the States, in the bare and pitiless Mojave Desert of southeastern California, his heart was broken wide open. The interlude was so brief and isolated a season in my father's life that it's almost possible to pass right along without mentioning it, except that it may just contain the key to everything that would follow.

On July 10, 1927, the *Empress of Russia* arrived in Vancouver. From there my father hopped a freighter headed to Los Angeles, California. I'm not sure why he chose Los Angeles, but it was a land of opportunity: clear skies and orange groves as far as the eye could see. The California economy was booming. In Southern California, and particularly in Los Angeles, the dipping-bird pumps of working oil wells were popping up all over the landscape. Oil drove the national economy, and my father was, or at least had been, an oil man. He may have considered getting back into the oil business. Los Angeles was the headquarters of Vacuum Oil Company, Socony's partner, as well as Richfield and others. And then there was Hollywood, a good place for dreams to take root. This is where a developer created the "Miracle Mile" and turned it into the shopping street of the stars, where L. Frank Baum had dreamed up the Emerald City and Dorothy, and where a young man named Marion Morrison changed his name and suddenly became John Wayne. Whatever the reason, something in my father seemed to subconsciously know that California would be the place where his destiny would unfold.

At the outset, Dad didn't seem to take advantage of any of the opportunities for connection, partly because, as he later admitted, "I was flat on my back and looking up." For him, it was a time to regroup, recharge his batteries, and figure out what he was going to do with his life. To the outsider looking in, he may have appeared all washed up. He was 40 years old and had arrived with only $24 in his pocket and the suit on his back. However, it didn't seem to bother him. He knew something would turn up.

In the beginning, he took whatever odd jobs he could find to make ends meet—bus driver, baby sitter, clerical worker—while he dabbled with his nutrition experiments. It was while he was a manager at a small hospital in Los Angeles that he received the initial correspondence of his divorce. Hester had dug deep in the past, to their argument over whether to move to Beaumont, Texas, as the grounds for the termination of their marriage. The final notice in July 1928 was returned unopened with a note that my father was "gone." It seemed to be proof that he wasn't going to lead the stable life she desired. Hester was awarded custody of the children.

This is when my father's vision quest began in an almost literal sense, in an austere place far removed from Los Angeles and Hollywood. Shortly after the divorce was final, my father took off to the desert to begin work as a statistician at the American Potash and Chemical Company in Trona.

Trona was a dusty town in a dead, desert landscape, on the edge of the Mojave Desert. Summer temperatures regularly registered 115°F. On the hottest days, the thermometer could soar to 125°F. Effective air-conditioning was as yet just a dream, and as for shade, only scrawny tamarisk trees and sagebrush could survive the salty soil. The bitterly cold winters weren't much better. Residents joked that Trona was a town of "too" seasons: too hot, too cold, or too windy.

The town itself was named after the sole reason for its existence: the soda ash used to manufacture such products as baking soda, glass, paper, and laundry detergents. The trona was mined from a lakebed, allowed to dry naturally, and then processed in the factory. Since

> "I have heard a story of a movie producer who had run through his second fortune. When his friends expressed condolences for his being ruined, he said, 'Heck, I'm not ruined; I'm just broke.' That goes for me, too."
>
> —Carl F. Rehnborg

it was a company town, employees were paid in scrip, usable only in the company-owned facilities. Most of the single men, like Dad, slept in barracks.

The work, for most men, was brutal and tedious. One resident remembered selling newspapers to them as a boy. "The look in their eyes said it all. This was damn hard work … and I feel something for all the men who ever worked the plant. It sure turned young men to middle-aged men in a hurry."

Most of the men found some solace with a cold beer in Austin Hall, with its poolroom behind the deep, shadowy arcade on the town square. Trona had a company store, a bar, a club, and a small weekly paper called the *Trona Pot-Ash* for reading enjoyment. Although my father didn't particularly care for beer, he did enjoy people and conversation. With few other places to go in town other than the barracks, he probably spent a fair amount of time in the club. While the men racked up balls for a pool game, he would speak about his days in China, about his ideas regarding nutrition, and about man's relationship with the universe.

Here, my father was doing statistical calculations. He was a cog in the wheel. The work wasn't particularly challenging. As always, he found comfort in his books and in his writing.

During this time, he wrote a letter to his sister Sallie in China. The letter just missed her. She had already left China for the States to prepare for one of Fuzzy's upcoming furloughs. Fuzzy got the letter, though, and enclosed it with a letter of his own and sent it on to his wife. Sallie received it in the middle of the night, having just arrived in Connecticut. She immediately sat down to dash off a reply. Her reply was like a lifeline:

> *Dearest darlingest Carl—*
>
> *You bet your sweet life I feel kindly to write! Bless your darling heart, I don't suppose anything came nearer making*

me weep for joy [than] hearing from you, and grief over the struggles you've had, than your letter did that I just got. It's 11 o'clock, I've just come back from N.Y. where I've been taking my driving exam & where I'm to collect a beautiful new Packard sedan tomorrow. This isn't a letter at all—you'll get one in a few days telling you all the dope—but this is just to tell you how gorgeously [underlined three times] happy you've made me. Your letter came enclosed in one of Fuzzy's.

And I [underlined twice] am enclosing some snaps of my sweet nipper—his name is Porter Davis & he was a year old May 15th. He is up in Fairhaven with Pump now & I'm motoring up Saturday with Chick (Pump's husband) in my lovely new car. Fuzzy comes in October via Siberia & we'll be West sometime around Xmas.

Carl, darling I love you so [underlined twice] much & am so happy to have found you again. I can't even tell you you're a bad brother for neglecting me for so long. More real soon, dearest--& in the meantime tons of love. From Sallie

Things were going well for the Vaughns. They had a toddler named Porter Davis who had celebrated his first birthday. Fuzzy was doing well at Socony. When he came to the States during his next furlough, they would be able to catch up in person. He and the family would drive across the country to California to settle in Fuzzy's hometown of Colton in San Bernardino County—about a three-hour drive from Trona.

Although my father was lonely, it was good to reconnect with his sister, and he realized things could be a lot worse. The Wall Street crash on Black Tuesday, October 29, 1929, put things in perspective. He knew he was lucky to have a job. And, with a regular income he was able to buy a car that he used whenever possible to escape the drudgery of life in Trona.

During the Thanksgiving holidays, he escaped by taking a road trip, which got written up in the *Trona Pot-Ash*. He left Trona on a Tuesday with some friends and made his way to Barstow, where he apparently met up with Sallie and Fuzzy. My father and his friends toured throughout Southern California into the San Bernardino Mountains to Big Bear, where the snow was already starting to fall, then south to the Imperial Valley along the Mexican border and over to the sleepy little coastal city of San Diego.

It was during this trip that he may have met a young nurse named Mildred Frances Thompson. Mildred was the instructor of nurses and the assistant supervisor of the

Chapter Eight: Desert Interlude

Cottage Hospital, a noted sanatorium in Santa Barbara. The details of how they first met are unclear, but what was very clear is that the 29-year-old Mildred and my 43-year-old father were soon deeply in love and talking about marriage. They were married on July 19, 1930, in Los Angeles, with Sallie as a witness.

Almost immediately the newlyweds faced a problem. There was virtually no family housing in town. The barracks housing was nice enough and cheap, but to find both privacy and some relief from the heat was virtually impossible. The plant manager and town manager lived in the only two-story houses in town. My father put his name on a waiting list for company housing. He also looked for work elsewhere, including writing a letter to the Pacific Commercial Company asking for a job in Asia. Although impressed with his resume, they had no openings. So during this time, my father and Mildred got used to the drill of weekend visits while she continued to work in Santa Barbara.

The next year, during the summer of 1931, Dad took a trip back East to visit his family in Bethlehem. He was able to catch up with 12-year-old Ned as well. Although he was delighted to see Ned, it was a painful reminder of how much he missed his children. It was also tough to see his father. Paul was very ill and it was clear that he wouldn't have much more time in this world.

Several months later, on September 11, 1931, at the age of 72, Paul passed away. His body was taken to the family's hometown of Huntington, Connecticut, and was buried in the town cemetery. Now, at the age of 44, my father had lost both his parents.

Just in time for the Christmas holidays, Dad and his bride got some good news. They had been assigned house number 19 on California Street in Trona. They could live together at last. They would be able to move in to their new home shortly after the New Year. They got even better news; they were expecting their first child.

They had much to be thankful for. My father had a job at a time of deepening economic depression, they had a baby on the way, a roof over their heads, and they were in love. Mildred was the love of my father's life and, for Mildred, it was mutual. My father was the kind of person who wasn't shy to show his emotions—whether he was angry or upset or gleefully happy—and he showered Mildred with love in a million different ways: little notes for no reason, unexpected presents, a tender touch, and constant reassurance of devotion.

Even a column in the *Trona Pot-Ash* noted how committed they were to each other.

That winter of 1932 was bitterly cold. Fortunately their new home was toasty warm with steam heat generated by the mill. But all was not well. On Tuesday, February 23, 1932, Mildred felt some pain in the middle of her abdomen, near her belly button. She was worried that something was wrong with the baby. After a few hours, the pain shifted to her lower right side. Mildred was examined by her physician, who concluded she had acute appendicitis. He operated on her two days later, and the prognosis seemed good. The baby appeared safe and Mildred's condition appeared normal aside from high blood pressure.

Then things took a turn for the worse. Mildred continued to feel abdominal pain. She was nauseous and so exhausted that she could barely move. She began to experience uterine bleeding. Apparently, during the course of her illness or treatment, she had suffered an infection. Mildred miscarried, and her bleeding wouldn't stop. The infection reached her urinary tract and shut down her kidneys. Mildred fell into a coma from which she never awoke. She died on February 28 at the age of 31.

The whole community was shocked. My father didn't even consider burying Mildred in Trona's dusty graveyard, a barren plot with random wooden crosses on the grave sites. After the funeral in Bakersfield, he took her to Santa Barbara to be buried. He never fully recovered from the loss.

On the drive back to Trona, alone all the way to the bottom of his heart, he told me that he had wept bitter tears, but finally emerged through them into what he later remembered as "the peace of nothingness." He marveled at the incomparably beautiful flowers, lush in their California rainy season greenery. It was less important that Mildred was gone than that she had existed at all and had shared her life with him. Somehow, on that mystical ride back home, Mildred came to him in a new form, a form that would never leave him, as a spirit of hope. Many years later, still trying to recapture the vividness of that experience, he wrote: "There is wonder and adventure in the highest degree in most of the elements of this affair of being a part of life in the universe." The myriad colors of flowers between the ocean and Bakersfield showed the beauty of existence and the power of living. The touch of her presence was right there, always with him, in the power of life itself. No matter how tough the going got, my father never again lost touch with that power.

CHAPTER EIGHT: DESERT INTERLUDE

On Monday, July 5, 1932, he left Trona for a month's vacation in Los Angeles. He never returned. During that month, he found work in the Payroll Department at Richfield Oil Company. It was a clerical job, to be sure, but it put bread and butter on the table while my father, tempered and strengthened by his season in the desert, was now ready to give his heart and soul to that passion that had so long been growing in him: finding a way to supplement the diet with all the vitamins, minerals, and other associated food factors necessary for optimum health. Now, more than ever, it seemed a way to honor the power of life.

*"The more original a discovery,
the more obvious it seems afterwards."*

—Arthur Koestler

Chapter 9 | From Stovetop to Storefront

Mildred was gone. My father dealt with the loss by throwing himself deeper into work, although not the work at Richfield Oil Company, but increasingly more to his real passion. His time in the desert and his time with Mildred had strengthened him. The famous quote from philosopher Friedrich Nietzsche, "that which does not kill us makes us stronger," was definitely the case for my father. He was ready to commit himself, heart and soul, to developing his food supplement.

During his spare time, he read all that he could about the new breakthroughs in nutrition; especially regarding those vitamins and other "unknowns" that are needed in very small amounts in human and animal diets. He was fortunate because the brand-new Los Angeles County Library was just blocks away from his "official" workplace. He spent countless hours absorbing the information tucked away in scientific journals, as well as clipping articles from newspapers and magazines for his scrapbook. The field of nutrition was buzzing with excitement and had started to gain momentum while he was down on his luck in Los Angeles and during his time in the desert during the late 1920s and early 1930s.

He discussed his ideas for a food supplement with his friends and acquaintances. One new acquaintance, also an employee at Richfield Oil Company, was a man named Spence Halverson. Halverson was an attorney who would soon become the manager of the Lease and Contract Department at Richfield.

Another new friend was a fellow inventor named Henry Stephens, who was working on a process to create frozen orange juice concentrate. Stephens was a kindred spirit and according to my father "a pioneer in that industry, contributing most of the

Did You Know

… in the span of three decades, starting in the early 1900s, all 13 vitamins were discovered? To today's observer, their discovery may appear straightforward. Science, however, has its own zig-zag approach to discovery. Along the way, certain compounds thought to be vitamins were debunked, while others were confirmed. For details, see Appendix 1: What's In a Name?

… in 1920, the final E on the coined word "vitamine" was dropped? Scientists discovered that not all vitamins contained the nitrogen-containing "vital" amine group.

methods that are in standard practice in fruit juice canning, such as irradiation in a vacuum and flash pasteurization of the canned product." The two spent countless hours together talking about their pet projects. And so the time went, weekdays at Richfield to make financial ends meet, and weekends and spare time with nutrition experiments and conversing with others about ideas, theories, and technologies.

Imagine Dad's surprise when a 25-year-old-woman with a long braid showed up on his doorstep in Los Angeles—with marriage on her mind. Well, she wasn't altogether a stranger. Evelyn Berg was a friend of his family back East. She had often babysat for Paul and Lillian's two busy youngsters and was also a friend of Sallie. Evie had met my father once or twice during his furloughs back from China and evidently quietly carried a torch for him. 'If ever he becomes available…' she had daydreamed. Hearing he was in mourning, she hopped a train to California, in spite of valiant efforts of her family to dissuade her. Now, here she was. Headstrong and spirited, as well as strikingly beautiful, she had her way. There was no record of how it happened, but within a short time they were married. Esther, one of Evie's two younger sisters, could see the appeal. She said years later, the Rehnborg boys "were all tall, nice looking. I could see why Carl would be attractive to Evie." He was confident, "he knew what he wanted and went after it. He got it."

It must have been a surprise for Evie as well, when she re-encountered my father. When she had last seen him, he was a dashing tai-pan, visiting from China. Obviously, she had heard that his business in China had been wiped out and about Mildred's fatal illness. She must have known that he was working at Richfield Oil Company. It's possible she thought he was working his way up the ladder, maybe toward a position similar to one that his brother-in-law, Fuzzy, held at Socony.

Dad's Scrapbook

My father kept a scrapbook with nutrition and health-related articles of interest. One such article he pasted in the book was from the December 1932 issue of *Scientific American*. The article described a study which documented that cod liver oil added to the regular diet cut the incidence of the common cold by 40 percent and decreased workplace absence by 50 percent.

Evie soon found out that during my father's time alone, he had been thinking about finding a way to supplement the diet. As the idea ripened, his experiments began taking up all of his evenings and weekends. It was "something I had to do," he told her and others, "because I couldn't do anything else." She soon found out that his job at Richfield, far from being a steady climb up the corporate ladder, was just a way to pay the bills so he could devote his time to his real passion.

Evie found work at a hospital in Whittier, but my father also got her involved in what he was doing in his spare time and convinced her it was going to lead somewhere. His reasoning would have appealed to a trained nurse like Evie: that inadequate soil, long storage times, food processing, and cooking all took away some of those factors that made food nutritious. According to him, "all these factors are necessary for full chemical supply of the living body." Not just vitamins, but also "plant auxina, chlorophyll, enzymes, and very many others not specifically named or even classified." He was convinced that the final answer was not yet in sight—that much more was involved than merely supplying a few missing mineral factors or the known vitamins. It was a dream, and he was able to convince even a headstrong, well-educated woman like Evie that he could make his dream come true.

So in 1934, when they were living in an apartment in Montebello, a city just east of downtown Los Angeles, she gladly joined in when my father took over their kitchen for nutrition experiments. Often they worked together side by side. It was a fun time for both of them, when anything was possible and opportunity was limited only by one's imagination.

Over the years, my father had been experimenting with developing a process to concentrate nutrient-rich plants. He would remove the water and fiber. What was left behind was a concentrate rich in naturally occurring plant components. He felt that the more nutritionally rich a plant was to begin with the better. Alfalfa was his first choice.

Vitamins were much in the news at this time. It was really the golden era for vitamin research. Scientists all over the planet were working diligently in their laboratories hoping to be the first to discover a new vitamin. In 1928, vitamin C and thiamin were isolated ... then vitamin D and riboflavin in 1932 and 1933, respectively. It was a race for discovery! Meanwhile, Henrik Dam had identified vitamin K in 1929 and named it after the Danish word "koagulation" because it was instrumental in blood clotting. He set out to prove that it could be isolated in alfalfa.

Alfalfa! My father knew he was on the right track. It had caught his eye on that very first cross-country train trip en route to China, nearly 20 years earlier. It was right in front of him all those years in China and at the Carnation factory. And those cows he had observed earlier, with shiny coats, were fed a diet solely of alfalfa. Here in Southern California, less than 10 miles away from where he was living, the fields were full of it.

He had already visited the owners of those nearby agricultural fields with an unusual proposal: he wished to harvest only the top four inches of the alfalfa plant, so the farmer could harvest the rest for hay. He would pay five cents a pound. And with a kitchen knife and some white flour sacks to hold the alfalfa, he would carefully cut the tips of the plants. After it was cut, he was eager to get the alfalfa back to his kitchen laboratory as fast as possible. Once or twice, he had set aside a few sacks for a while and opened them later only to find them full of hot, whitened, decomposing alfalfa. Freshness clearly required speed in processing.

Back in the kitchen, he tried different experiments with the alfalfa. In one experiment, he used a meat grinder from Sears to get fresh juice. He found that it "fragmented the plant material without mashing it." He then squeezed the alfalfa in a press to get the juice, which was mixed with an equal amount of a solvent mixture. He continued this process until the plant material was colorless and he was left with a jar of green juice. The juice was then put into a rudimentary still, which he created himself out of various jars, tubes, and kitchen pots. He pumped air out and created a vacuum like the one Carnation used to produce its evaporated milk, then using a very low heat, so as not to damage those

Did You Know

… in 1928, the Hungarian biochemist Albert Szent-Györgyi isolated vitamin C? At the time, the compound was named hexuronic acid.

… in 1931, the Swiss biochemist, Paul Karrer, established the correct formula for vitamin A and its chief precursor—beta-carotene?

… in 1934 vitamin C was synthesized in the lab? It was the first artificially synthesized vitamin.

… George Whipple, George Minot, and William Murphy from the United States proved the value of iron for making red blood cells? In 1934, they received the Nobel Prize "for their discoveries concerning liver therapy in cases of anaemia."

… in 1968, USDA researchers found that the tips of alfalfa are more nutrient dense than the base of the plant? The Nebraska study found that the top half of a full bloom alfalfa canopy is richer in digestible nutrients than the bottom half of the plant.

---

precious vitamins and associated food factors, distilled out nearly all the solvents for reuse in later experiments. What was left behind was a pure alfalfa juice concentrate.

Besides concentrating alfalfa juice, he would also dry the alfalfa by placing it in the oven at a low temperature. After it cooled, he would grind it up with a mortar and pestle and then use solvents to extract the nutrients from the powder. This became his base material. He turned the powder into a solution, mixed it with a little of the fresh juice concentrate, and put it into bottles with dropper caps.

He also experimented with extracting vitamin E from wheat germ. Since vitamin E is a fat-soluble vitamin, it required a different solvent for extraction than the one he used for alfalfa (and the extraction of water-soluble vitamins). Initially he used ether as the solvent, making the apartment smell like the hospital where Evie worked. Later, he would use primarily alcohol. He was always experimenting.

My father was the first guinea pig for his food supplement, which he would add by drops to his food or drinks. Evie tried the concoctions out, too. He enthusiastically gave it to their friends, but it was far from a done deal. People thought he was crazy; his friends didn't seem to share his enthusiasm. Often, he would sneak a peek into their medicine cabinet and would see the bottle there—unopened. It later dawned on him that many people don't value what they get for free. He mused, "… if I charged for it, they might use it." And that's what he did. No one, however, beat a path to his doorstep.

It might have gone on that way indefinitely. For some inventors, that's how it works: great ideas and dreams remain weekend experiments in the kitchen. But in 1935, in one of those once-in-a-lifetime lucky breaks, one of those bottles of giveaway samples made its way to Dr. Walter Scott Franklin, and the picture changed.

It was Henry Stephens, my father's friend who was working on his own process to create frozen orange juice, who introduced him to Dr. Franklin. Dr. Franklin's wife suffered from migraine headaches. Yet when she tried my father's food supplement she felt better. Dr. Franklin became an instant convert.

Franklin was a well-positioned supporter, a successful and respected member of the medical community. He had been the head of the Department of Ophthalmology at the University of California Medical School before taking early retirement to manage a very successful citrus and walnut ranch in Goleta, just west of the city of Santa Barbara. He was a member of just about every medical board you could imagine, but also kept a practice in Santa Barbara as a general practitioner.

That spring, Franklin decided to back both Stephens and my father in their respective projects. It was verbally agreed that the new company would be called Vitamin Products Company, and it would be a three-way partnership with Dr. Franklin contributing cash, my father time and completed work and Stephens "mainly interested in what was going on," as my father put it. For the next three years, Dr. Franklin would become my father's most steadfast supporter, not only birthing the fledgling company, but keeping it afloat for those early years until it could begin to take hold of its own.

Dr. Franklin would advance Dad $100 at a time to develop his food supplement (equivalent to about $2,000 today). With money coming in, my father could really get serious about his passion. He rolled up his sleeves and got busy. He rented a storefront that he called "the shop," and set it up with his basic equipment. It was close to his apartment and located at 5917 Whittier Boulevard in the city of Montebello. He started writing checks for all kinds of expenses: pipes, rubber tubing, gaskets, milk cans, and a garbage can to cobble together an apparatus for extracting and concentrating his food supplement. He bought a big commercial meat grinder that weighed several hundred pounds and had it delivered to the shop. He hired plumbers and sheet metal workers to build some of the equipment to his specifications and a carpenter to put together the workbenches and cabinets. He bought gallons of alcohol, 45 pounds of wheat germ, and dozens of bottles. He continued collecting alfalfa, 60 pounds or more on each trip and hired kids to help him fill the sacks.

On June 6, 1935, my father wrote a check to register Vitamin Products Company. One month later, he registered VITAMIN as the company's cable address, which must have been a real coup, establishing Vitamin Products Company as *the* vitamin company, at least as far as telegrams were concerned.

Did You Know

… in September 1934, Carl Rehnborg introduced what is believed to be the first multivitamin/multimineral food supplement in the North American marketplace? However, no one beat a path to his doorstep.

Vitamin Products Company became a family project. Rising at five in the morning, Evie and Dad would hitch a trailer to their car and head out to the alfalfa fields together. Evie enjoyed working with my father, while he thought of it as "one whale of a good time." A photograph shows Evie smiling in the alfalfa, holding a special harvester Dad had rigged together from a scythe and chicken wire, which allowed him to reap the alfalfa faster without any of it touching the ground. Dad cut the alfalfa and dumped baskets full of it onto clean sheets. Once full, Evie tied them up in bundles. They loaded up the trailer with the alfalfa and rushed back to the shop.

At the shop, the alfalfa was placed onto wooden drying trays and then rolled into a gas dryer. The dryer heated pipes in the drying space, which created a dry but not hot environment. When the leaves were almost dry, my father would grind them in the big grinder and then load them into five-gallon milk cans. He then passed a solvent through the plant material in stages—through four or five of the milk cans. In the last step in the process, the finished material was placed in a vacuum still, also made from a large milk can, to evaporate the solvent, which then condensed into another milk can. My father knew the exact temperature at which the solvent would boil off, yet leave behind the nutrient-rich material. This process was similar to the petroleum fractionating process he had studied during his training program at Socony. His previous work and training was coming to good use. The whole process would take at least a day or two. While waiting for each step to finish, he would read or, if late at night, nap.

While at the shop, he would take inventory of his needs. He continued to buy materials for the shop—Pyrex test tubes, Y connectors for flasks, clamps, gaskets, bottles, more bottles, another milk can, and a coffee maker. He bought a desk and chair, chemicals from an industrial supplier, and an expensive pump on credit. He rented a typewriter and hired a woman to do some typing, preparing explanations of the process and theory behind the product to show investors. He also took the document to a law firm to see about applying for a patent.

After trial and error, he was pleased with the product. He bottled it in two-ounce bottles and hand-glued labels on them. It would help to have a catchy name for the product.

The product was a solution that contained six known vitamins. Dad and Evie spent a lot of time brainstorming the name before settling on VITA-6 (for the six vitamins it contained). However, the name didn't last too long because soon there would be at least six B-vitamins alone. By 1937, the name had transformed into VITASOL.

My father was wildly excited and sure it would eventually be a million-dollar business. In the short-term, he felt that within a couple of months he would be selling enough products to carry expenses. He started out selling it to friends and acquaintances and soon developed a small, but faithful, route of customers. Some of them felt good enough about the product that they asked him to talk to their friends. He was having a hard enough time as it was keeping his job at Richfield and making batches of solution. He suggested that his friends tell their friends about the product. If they bought some, he would pay them a commission.

He came upon the realization that a satisfied customer was the best salesperson. He had one of his regular customers, Alma Stewart from Pomona, California, to thank for that. As she told him, "Carl, I've been using this product for several years, and it's just made a tremendous impact on my life. I've heard you telling me about your challenges in trying to sell the product at retail,

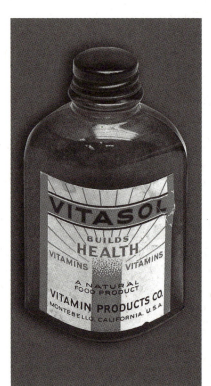

VITASOL, circa 1937. One of my father's earliest food supplement products.

and all your efforts at trying to get people to back you. I think I could sell your product. You know, I've never sold a thing in my life, but I think I could sell your product."

He gave it some thought and told her, "I tell you what, Alma. I have been thinking about this. I figure I've been spending about 35 percent of my time with my little route of customers I have been building. I'll give you a 35 percent discount on the product, and you can mark it up to whatever you want, and we'll see what you can do."

CHAPTER NINE: FROM STOVETOP TO STOREFRONT

It turned out that Alma soon became an even more successful distributor than my father. As a satisfied customer, her enthusiasm naturally shined.

Every day was a new day, full of possibilities. When my father was not at his "official" workplace (at Richfield), making product or sales rounds, he was talking to various organizations about nutrition. He would visit small stores, pharmacies, cafes, and even bars in hopes that they would carry his product. He thought drugstores were the most logical place. He imagined the thousands of pharmacies around the country, all stocking VITASOL solution and selling a dozen or more bottles a month. It could be a huge business, but more importantly, he could help people nationwide achieve good nutrition. He figured that pharmacists had a built-in credibility with their customers. However, the question was whether the pharmacist would take the time to explain the concept of food supplements to their customers. That part was critical. My father knew that the VITASOL product wouldn't fly off the shelves without some help. Meanwhile, he traveled throughout Southern California and even up to San Francisco to deliver his bottles. The Sir Francis Drake Pharmacy took a dozen on consignment. It was a high profile location in San Francisco. He crossed his fingers.

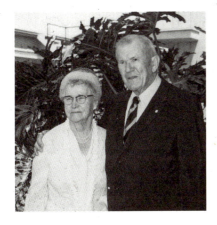

Alma Stewart and my father many years after Alma first began selling his food supplement, August 1963.

It was a different world when it came to health and nutrition. Nutrition was just in its infancy. The concept of dietary supplementation was novel. People didn't know much about it. There was no such thing as the Recommended Daily Allowances (RDA); that wouldn't happen until 1943 when the Food and Nutrition Board would introduce the first printed version. As my father put it, no one, including himself, knew how much of the accessory food factors were necessary just to stay healthy or overcome what he called "deficiency effects." He felt, "I was alone in believing that all plant factors were necessary." It was just a theory.

For many people, the thought that other elements, valuable to good health, might be missing from the diet and that they might be available from fruits and vegetables (or even more strangely, from something called a "food supplement") was incomprehensible. Besides, the benefits of his product were not immediately apparent. The VITASOL product didn't cure anything. With the exception of individual nutrient deficiencies, the results usually appeared over time, in a reduction of common complaints. The true value of the product required regular use and commitment—a tough, undemonstrable sell.

My father's approach to making the VITASOL product was to combine some of the foods that were known to be good for you and make them into a liquid form—placed in little dropper bottles. You could just put a few drops in your milk or on your rice to help balance the diet. However, he didn't quite sell it that way. He was thinking like an inventor. He presented the problem to the public like he had previously to Evie: damage to heat-sensitive vitamins from cooking and processing, loss of vitamins from storage, limited amounts of certain vitamins in the average American diet, and so forth. And then he presented the solution: VITASOL product, a supplement designed to help bring the diet "back into balance." But the whole sales process was overwhelming to a population that, for the most part, had little understanding of chemistry and nutrition. If you failed to understand the logic behind the product, you failed to buy the product. If your stomach was full and you had enough to eat, why did you need a food supplement, especially when it cost half a day's wage? It was just unnatural to add something to your food, and why should you, if you weren't sick? My father was faced with the necessity of not just growing a business, but growing a market.

There were a lot of objections to overcome. He did what he could, but working full time at Richfield and with so much of his "free" time spent running around on errands and making and distributing the VITASOL product, he was in a bind. The company was not self-supporting as he had imagined it would be at this stage; he even had to ask his younger sister Pump to float him a loan so he could pay his bills.

Although his finances were precarious, he felt it was time to take a leap of faith. He quit his job at Richfield Oil Company in August 1935 so that he could devote himself completely to his business.

People thought he was crazy. Only two years earlier, 25 percent of the nation's workforce was unemployed. My father didn't care if it was the middle of the Great Depression. He said, "I had to break away from everything else and do this one thing." He looked around for a way to break into the routine, but there wasn't an easy way. "I found I could not give up the experiments, so I left the Richfield Oil Company." He now had the opportunity to dedicate himself wholeheartedly to the subject that had fascinated him for so many years.

CHAPTER NINE: FROM STOVETOP TO STOREFRONT

My father took the plunge, although gently by first paying off old debts at the Whittier Merchant's Credit Bureau and the last installment on a new radio before quitting his job at Richfield. He knew he had Dr. Franklin's promise of financial assistance. And Evie was there, by his side, to support him and his decision.

That summer, my father had also met a man from Ohio who would soon be returning home. Sam Wales was a pioneer in electrical engineering and saw the potential of my father's nutritional products. He asked if he could be his first agent to represent the company on the East Coast. With Wales back East and Dad, along with a handful of distributors now, out West, the beginning of a distribution network was taking shape. The pieces of the puzzle were coming together.

On the whole, my father and Evie had a lot to celebrate that Christmas of 1935. Although finances were extremely tight, Dad had a half a dozen distributors and could even call his business nationwide. Evie also had her share of wonderful news. Early next year, the Good Lord willing, they would be blessed with a child. Things were turning around.

> "A position is a position, but this is independence and interest and ideals all rolled into one. I have never done anything in my life that I liked more to do than this job of making a product which actually benefits those who use it, and seeking always to improve the product... My heart is tied into this little business, more completely than I can possibly tell you. There is something grand and lovely in the thrill that comes from seeing people who are under par come up with clear eyes and a new joy in living."
>
> CARL F. REHNBORG
> DECEMBER 10, 1935
> IN A LETTER TO SAM WALES

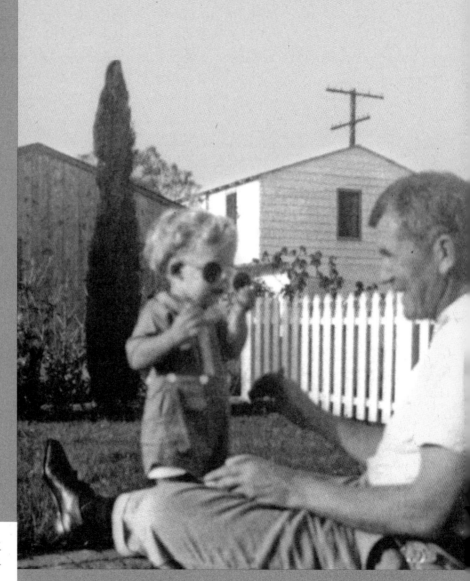

"... I had to stay with the equipment for literally several days, napping instead of sleeping. And when I napped it was because the process was at a stage where it could proceed by itself."

—Carl F. Rehnborg

My father and me in Balboa Island, California, 1937. He always took great interest in my accomplishments.

Chapter 10 | Burning the Midnight Oil

The next few years proved to have a steep learning curve. For, as anyone who's ever launched a business knows, it's a huge leap to go from an interesting part-time hobby to a thriving, full-scale business. Success demands attending to all critical aspects of the business operation: R&D, manufacturing, marketing, distribution, and financing. Certainly, it's a 24-hours-a-day, seven-days-a-week sort of demand.

On top of starting his business, my father also started his new family. On February 5, 1936, Evie gave birth by Caesarian section to a nine and three-quarter pound son. As you might have guessed, that son happened to be me. Dad and Evie named me Carl Reinhold Rehnborg, but one of the attending nurses, seeing how big I was and the fact that I had long dark curls, nicknamed me Samson. That name stuck as Sammie.

It was a happy time for our family. We had moved to Balboa Island—a small beach community about 90 minutes south of my father's shop in Montebello. Here my parents could take advantage of the low rents during the town's slow winter months, as well as be close to the ocean. We lived in what my father called "a grand little house," which was only a stone's throw from the beach.

My father was busy—every day brought something new. He spent much of his time at the shop. The concentrate was time-consuming to make, and he found himself up at all hours of the night moving it from one stage in the process to another. Often he would nap on site. Thankfully, he could. All the basic living necessities could be found in the rear of the shop: a pull-down bed, a toilet, a sink, and a two-burner gas plate, as well as a card table and two straight chairs.

The R&D and manufacturing aspects, which always appealed most to my father, continued to improve. Besides the VITASOL product, he created others such as Vitamin E Concentrate (with B&G Proportions) and VITAPHYLL (a chlorophyll-rich product that came in two-ounce bottles). He also created a skin renewal cream with added vitamins, as well as a product designed for prostate health.

However, the big challenge was to make the VITASOL product even more concentrated. He figured he could achieve this by converting the liquid concentrate into a capsule or tablet. To do so, he reconfigured the vacuum-distillation apparatus. He added solvents to the plant material and then boiled them off at a very low temperature. What was left behind was a "syrupy or tarry concentrate" in which he mixed dried and powdered alfalfa, wheat germ, and citrus fruit concentrates with a binder of powdered acacia and finely ground alfalfa or parsley. He placed the mixture on trays in the dryer. Once dried, he ground the material and passed it through finer and finer screens until he was satisfied.

The mixture was then placed in hard, two-piece gelatin capsules. With a spatula in hand, he worked the concentrate mixture into the bottom piece of the capsule. When he placed the top piece on, the powder would appear to explode from within, filling the capsule with the emerald green powder. He then dropped the capsules into a pan and sifted them to remove tiny bits of excess powder.

He described the process years later:

> *To fill capsules, I had a brass plate bored with 100 holes, into which the lower part of the capsule would fit. The plate was raised on blocks so that the bottom half of the capsule which was to be filled was flush with the brass plate. Then I weighed out a measured quantity of my formula, sufficient to fill 100 capsules, and put it on the plate and worked it into the capsules with a spatula. Next I took out the blocks that held the plate up and the bottom parts of the capsules with their little cups of concentrate would show and I would carefully put on the other half of the capsule.*

The new, concentrated product Dad was working on was given the name VITASOL tablets. To his surprise, sales didn't skyrocket. Food supplements, he found, were proving to be every bit as difficult to sell as milk to the Chinese—probably even tougher. Remember that case of VITASOL solution that my father left on consignment at the Sir Francis Drake

Did You Know

… in 1933, the brilliant Austrian chemist, Richard Kuhn, along with his research group, began their investigations to isolate 1 gram of a pure yellow substance from 5,300 liters of nonfat milk? This "beautiful yellow substance," as Kuhn called it was none other than the important B-vitamin, riboflavin.

In December 1936, Dad developed a concentrate of riboflavin from skim milk using the process developed by Kuhn; however he experimented with a more reasonable 40 quarts of milk, which yielded about 10 milligrams, enough for roughly a six-day supply for one adult.

Pharmacy in San Francisco? A year later, they returned 11 of the 12 bottles. Other pharmacies had similar success rates.

Without adequate marketing funds, the product languished on the retail shelves. Dad soon realized that the best way to promote it was by using a one-on-one approach. That way he could explain the product and its benefits, and answer any questions that might arise. For the most part, it was this one-on-one approach that allowed him to keep his business afloat.

However, even with my father's group of loyal supporters, the bills kept adding up. To make ends meet, my parents had to give up their home on Balboa Island and we moved into the small back room of the shop. The rent of $25 a month for the house was just too much. My father also took out a loan for $50 from the bank to help cover the family's living expenses.

Around Thanksgiving of 1936, when things were looking particularly bleak, my dad's luck began to turn. Knowing how tenuous my father's finances were, his East Coast distributor Sam Wales wired him $100, which promptly went for back rent and other expenses, and mailed a check for another $25 two weeks later. But Sam Wales was sending more than money. He was sending both encouragement (for a possible business deal) and a vote of confidence in my father and his business. As Dad wrote a couple of years later, Sam Wales had never given up the idea of creating a fully funded company to make and sell food supplements. My father began calling him Sam "Helping Hand" Wales. He cashed that $25 check and promptly went out and bought 250 pipettes and some sulfuric acid for a new product he was working on.

As Christmas approached, the deal that Wales referred to came through, allowing my father to pay off his creditors.

Around that time, my father changed the name of his company. He found out that the earlier name he had chosen, Vitamin

Products Company, was not available for a national trademark. With that knowledge, he changed the name of his company to California Vitamins, Inc. And so, on December 19, 1936, California Vitamins, Inc. was capitalized. My father could breathe again. Best of all, our family was able to move back to Balboa Island, to an apartment over a garage.

1937 was a new year, and my father was off to a bright start. Every day, he crammed in as much work as he could. He picked up printed labels, bought some corporate books, and ordered new stationery. He had an accountant look over the books to set up his accounts for the new corporation. He bought 20 gross (2,880) bottles and paid the deposit for another 20 gross in January. He ordered a design for a new carton for the skin cream he created and hired a woman to help package the big orders he anticipated would come.

It wasn't unusual for him to work 17- to 18-hour days, and the long drive between home and work didn't help. So it turned out to be a blessing in disguise when the new owner of the property on Whittier Boulevard in Montebello wanted her shop back. My father befriended the owner of Richardson's Boatyard, right around the block from our home on Balboa Island. He asked "Rich" Richardson if he had some room in the back of his boat shed to lease out. Rich said, "Business is kind of slow." Yes, he did have some room and would appreciate the $50 monthly rent. A deal was struck.

On March 31, 1937, my father had all the equipment and materials from the shop on Whittier Boulevard loaded into a moving van and hauled down to Balboa Island. He tipped the driver and, with the help of Rich's teenage son, Ed, moved it all into the shop. The corporate and manufacturing headquarters of California Vitamins, Inc., officially took up residence in Richardson's Boatyard on Marine Avenue.

The boat shed was on one of the biggest lots on the island. A bank of enormous windows flanked two huge front doors, which would swing wide open to allow boats in and out for storage. A loft over the front office stored the sails. The building itself was free of interior posts, giving the interior an expansive feeling. In an unused portion at the back of the shed, about 200 square feet or so, my father set up shop.

By this time, vitamins were in the world news. Two biochemists had shared the Nobel Prize for Chemistry in 1937. Paul Karrer, of Switzerland, won it for describing the structure of vitamin A and for his work on riboflavin (vitamin B2), carotenoids, and flavins. Norman Haworth, from the United Kingdom, was awarded the prize for his work on determining the chemical structure of carbohydrates as well as that of vitamin C. Eli Lilly & Company and other big companies were beginning to take interest. My father was still leading the way to consumers with his products, but his earlier cash infusion, with the Sam Wales connection, had already dried up and his marketing edge was at risk without adequate capital.

In September 1937, R. Templeton Smith walked into the picture, like a knight in shining armor. He had come onto the scene, done his own investigating, and was prepared to make a commitment. Smith, a colleague of Andrew Mellon, the east coast financial magnate, was a vice president at Mellon's Pittsburgh Coal Company. According to my father, this deal "had substance." Not only did Smith want to invest his own money into the company, but he wanted to act as president and manager. He planned to sell off some of his miscellaneous holdings and put the money into California Vitamins, Inc. With someone of Smith's caliber leading the team, the business might at last fulfill its potential. The company was recapitalized, and the previous investors were bought out.

With Smith's involvement, there was now money available to make a real production facility. My father threw himself into his work with renewed spirit and energy. Things looked really good. The Dow Jones Industrial Average was sky-high, bumping against 190. It looked like it might even pass 200. At the end of September, Smith visited the factory in the boat shed and went over the product and process with my father.

After Smith's visit, my father prepared a document detailing the process, including all the materials used. He wrote that there had yet to be a production line, just small-scale laboratory production. He thought they might be able to patent the process. He described everything about it—how alfalfa was prepared for extraction; what vitamins were expressed at each stage of the process; how the larger dryer would be designed; how the low temperatures protected the heat-sensitive vitamins; how wheat germ was processed for vitamin E, citrus for vitamin C, and yeast for the B vitamins; and why using extractions was better than only using refined or synthetic vitamins. He described the leach process, the evaporation of solvents, the stability of vitamins in a vacuum, the fractional distillation, the vacuum distillation, the recovery of solvents, the preparation of concentrates, and the grinding process of the vacuum-dried concentrates in preparation for capsule filling.

Thanks to Smith, there was money available to turn the boat shed into a real production facility. My father had plumbers install sinks and drains and rough-in

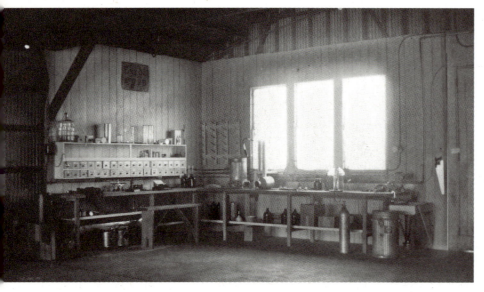

My father's laboratory located in a boat shed on Balboa Island, California, January 1938. Here the company took up residence from March 1937 to June 1939.

connections for a shower and darkroom. They installed water, gas, and vacuum lines to the workbenches. The electricians improved the wiring. The carpenter built shelves and a table for the grinder. My father took photographs of the operation; sun sparkled into the corner of the room.

The dehydrator at the boat shed was on almost constantly when the plant material was drying. Its fan vented onto a lane outside the shop and became a kind of conversation piece for people passing by, but because it was so noisy, it was hard to talk. A young newlywed named Leverne Parker, who lived down the street, would pass on her way to the post office or market. She was curious about what was happening inside, so she stopped by one day to chat. Leverne liked my father from the day they met.

"How about coming in and filling some capsules for me sometime?" he asked her.

"Well, sure! I'd be happy to if you'd show me what you want."

So he showed her how his process worked. The shop and the machines were spotless, and Leverne thought the shop smelled nice, "like on the farm," because of the alfalfa.

It was Leverne's job to fill the capsules. She was amazed how much of the fine powder could fit inside each capsule. It wasn't a full-time job. When my father needed some capsules filled, he would just walk down the alley and tap on her door. Her friend Bea joined her for a while.

"Verne, can you come over and fill some more capsules for me?" he'd ask.

"Sure," she'd reply, "as soon as I finish doing the dishes."

The two of them, Leverne and Bea, would sit there at the bench filling capsules for hours. When they had finished a batch, they would let my father know. He would take the capsules away and they would begin the next batch. She liked the work and she liked conversing with my father. However, most of the time, she was focused on her task. She

Chapter Ten: Burning the Midnight Oil

hardly noticed what was happening behind her back when Dad filled the racks with alfalfa to dry. She didn't notice what my father did with the capsules once they were filled—how he took the capsules, sifted off the excess powder, and placed them in glass bottles with hand-glued labels; or when he added an extra step of immersing the bottles in nitrogen before putting on the tops to better preserve the nutrients.

Ed Richardson, the boatyard owner's son, had his own theory about what was being manufactured in the boat shed. He saw alfalfa go in the door and little green pills come out. He assumed my father was making rabbit feed since he had seen his uncle feed little green alfalfa pellets to his rabbits. My father reminded Ed of a professor because of his quiet, yet forceful nature. Ed respected my father as did many of the folks who lived nearby who admired him for his dedication to what he was doing.

With funds from Templeton Smith, there was even money available to contract with a man named Bucklin to turn some of the dried concentrates into tablets. My father continued with the R&D aspect of the business, experimenting and developing his first separate mineral product. He mixed minerals such as calcium, potassium, and magnesium and combined them with various acids to wind up with a "modified Osborne-Mendel salt mixture," as he described it on a label. He also developed a process for concentrating vitamin C from lemons.

The best part was that Templeton Smith appeared to have been as interested in the science behind the company as my father. Smith sent Dad a note enclosing a clipping about a "life organizer" adjunct to chlorophyll "which has to it the same relation as globin has to hemin in hemoglobin of the blood corpuscles." The next day, Smith sent another note to say that the test tablets appeared to weigh less than they should have. Dad wrote an angry comment in his journal: "Damn Bucklin and his air-drying!"

It looked like the corner had finally been turned. The influx of money from Templeton Smith covered both the business expenses as well as an actual salary for my father. For the first time, my father could also give Evie considerable money for household expenses. In his journal, he occasionally began drawing a tiny circle and writing in tiny letters, "Afternoon Club," of which Evie may have been the only other member. Things appeared to be going well at home.

"Never, never, never give up."

—Winston Churchill

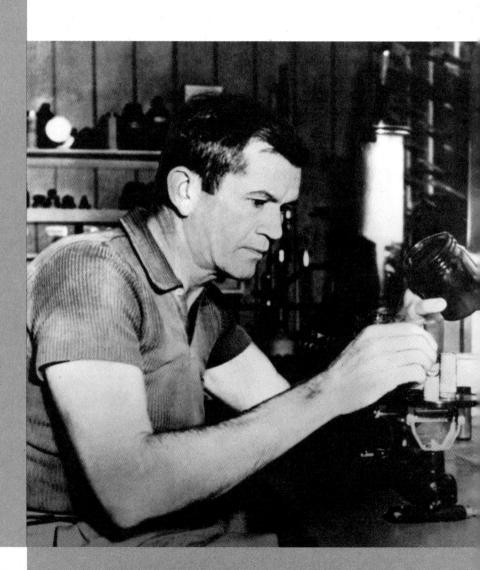

My father, "head vita-man," working in his Balboa Island laboratory, October 1938.

Chapter 11 | Vita-Man

At the end of the year, just two days before Christmas 1937, my father's sister Sallie and the rest of the Vaughn family arrived. They planned to live on Balboa Island during Fuzzy's furlough before leaving for his next assignment in Shanghai. By this time, they had three children: two boys and one little girl named Sara who was about six months younger than me and who gave Evie her new nickname: "Aowan."

The Christmas holidays with the extended family appeared to have inspired my father even more. He wrote down a plan to extract vitamins A and D from plankton. Why go to sharks and codfish when you can go straight to the source? The ocean was teeming with plankton. He also made a wish list for the company: another lab bench and sink, spectrographic equipment to determine chemical composition of materials, and a tableting machine of his very own.

His ideas continued to flow. He made some more notations about vitamin A and vitamin D extractions from plankton. He read an article about another company that was making a product from dried whey, which was similar to one of his earlier experiments in which he concentrated skimmed milk.

That winter, a huge storm blew in from the Pacific, pouring rain and raising a flood tide that inundated the little island of Balboa. Some of Leverne's friends got a surprise when they woke up in the morning and put their feet down in a few inches of water.

Like the weather, the stock market had turned brutal. The Dow had fallen to 121. The stocks that Templeton Smith had planned to sell to raise the capital for California Vitamins had fallen even further. To continue with the project would cost him twice what he had anticipated. Reluctantly, he withdrew. The timing just turned out to be off for Smith and my dad. When the stock market recovered, Smith went on to found Ben Venue Laboratories, a company that today manufactures more than 800 pharmaceutical products.

Although it was a bitter blow, something remained. Encouragement and belief go a long way for a man like my father. Smith believed in him and had sparked a creative surge that just wouldn't stop. They were of like minds. They both saw a need and hoped to fill it. The timing was just off. And during that brief time as an investor, Smith had made possible a complete production line for small-scale manufacturing. Dad could contract the facility out to other companies to improve cash flow, while continuing to work on his own products. The rent was paid up and my father's ideas just kept coming.

As Dad's ideas flowed, he wrote about them in his journal. He was contemplating a way to encourage people to take their mineral supplements. He figured that most people added salt to their food. What if you added minerals to the salt? He tried combining salt with his "modified Osborne-Mendel salt mixture" in a three-to-one ratio. According to his notes, it had "a definite and pleasing flavor in foods. At the average salt intake of six to 10 grams (per day) which is a civilized habit, it will furnish 1 ½ to 2 ½ grams of the comprehensive accessory supply." It was a little acidic and appeared to react with the metal cover of a salt shaker. But, he figured it was a patentable idea and it could be sold in glass shakers to get around the acidic taste.

The next day he had an idea for what he called "VITAPOTENT" foods in a can. He wrote:

> *It should be quite possible to add vitamin potencies, such as B&E crystals, carotene, and G concentrate, to foods and fruits, flavoring where possible with the 'mineralized salt' to make these foods adequate sources for an optimum vitamin and mineral intake.*

Fortifying food products wasn't an entirely new idea. Iodine had been added to salt since 1924 to prevent diseases like goiter, and vitamin D had recently been added to milk to help prevent rickets, but no one had apparently proposed vitamin-fortified packaged foods before.

While he noodled over all these developments and ideas, his bank account dwindled to a balance of $7.17. While his situation may have seemed precarious to most people, he

Chapter Eleven: Vita-Man

knew that something would turn up. Kay Hosking, a local distributor, continued to sell quite successfully and reliably to her customers in Balboa and the surrounding area. In addition, another deal was beginning to emerge. A company in Long Beach called Ferri-Min was interested in adding a vitamin product to their line and had approached my father about becoming their major supplier in January 1938.

Even at the start, my father was uncharacteristically cautious and wrote the following in a letter to make sure that he didn't reveal any of his manufacturing secrets:

> *I had slowly learned to be more cautious, so I agreed only to furnish them with an unbranded product, and did not, at any time, disclose any details of process to them. In our common interest I went each week to talk to the groups of salesmen and prospective customers who met at their offices. They had a quite worthless mineral solution, and later a 'desert clay' which was 85 percent clay and sand, with traces of other minerals, and they would not use the mineral mixture I offered them, but they bought vitamin tablets.*

The initial meetings with the two partners, McIntyre and Moody, looked promising, and orders were real—with a request for "super-potency" vitamin B tablets.

Business was starting to gather some momentum with various distributors asking my father to create special preparations for them that they could sell under their own label. A woman named Ada Alberty, up in Hollywood, asked him to provide a month's supply of vitamins and minerals in separate plastic containers. Even though this kind of private-labeling work could bring in thousands of dollars, he was uncomfortable with it.

Meanwhile, Bucklin and his tablet machine turned his concentrates (powders) into his first packaged vitamin and mineral tablets. By April, Bucklin was churning out 10,000 mineral tablets at a time. Meanwhile, Dad had perfected a version of skin cream that could be put in tubes. He was tossing around ideas of developing a vitamin G concentrate made from skim milk or whey. And, he was perfecting a new marketing technique as well: giving talks wherever he could, to whatever groups might be interested in his message.

In April of 1938, my father spoke to a Mrs. Reed's group at the Rainbow Tea Room where he met a Long Beach widow named Lela H. Calcote who made her living through a small real-estate empire. She took an immediate and sparkling interest in what my father was doing. She was a rather unconventional woman, strong-willed and gruff, who wore slacks and cut right to the chase in conversation. Could she perhaps come by the shop and have a closer look?

The following week, she and Mrs. Reed arrived to tour the shop and ask questions. They were curious about whether there was any connection between vitamin and mineral rations and sexual desire. Either remarkably naïve or remarkably sophisticated, my father sat them down and gave them a detailed explanation of the modest limits of vitamin products, which were, after all, food supplements, not miracle products. The women were much enchanted, and some of the energy of the encounter must have sunk in for my father as well. At the next sales meeting in Long Beach, Lela Calcote must have been there, for my father wrote the tiny letters LHC at the top of his journal page.

A couple of big orders came in: one for 25,000 capsules for Mrs. Alberty and a request for an estimate from Ferri-Min on 20,000 capsules for a new synthetic and purified vitamin pill. In a temporary cash-flow crisis and facing these large orders, my father again turned to Dr. Walter Franklin for help, but this time Dr. Franklin turned him down.

Then the dark side of the Ferri-Min connection began to show itself. Who actually owned whom? To my father, it looked like a distributor arrangement. To the Ferri-Min folks, it looked like a buyout. They tried to pressure him to combine with Ferri-Min to form a single corporation by withholding payment for the product they had contracted out to him. Dad wanted to stay independent. The whole situation made him increasingly uneasy.

To top it off, he discovered that Ferri-Min was selling another manufacturer's very inferior B-vitamins under his label. It was unpleasant news, especially on the day before his birthday. He would be turning 51. He was furious with Ferri-Min's duplicitous tactics, but at loss for how to handle them. With Franklin out of the picture (at least temporarily), how could he afford to shut off sales to Ferri-Min and go head-to-head with them in the market? He would need a backer.

"I'll be your backer," said Lela Calcote.

My father leapt into action. They rented an office in the Hartwell Building in downtown Long Beach, overlooking the ocean, ordered a set of low-cost black and white labels for the interim, and shopped for office furniture and rugs. They created a second company, California Vitamin Sales Company, to distribute the vitamins. On June 22, 1938, California Vitamin Sales Company was incorporated. The company was owned 75 percent

Did You Know

… on June 25, 1938, the U.S. Food, Drug, and Cosmetics Act was passed and signed into law? The new law banned any false and misleading statement, whether it was a direct statement or an omission of warnings when a product might be hazardous. To enforce these new requirements, the U.S. FDA was given the authority to seize a product, take criminal actions against manufacturers, and issue injunctions to prevent them from making or distributing a product they deemed dangerous. The law was intended to protect consumers from snake oil salesmen as well as dangerous drugs—such as acetanilide, which had been proclaimed as safer than aspirin but turned out to have deadly side effects.

by California Vitamins and 25 percent by Lela. It was agreed that the principals would divide the profits equally. Lela became the business manager and my father was the advisor, lecturer, plant manager, and research chemist. They hired two new sales recruits, Ray Burlingame and Ralph Hoard, who would get one-year contracts to manage the company's sales.

Part of the plan was to have a doctor on staff who would examine patients and make recommendations as to any vitamin deficiency that could be corrected. This was initially part of Hoard's job, but with the new Food, Drug, and Cosmetic Act of 1938, Dad felt that Hoard's background as an osteopath rather than a medical doctor would cast doubts on the validity of the business. Dad wrote that it "would call three strikes against us before we start." So they soon hired a physician to help with the exams.

With the establishment of California Vitamin Sales Company, Dad cut ties with Ferri-Min, but some of the Ferri-Min sales representatives eventually decided to come over and join his team. He also discovered that Bucklin was the one who had double-crossed him. Bucklin had gone to Ferri-Min claiming he knew my father's formula and could make a substitute product at a lower price. However, it turned out that Ferri-Min was actually paying Bucklin a third more to buy the substitute tablets. "They are stupid as well as crooked," my father wrote in his journal.

The new business held its first sales meeting on June 28, 1938 and officially opened its doors on July 4. Twenty-five people showed up for the first meeting—already an improvement over Ferri-Min. Not only did my father have a new sales force to handle distribution, he also had a new product to introduce. It consisted of three parts—a bottle of soluble vitamins, 31 "High B" capsules, and 31 mineral capsules. This was the first full-spectrum vitamin and mineral product, containing not only the known, synthesized or purified vitamins, but also the unknown factors contained in my father's natural extract.

Altogether, Dad had about 40 distributors, most in Southern California. The new team was working well. Every day something new and exciting was happening.

At about this time, my father wrote up a basic sales plan for the company. It was called the *Ladder for Salesmen*. Dad had found over the years that a satisfied customer was the best salesperson for his product, and he wanted to find a way to motivate them so they could build their own sales force. The *Ladder for Salesmen* did just that. The sales plan consisted of four levels: junior salesman, senior salesman, junior dealer, and field dealer. As salesmen moved up the ladder, not only would their discount increase, but they would also earn higher bonuses on sales over a certain amount and an override on sales by the people they recruited. For example, a field dealer would get a discount of 40 percent, plus an override of 5 percent based on their sales force's revenue.

By the fall of 1938, things were moving along, slowly but surely. There was a big break when my father was interviewed by Bob Swanson in October for an extended news article in the *Santa Ana Journal*. Swanson wrote:

> *Vitamins have been a popular fad for years, but no one knows exactly what they are. No one has ever seen a vitamin, or held it in his hand…*
>
> *One of Orange County's most unusual industries is the making of vitamin and mineral concentrates used to supplement the diets of the modern civilization. It's located on Balboa Island, and head vita-man is Carl Rehnborg, who organized California Vitamins, Inc., two years ago.*
>
> *Rehnborg says his factory operates just like a "human stomach," with the products being reduced from natural substances. Just how he does it, of course, is his trade secret. He makes the concentrates from rice hulls, wheat hulls, wheat bran, yeast, citrus fruits, and many types of green materials, such as alfalfa.*

My father told Swanson that vitamins aren't food, but are *in* food and essential to the processes of life. Swanson wrote:

> *Rehnborg says vitamins are to food what a spark is to gasoline. If you don't "feel like kicking the ceiling off every morning," Rehnborg claims, then maybe you need some vitamins that*

Did You Know

…during the mid-1920s to mid-1930s, the majority of vitamin discoveries were made? However, for many vitamins, it would be another decade until synthesis was achieved. Dad's food supplements naturally contained vitamins, some of which, such as folic acid, had yet to be isolated.

For specific dates of discovery and synthesis see Appendix 2: Nutrition and Nutrilite Timeline.

are missing in your diet. Although he isn't pushing it as a cure-all, Rehnborg points out that an adequate amount of vitamins will help practically anything that isn't an infection.

The article mentions that my father's concentrates have more than just vitamins:

Besides the vitamins, there are minerals and unclassified factors such as auxins, chlorophyll and others.

As a fad, he explains, most people have thought of vitamins as a separate, tangible "something." Actually, he says, [it] is the interaction of vitamins with the other components that makes food.

The article was an excellent summary of what my father had been saying to his audiences around the Southland. He clipped it out and posted it into his scrapbook. He continued to work and read at a prolific pace. He read an article about "macro molecules" in tobacco mosaic disease, which aren't really alive but could still kill plants. The macro molecules themselves could be destroyed by a natural enzyme like pepsin. This was yet more evidence of nature's method of fighting diseases in plants.

My father needed the distraction of reading because, as would soon be made clear, things weren't going well at home. For six years, Evie had taken up the slack, supporting the business as best as she could. She had endured poverty, but perhaps even tougher was that my father was never home. He was consumed with the business. She could see my father was in his own world, filled 24 hours a day with his dreams and his business friends.

Even though it was fulfilling, the hard work took its toll on Dad, too. He worked on Thanksgiving Day and the day after. The next Tuesday, he noted in his journal that he had ground salt endlessly. He wrote a long letter to Sam Wales and gave a talk to a thin crowd at Long Beach.

At the end of the year, the inevitable happened. The entry in his journal is succinct, but poignant:

> *Aowan & Sammie left on the SP Californian at 8:05 PM for New Haven, where they will be arriving at 10:50 AM Saturday.*

Evie wasn't coming back. My parents had been together for six years. It was a momentous six years, which saw the birth of a company, a product, and a son, me. Although she believed in my father and his food supplement, which she continued to take faithfully, she had had enough. There were too many uncertainties. She finally left, taking me with her, in much the same way that she came.

Dad stopped by his friend Matt Cox's gasoline station one day with tears in his eyes, all choked up. Things weren't going the way he had expected; Evie had left and she had taken me with her. He had run out of money and didn't know what to do. "Matt," he said, "you're the only merchant that wasn't on my doorstep when I left home this morning." It was like a chain reaction. Everyone was calling in his lines of credit.

Matt told my father that he admired his grit and tenacity as well as his generosity, giving many people on the island his food supplement for free. He never seemed to give up. Even with all his setbacks, he seemed to have confidence that he was on the right track. But the tears were real. Everything seemed to be coming down at once.

Chapter Eleven: Vita-Man

"We are made of nothing but what plants provide and of other substances available in the air and water of the earth, and so we are inescapably in and of the earth, and in and of the universe. If we cannot get what the plants provide, we cannot live."

— CARL F. REHNBORG

One of the many fliers promoting my father's presentations, 1939.

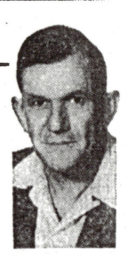

HEAR
CARL F. REHNBORG —
TUESDAY
February 21
Ebell Theater
HOMECRAFTERS COOKING SCHOOL

● The Relation of

VITAMINS and MINERALS to
HEALTH, HAPPINESS BEAUTY

FOR more than twenty years, Carl F. Rehnborg has been engaged in active research of the relationship of *Vitamins* and *Minerals*, of the right order and in sufficient quantities, to the properly balanced diet.

His talk will prove most interesting and instructive, providing opportunity for listeners to ask questions concerning this timely and vital subject. And he will explain the theory and successful practice of providing for dietary deficiencies through the use of—

CALVITAMINS
Vitamin and Mineral Food Supplements
California Vitamins, Inc.
East Seventh St. at Atlantic Ave.   Telephone 664-96

Chapter 12 | The Birth of NUTRILITE

Dad dealt with the loss of Evie and me in much the same way that caused it: by burying himself deeper into work. He was determined to make a go of it. "I am persistent, and I had my teeth in this thing," he had written. Alone in the boat shed, he thought about his New Year's resolution for 1939. Even though he was already working 11- or 12- or even 17-hour days, he wrote in his journal that he needed to buckle down. He vowed to do more: "more system, more do-it-now, more hours at work." For the first time, he broke down the cost of each batch in his journal, so he would know exactly how much each capsule cost. In order to determine labor costs, he began timing Leverne while she worked. While he did, it became clear why she hardly noticed what he had been doing. She was too busy filling hundreds of capsules by the hour!

If she had turned around, she would have seen him mixing together hydrochloric, phosphoric, and sulfuric acids in a jar. In another jar, he was dissolving alum and potassium iodide in water, and then adding the mixture along with citric acid and some extra minerals to the first jar. This is what the reporter from the *Santa Ana Journal* referred to when he described the factory as being like the "human stomach." The smell of the acids lent a pungent and irritating aroma to the shop until they had combined with the minerals. He would let the batch bubble while he calculated the cost: $4.33 for the material, $2.40 for tableting. He made these kinds of calculations over and over while he perfected the process.

While working with all the acids, my father had to be careful. Some of his experiments were dangerous. In one, he tried to extract vitamin K by boiling dehydrated plant material in isopropyl alcohol. "I did the heating over a gas stove," he noted in his journal, "with constant gentle stirring (and great care not to spill any over edges), with CO_2 [carbon dioxide] tank handy, and with considerable trepidation—but no accident."

Quality was always on Dad's mind. Back before he even began to get involved in the food supplement business, he noticed the high quality of the product and manufacturing standards of his former employer, Carnation. It was something that was very important for him too. During his time in the solace of his laboratory, he looked for ways to preserve the nutrient content of the products he made.

As vitamins were being discovered and soon to be manufactured in bulk, my father began to add crystalline and purified forms to his products. He knew his food supplements naturally contained vitamins, minerals, and associated food factors, but to assay for them would be cost prohibitive. By adding nature-identical vitamins from commercial vendors, he could claim these nutrients on the products' label, while simultaneously boosting nutrient potency. The prices from wholesalers for crystalline or man-made vitamins were, unfortunately, sky high. Fortunately, although California Vitamins wasn't the million-dollar business my father had imagined it would be, his volume had grown enough to convince Merck, the big pharmaceutical company, to begin selling to him directly, which allowed him to get a substantial savings when purchasing large lots. Every increase in savings, he figured, made it more likely for his business to become self-sustaining.

Meanwhile, my father continued experimenting with other things in the R&D arena such as vitamin-fortified candy. It was at least one way to get children to eat their vitamins. He introduced the candy in early February 1939, at 75 cents per jar.

Sales slowly trickled in, although money remained tight. Dad was late paying rent and two months behind in payment for the utilities. He managed to send nominal amounts to Evie in Connecticut, but was looking for savings anywhere he could get them. The local pharmacist let him pay his account through products.

It was a tough time for many. Not all of my father's customers were promptly paying their accounts either. He found himself standing on the doorstep of an island neighbor waiting while her maid was sent with five dollars due that day, overlooking the 10 dollars past due.

Looking for ways to trim expenses further, on March 31, 1939 my father moved out of his Balboa apartment and into the boat shed. He lived like a monk; no frills, no

Did You Know

… in 1940, the American biochemist Edward Doisy synthesized vitamin K for the first time? It's abundant in alfalfa.

… by 1939, seven vitamins had been synthesized? They were vitamin C, thiamin, riboflavin, niacin, vitamin B6, vitamin D, and vitamin E.

Journal Notes

From the start, Dad developed his food supplement to help "balance the diet." They were not intended as a cure-all—which some manufacturers were claiming for their products. His approach was simply and poignantly illustrated in this journal entry written on January 16, 1939:

"Saw Dr. E. J. Stren, Fullerton, concerning a child of 3 years with inoperable cancer. Mr. and Mrs. Rogers took me to see her. The doctor thought it a good idea to let the child have (regular) capsules (& some minerals) so I made the parents a present of the material. I think, however, the case is entirely hopeless, and I have never seen anything more pathetic and distressing than that baby." He noted under this entry that the child died two weeks later.

---

entertainment except the radio, no bed, but he did have a cot. He also had a shower and toilet, which he had installed two years earlier. But what he really needed was not so much trimming costs as increasing sales. It was the marketing aspect that continued to plague him. The sales manager Ray Burlingame, who had entered the field with a flurry of excitement about the time that California Vitamin Sales Company (the distribution arm of California Vitamins), had begun operation, turned out to be less and less effective. Another one, named Whitlock, washed out even faster. The missing link in the chain kept proving to be someone who could effectively drive sales.

My father received some help on this front from the strong political and emotional bond that was forming between the United States and China in the late 1930s. During this time, there was a growing fascination and sympathy with things Chinese in American popular culture. Dr. Fu Manchu, Charlie Chan, the actress Anna Mae Wong, and the comic strip *Terry and the Pirates* all gave popular expression to the continuing interest in China. While a daring and imaginative radio series reversed the pop archetype by suggesting a Chinese influence working within the United States. *The Shadow*, with a title character originally portrayed by Orson Welles, broadcast weekly episodes in the life of the American Lamont Cranston who, "while in the Orient, had learned the secret of how to cloud men's minds so they cannot see him." *The Shadow*, with its eponymous hero's unnerving laugh that baffled and disarmed evildoers week after week, attracted and sustained a national audience from 1932 until the postwar dominance of television spilled over into comics and pulp novels.

Among the beneficiaries of this increased American interest in and respect for the Far East was my father, whose life and work had been an embodiment of American-Chinese cultural interchange. His lectures, given to promote interest in his products and in nutrition as a means of maintaining good health, acquired the added appeal of adventure and intrigue. People, who might have otherwise been indifferent to vitamin research or the use of food supplements, found themselves acquiring useful information they'd never expected from going to hear a real-life version of Lamont Cranston.

At the Bellflower Junior Chamber of Commerce, the Homecrafters Cooking School in Long Beach, the Los Angeles Kiwanis Club, and the Lions Club, Dad spread his message, running a kind of China mission in reverse, bringing the saving word of good nutrition to America. "Mr. Rehnborg," reported one newspaper, "interested himself in the scientific study of vitamins and their close relation to health nearly two decades ago while employed in China as a representative for a large American canned milk company, and has since become recognized as an authority on the effects of proper dietary balance among a people said to be suffering widely from food deficiencies."

His only rest came when he took an occasional Sunday off. On one such day, he drove up to Mount Palomar, high in the San Gabriel Mountains, to see the observatory dome for the 200-inch telescope being built there. It would be the largest telescope on Earth. He probably wondered what his own father, who had loved pointing out the constellations and the planets to him when he was a young boy, would have thought of such an impressive instrument.

Meanwhile, the procession of potential sales managers continued to flow through the office, none of whom seemed to be the right person for the job. Many came out of the "hard-sell" arena. Dad would explain the product, and they would say, "Don't worry about it. I don't have to eat this product. I can sell anything." The hard-sell approach would infuriate my father.

Between interviewing potential sales managers, making more product, and speaking to groups, Dad was trying to unify his collection of products into an identifiable product line. He did this by creating a product line based on nutrient potency. One product he called MAINTENANCE. It was intended to provide enough nutrients for a maintenance-level diet and sold for $2.50 for a month's supply. The second was named STANDARD and it retailed at $7.50 for a month's supply. The third was a HI-B for $10, and finally the

Chapter Twelve: The Birth of Nutrilite

SPECIAL for $15. My father's goal was to adjust the potencies of each version to be somewhat proportionate to the price.

In order to comply with the new 1938 Food, Drug, and Cosmetic Act, my father drove up to Los Angeles in March 1939 to visit the local FDA office for advice on the new labels he had designed. The local representative suggested that he send a couple of the labels to his office and four to the main office in Washington, D.C., along with a letter "for a ruling."

The labels landed on the desk of George Larrick, a dapper man with a clipped mustache and slicked-back hair. He was an assistant commissioner at the FDA. He had joined the FDA in 1923 and spent most of his time as a chief inspector. His job was to visit factories to ensure that they were clean and well run and to review labels to make sure they conformed to the law. Larrick considered himself trained to distinguish between suspicious products and those products that didn't require any further investigation. Larrick looked over the submission submitted by my father and determined that the label was entirely proper.

The evening after the visit to the FDA, my father and the "whole crew" attended a lecture by Dr. Frank Warren who was a merchandising counselor for a nearby dairy. Would he be the man for the job to help get California Vitamins on the map? With high hopes, Dad and Lela set up an appointment for the following week to discuss business.

Dr. Warren swept into their Long Beach office and liked what he saw. "I'm a gambler," he told them, and he agreed to lead a series of weekly meetings for free to demonstrate how powerful his training sessions would be. If California Vitamins could round up 50 to 75 prospects each week, he would instruct them in sales methods and products. If the arrangement was successful, they would repeat the process in Los Angeles, at which time his services could be secured. However, before his services as a sales manager were put into action, Warren announced he had found another man for the job … a friend and longtime associate named Jack T. Harvey.

When Dad and Lela met Harvey, they both were so impressed that they hired him on the spot. My father, so excited that he was the one, sat down and wrote Harvey a very long letter detailing the whole history of what had brought him—and the company—to this point. It was a vintage document that not only reviewed the history going all the way back to the days in China when foreigners had to take furloughs every year or so to combat what my father believed were vitamin deficiencies, but also described much of his philosophy on nutrition and well-being.

His goal, as he explained to Harvey, was to create a supplement that would work with the average Joe's diet of hamburgers and canned beans and "make that diet effectively natural," allowing the body to function the way it was designed.

He explained that the original idea was to take the most nutritious plants and remove all the things that added bulk and volume, like fiber and water, leaving a concentrate consisting almost completely of nutritious elements. He made both a "base material" that contained the full line of plant nutrients and special concentrations that contained more of certain vitamins. Purified and synthetic or man-made vitamins were added to this as reinforcement.

He explained that although "our salesmen have accepted the word 'synthetic' as signifying inferior," this really *isn't* the case. The synthetic vitamins are fully effective against deficiencies "for particular values they contain," but they don't necessarily contain all the fractions, for example, of the B complex or any of the associated food factors that he believed were necessary to provide optimal value and complete balance. But, he explained, those "reinforcements" were the only forms that were easily measured and could be claimed on the label.

He went on to write, "The actual potencies of our product are complete for all of the vitamin fractions, and approximately 30 to 35% higher than the 'declared' values. I think that I have made clear that it is this inclusiveness of all factors to which our product owes its special characteristics."

He wrote about his experiments with extractions and concentrations and his reading on the chemistry and science of nutrition, but glossed over his struggles since returning from China. He admitted he was not a "scientist" and that "most of our conclusions about our product are speculative," even if the basis was the result of sound, scientific research.

He wrote about his partnership with Henry Stephens and Dr. Walter Franklin, about Sam Wales and his various attempts to get East Coast funding for the business, and his disappointment when the partnerships and funding fell through. He also wrote that the only plan that had substance was with R. Templeton Smith, which also fell through, and the troubles with Ferri-Min. My father wrote:

> "… I was told by enough people to make it sound convincing that I was a fool and I did not doubt that I was exactly that. I did, however, have the idea, or rather hope, that within a few months I could make the idea 'click' commercially, but instead I practically starved to death for three years. So did my family, but no one suffered harm to health. As a detail, a perfectly sound subsistence level is possible at the smallest cost, provided the supply of 'accessory factors' is always maintained. The difficulties, as a matter of fact, were in no way great enough to cause self-pity. They mainly concerned amusements and new clothes …."
>
> —Carl F. Rehnborg, May 2, 1939; in a letter to Jack Harvey

I was quite sure that within two months I would be marketing enough product to carry expenses. Of course I did not, and so went on and on, each month expecting next month to be much better. It finally took three years to reach the point of opening the office at Long Beach. While all that time was used to improve the product, and I did not on any one day worry very much about what was to happen the next day, and while that long struggle makes good "copy", you will see, even if I did not explain it, that there was no time when I did not believe that a month or two more would turn the corner …

He also admitted that, "The present status is that the corporation is a shell with no contents. It has a name and charter but no assets and no liabilities."

"Finally," my father confessed, "I realized two things: First, I could not hold my own with promoters … and promoters were not interested in what I was trying to do, but only what they were to get out of it personally. Even at that I had drawn rather poor promoters. Second, I recognized that I would have to work it out the long way and just saw wood until the right man came into the picture and took hold."

"This is the point at which you pick it up," Dad wrote to Harvey. "I cannot tell you how happy that I am that someone of organizing ability and strength and fineness of character has finally taken hold of it, and that I may retire to my fairly important but unobtrusive corner and just make product."

As it turned out, the timing was right. The old product labels ran out by the end of May, so it was the perfect time to start with a clean slate: a new company name, a new board of directors, a new vision, a new energy. And my father had the perfect name for the company—Nutrilite. Over the past few months, he had been

From *Science* magazine, June 15, 1928. [Reprinted with permission from the American Association for the Advancement of Science.]

SCIENCE

Vol. LXVII   June 15, 1928   No. 1746

"NUTRILITES"

The term "vitamine" was introduced by Funk to designate those unknown factors in nutrition which were thought to prevent various diseases. This term with a modified spelling has become widely adopted in spite of its obvious defects. The term has been applied in some cases to unknown substances which in small amounts are effective in the nutrition of fungi (including yeast), bacteria and other organisms. At present, however, the tendency is to restrict the use of the word "vitamin" entirely to substances concerned in *animal* nutrition.

The word "bios" was introduced by Wildiers to designate an unknown substance which in small amounts stimulates yeast growth. The word "auximones" was likewise introduced by Bottomley to designate substances of a similar nature which were thought to be effective in the nutrition of certain green plants. It is increasingly apparent that there are unknown factors which function in the nutrition of many types of organisms. It is also obvious that there is need for a general term to designate these factors. Otherwise it will be necessary to invent new names for substances found to be effective in the nutrition of bacteria, molds and other forms of life. None of the terms in use at present applies.

It is suggested that the word "nutrilite" be used to designate all those vitamin-like substances which in small amounts function in the nutrition of organisms in general. The term has the advantage that it indicates that the substances function in nutrition, but does not indicate in advance of our knowledge *how* they function. The term makes no extravagant claim as to the indispensability of the substance or to any peculiar relationship to life, as unfortunately the terms "vitamin" and "bios" do. In form the new word is similar to the word "metabolite." There is a closely related word already in the dictionary, "nutrility," which pertains to nutrition, but is rarely used.

We may then define a nutrilite as a substance, other than the well-recognized nutrients, which functions in small amounts in the nutrition of organisms. It is to be expected that borderline cases will appear in which it will be difficult to decide whether or not the material in question should be regarded as a nutrilite. This will not seriously impair the usefulness of the term, however, since a similar situation exists in the case of many words such as, for example, "carbohydrate" and "alkaloid."

Roger J. Williams
University of Oregon

---

looking for a more distinctive name, anyhow. And he had found it buried in a 1928 issue of *Science* magazine. The word "nutrilite" had been coined by Roger Williams of the University of Oregon and was used to describe vitamin-like substances other than the well-recognized nutrients, which in small amounts function in the nutrition of organisms. What could be a more appropriate name for the new company? He liked the name so much, he always wrote it in capital letters … NUTRILITE. He wrote to Roger Williams and asked if he could use the name.

While noodling over the idea for a new name, he experimented with adding parsley to the basic alfalfa extract, noting that the parsley mixture "leaches with a far better color

Chapter Twelve: The Birth of Nutrilite

> **MONDAY, APRIL 3, 1939**
>
> NUTRILITE, & NUTRILITES, Inc.
> (Thinking this over for a week, and like it better every day.)
> We have been groping for a better word to express "Vitamins, minerals, and other organic association factors".
> NUTRILITES is such a word. Quoting R R Williams
> "Among the substances which are regarded as functioning as nutrilites are
> — thiamin
> — riboflavin
> — vitamin C
> — biotin
> — pantothenic acid
> — nicotinamide
> — auxin A
> — auxin B
> — hetero-auxin (β indolylacetic acid)
> — inositol
> — folliculin
> — etc."
> Probably chlorophyll, carotin, & others will be added, and Williams says of these that "some are not yet isolated and therefore cannot be regarded as fully established entities".

Carl Rehnborg's journal entry, April 3, 1939. My father contemplates the idea of using the name Nutrilite for his business.

and strength." Parsley was also a tremendous source of vitamin A and a good source of vitamin C.

Williams wrote back, "No one in the nutrition world has seen fit to embrace my term, so I'm more than willing to let you use it," so my father decided to trademark the name. And so, on May 29, 1939, application for incorporation was filed and Nutrilite Products, Inc. (also known as NPI for short) became an official entity, with my father as president, Jack T. Harvey and Dr. Warren as vice presidents, and Lela Calcote as secretary and treasurer. Harvey was also appointed as general manager.

Handling the incorporation papers this time was a new face: Lester Lev. Dad's longtime lawyer friend, Spence Halverson, who had worked pro bono for my father from the start, had become too busy with his recent appointment as head of the Lease and Contract Department at Richfield and passed the job on to a fraternity brother who had recently graduated from law school at the University of Washington. Les was a very tall and thin man, "starving to death, practically," as Les put it, and in those days of the Depression was eager for the work.

At first, Les was dubious about the company. What was he getting into? The way Spence described my father, Les didn't think Dad had more than 25 cents in his pocket. Nevertheless, he went down to meet him and to inspect the "factory." His memory from much later vividly captures his less-than-impressed first impression about the operation:

His equipment consisted of two picnic tables with attached benches and a big milk can of about 10 or 20 gallons, a galvanized milk can, and a steel slab about a foot long or maybe a little longer, and about an inch or inch and a half deep, with 31 holes in it. And the way Carl made products then, he'd buy capsules, pull them apart, open them up, put one in each of 31 holes, that's for a 31-day supply, and then he would mix his ingredients and put it on top of this slab and then scrape it with a knife back and forth and then fill up the capsules, and then he'd pull them out and put them together. All by hand.

But Les and Dad hit it off. Les also liked Lela. He thought she was rather mannish, but as honest as the day was long. According to Les, "She was outspoken; if she didn't like you, she would let you know. But if she liked you, you'd know." Les could also see that my father really believed in what he was doing. There was something he found in his spirit that was contagious. Les took on the project. On June 30, 1939, Lela wrote a check for $69.56 to pay for his services for incorporating Nutrilite Products, Inc. It would be the first in a longstanding series of exchanges over the next five years. Les would prove to be not only a loyal and indispensible player in the story of Nutrilite, but also a close personal friend.

That summer, Dad's hopes for Jack Harvey really seemed to be panning out. The contrast between him and the earlier sales managers was palpable. Sales were up, and Harvey was thinking long-range.

Harvey wanted to prepare a standard sales manual. He also felt that the manufacturing and sales component should be consolidated into a single location. Drawing on Lela for a $2,000 contribution, manufacturing and sales were consolidated and moved to a central location in Los Angeles on Slauson Avenue, between Normandie and Western, near the University of Southern California campus and Watts, with the main Santa Fe railroad line running parallel to the street. The new headquarters was roomy enough to include offices, a laboratory, storage space, and a lavatory. However, this time, my father's household goods were not part of the new installation; for $5 a month he had found a small room in a house only a few blocks away.

On June 29, 1939, the moving van pulled up to the sail loft. Milk cans, benches, condensing coils, and the old Hobart mixer got loaded into the truck and were transported up to Los Angeles. There was a sour note to it, however. From the Balboa Island side of

CHAPTER TWELVE: THE BIRTH OF NUTRILITE

things, it looked and felt a bit like a Depression-era disappearing trick. My father had left on short notice and was not quite current with the rent. The only way Leverne knew that he was gone was that Dad wasn't coming around asking her to fill capsules. It was an awkward departure; one that evidently troubled my father. He would eventually make good.

The head of steam generated by the new Nutrilite team began to make itself known in all sorts of ways. They decided to systematize and label the product line. There would be three products and three "potencies," designated as No. 1, No. 2, and No. 3. They felt that this would further help to avoid the "prescription" implications of titles such as "REGULAR" and "SPECIAL" that could be a potential issue with the new Food, Drug and Cosmetic Act.

Then suddenly, the Jack Harvey bubble burst. In less than six months, he was gone. In Dad's journal entry for September 11, 1939, he summarized the drama succinctly:

> *Directors' meeting at 3:00 PM at which Mr. Harvey resigned, as vice-president and manager and as member of the board, without prejudice to his "claim;" as to his compensation in addition to salary.*

Evidently, it had been yet another takeover in the offing. My father had assumed that with sales in the hands of take-charge Harvey, he would be free to concentrate on production and research. He quickly came to realize, however, that Harvey planned to take charge not just of sales, but of the entire company.

During his employment with NPI, Harvey had been lining up his distributors, making arrangements with some of them as if he were the owner of the company or in the position to make such arrangements. It later came out, as my father listened to stories, that Harvey had in fact been presenting himself as owner of the company. Hypersensitive to these maneuverings from having nearly been burned with the Ferri-Min people, my father acted quickly and Harvey was asked to leave.

This was the last mention, in Dad's journal, of Jack Harvey and his longtime associate Dr. Frank Warren. Another team of sales managers had washed out. Henceforth the company would be run as a tighter partnership. On April 14 of the following year, Dad and Lela filed to have NPI dissolved. Now they would have a partnership and no need to worry about someone trying to take over the company. As Les commented about the string of failures with sales managers, "Oh hell, they all talk big, but they all wash out."

The abrupt departure of Jack Harvey from the scene had left my father and Lela Calcote as close working partners. They had been spending increasingly more time together. Dad and "Cal" gradually drifted into a relationship.

With Harvey gone from the picture, my father once again became the company's de facto sales manager, trainer, promotion director, distribution manager, deliveryman, as well as factory manager and research chemist. Also added to the list was stock boy, and in an effort to add "more system" he vowed to take regular inventories at the end of each month, getting off to a bumpy start by doing the September inventory in October. Over the years, he had developed a surprisingly large product line, including not only the three numbered products (No. 1, No. 2, No. 3), but also 10 more, with a laxative and two skin creams among them.

The work had become his life, not only during the day, but also at night. Even with the help of a hired hand for the evening shift, he was still up regularly tending to the dryer or working on one thing or another.

At the end of 1939, my father traded in his old car for a new 1939 Ford Deluxe Coupe and broke it in on a leisurely drive up to Santa Barbara for a sales meeting. However, he noted in his journal that the attendance was not so good. Unfortunately, this kind of thing seemed to be happening over and over again.

In the early 1940s, Dad was approached by Faraon Jay Moss, a Hollywood advertising and merchandising counselor, about developing a marketing plan. The initial connection had actually been made by Harvey, who had given them the impression that he was the owner of the company—but no matter, an opportunity is an opportunity. Moss and his associate Allen proposed a $100 monthly retainer in exchange for turbocharging Nutrilite's marketing by developing a set of training and promotional materials.

Out of this encounter emerged one of Nutrilite's first pamphlets. The pamphlet was entitled *Stay Well!* and proclaimed the dawn of the vitamin age. The pamphlet stated:

> *All this knowledge is not a 'fad,' but a new way of living for all mankind. ...It has to do with "accessory food factors" so small that they escaped attention until the science of chemistry and endless patient research disclosed their existence and their nature—the minerals, the vitamins, and other 'nutrilites'.*

Chapter Twelve: The Birth of Nutrilite

> ...We have adopted this word, which lay dormant in chemical literature, to express the inclusive nature of our products.

The pamphlet draws the very important conclusion that is the real basis of my father's work and the Nutrilite philosophy:

> But a host of people are not quite well. Their degree of deficiency is not sharp enough or specific enough to call by a name. They are only listless, or very easily tired, or have miscellaneous discomforts—they do not abundantly enjoy being alive. These are the people to whom the adjustment of nutrilite supply can mean the most, because of their subnormal state is so unnecessary and so readily corrected.

It goes on to state:

> The best method is to combine ... the use of fewer refined products and more of natural and uncooked foods, especially fruits and leafy vegetables and dairy products [with] a diet supplement such as NUTRILITE which contains not only all the commercially available vitamins, but also plant concentrate that supplies substances which enhance the effectiveness of the vitamins listed as potency.

In short, the pamphlet concludes:

> If you are tired or 'run down' from an incomplete diet ...TAKE NUTRILITE.
>
> If you suffer from any of the numerous ailments resulting from dietary deficiencies ... TAKE NUTRILITE.
>
> If you want to make certain that your diet contains the listed substances so necessary to maintain health and vigor ... TAKE NUTRILITE.

And most likely on the advice of attorney Dick Addison, an expert on food and drug regulations and familiar with the 1938 Food, Drug, and Cosmetic Act, the brochure concluded with the following:

> NUTRILITE, in capsules, with the supplemental mineral tablets, is offered strictly and only as a food supplement. It is not a drug or a medicine and no therapeutic claims are made for it, although the 'therapeutic value' of vitamins is undisputed. NUTRILITE is designed to aid in a return of the depleted organism to chemical balance. With its use, ailments resulting from dietary deficiencies for the NUTRILITE factors tend to disappear—and that disappearance is a return to health.

Moss and Allen continued working on marketing materials for NPI. They placed an ad in the *Los Angeles Times* to recruit new salespeople … however, nobody showed up. Dad submitted the new brochures to the FDA, where once again they landed on the desk of George Larrick, Assistant Commissioner.

At the suggestion of Moss and Cal, my father attended an introductory meeting of a Dale Carnegie sales and public speaking course. Cal felt that such a course might help my father deal with distributors who were from the hard school of sales. She felt that such a course might help him from losing his patience when dealing with distributors who pushed the product aggressively without really understanding it. My father wasn't that impressed with the course—"a nice racket," he called it. By this time, he was already a competent speaker. But there he met a skinny psychologist with a penchant to wear clerical black, who would soon figure prominently in his life. Dr. William Casselberry was a Stanford-trained psychologist, who had earned his doctoral degree just in time for the bottom of the Depression and had wound up cobbling a livelihood together, the centerpiece of which was his own radio talk show called *Problem Solving*. While the show was not hugely popular, he had stuck it out for eight years, while also writing a book on psychology that he sold through his radio program. It turned out he had been reading about nutrition for nearly 30 years—longer than my father, actually. When they met at the public speaking course, Casselberry was fascinated. Nutrilite Products, Inc. seemed to be the only company making a food supplement that contained not only vitamins and minerals, but also associated food factors. He felt there was something intriguing about the way my father sold it; letting the salesmen recruit others and then giving them a cut of their sales force's revenue. Casselberry signed on immediately as a distributor.

During this time, there was an awakening interest in the value of nutrition—an unanticipated effect of the outbreak of World War II in Europe and the increasing concern for the defense of the United States. The prospect of mobilization in some form, military service, rationing, increased physical and mental stress, and the value of being prepared generally raised questions of health and nutrition in the public consciousness. Newspapers and magazines ran articles stressing the benefits of good nutrition and detailing the state of vitamin research.

For the manufacturer of a multivitamin food supplement, such articles constituted

Did You Know

… what was said about vitamins in the 1940s? An article in the *Los Angeles Times*, co-authored by a well-known biochemist, related the list of known vitamins to specific human illnesses:

Vitamin A: For night blindness, certain skin diseases

Vitamin B complex I (consisting of some 15 related vitamins): For pellagra and deafness caused by deterioration of the auditory nerve

Vitamin B1: For beriberi, certain heart disturbances, nerve diseases of alcoholism, facial neuralgia, cirrhosis of the liver, and sciatica

Vitamin C: For scurvy, pyorrhea, rheumatic fever, cataract, insomnia, and inflammation of bone marrow

Vitamin D: For rickets, nervous spasms, softening of the bones, acne

Vitamin E: For sterility, muscle weakness, diseases caused by degeneration of nerves

Vitamin K: For hemorrhage

---

a promising sales tool for using a supplement as part of a normal diet to preserve and maintain overall good health. However, it also presented a dangerous temptation to market one's product as a cure-all. It was a temptation some manufacturers found difficult to resist.

ALL Vitamin Tablets, manufactured in Cincinnati, Ohio, advertised its vitamin product as preventing colds and improving appetite, skin tone, teeth, and "parenthood," while Vita-Diet, produced in Pasadena, California, was promoted with the claim that "normal" good health was actually only mediocre health, while "buoyant" health or fitness was achievable only through vitamin supplementation.

It seemed only a matter of time until the grandiose statements of some multivitamin manufacturers, in what was still a New Deal era of activist regulation, would provoke action by federal authorities.

More ominously, the giant manufacturer Miles Laboratories had introduced its own multivitamin product with the simple yet descriptive name One-A-Day™.[††] It was an impressive endorsement of my father's original thinking. It also marked the arrival of a new competitor from a company that already had almost universal retail distribution.

No record exists whether my father had heard of this new product when, in March 1941, he zeroed in on the concept of "a one-a-day vitamin capsule, to be sold at drug-store lunch counters and other eating places at 10 cents." It could be dispensed like gumballs. Stick a dime in the vitamin machine, turn the crank, and out pops your vitamin. He even suggested a line for the counter card: "Have you had your vitamins today?" The dime-a-day Nutrilite version contained what he was calling the NUTRILITE extract, in addition to 10 vitamins and "wheat germ oil as antioxidant."

[††] One-A-Day trademark is Bayer Healthcare LLC, Morristown, New Jersey.

About this time, he was also beginning to seriously think of ways to promote a concept that had been bouncing in his mind for a couple of years. The product would eventually be called OLD SETTLER. It was a high-potency vitamin B tablet geared to drinkers and was intended to be sold in bars. Besides B-vitamins, it also provided calcium and magnesium in a base of plant concentrate. My father thought of ways to promote the product and even created a poster to be placed in bars. The black, white, and orange poster showed an old settler in a cowboy hat, big handlebar mustache, and a bandana around his neck cheerfully advising a clean-cut young whippersnapper with a miserable expression who was holding an ice-pack to his head. His advice, "Never start out unless you are all prepared. Before you start, use two capsules. 25¢." The product turned out to be enormously successful. Before it caught on, however, the local government, inundated with complaints that it made drinking too pleasant, banned its sale in bars. Dad shelved the idea.

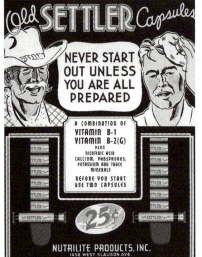

Poster to promote OLD SETTLER capsules, circa 1940s. OLD SETTLER was a high potency B-vitamin product that was sold in bars.

On May 28, 1941, around the same time that the first U.S. ship was sunk by a U-boat and President Roosevelt proclaimed an unlimited national emergency, my father left a short entry in his journal:

Sammie & Cal left for New York & New Haven by way of New Orleans at 8:15 PM.

It had been over two years since Evie had left California for good. During that time, I would live with both of my parents—shuttling between California and Connecticut. It was tough on both of them. A friend said that it "just killed his soul" when Dad had to send me back. The same was true for Evie.

For my father, it didn't take too long to come to the realization that he wanted custody of me. He was determined not to let fate repeat itself. He had already been separated from Ned and Nancy; he was resolute it wouldn't happen again.

When Evie initially returned to her childhood home at the end of 1938, her family was never sure what had gone wrong between her and my father, but it was clear that something was radically wrong. Evie's younger sister, Esther Berg put it this way:

They were totally unsuited for each other: she was too young, he was too old. She was the oldest: she bossed us around a little bit. Maybe she got out there and she couldn't boss Carl around; who knows?

Chapter Twelve: The Birth of Nutrilite

Bolstered with the additional resources at his disposal from Cal and the gradual building sales of food supplements, my father hammered the point with Evie that I would have a better life in California and a better education because he could afford to send me to private school. When an amicable resolution to the problem did not seem to be emerging, divorce papers were filed with my father demanding full custody. There are conflicting stories about the divorce, as there always are, but the one thing that was reasonably clear is that it was painful. One version states that it was Evie who pushed for the divorce, but my father would only grant it if she gave me up. The other version is that my father wanted it badly and brought to bear on it the full force of what he already had in abundance: his steel-edged will. In either case, the process must have been difficult for Evie. In those days, the only way in which custody would go to the father is if the woman could be proved to be an unfit mother. The details are unclear: whether Evie actually came to court in California and testified that she was an unfit mother, or whether she simply lost heart for the whole adventure. At any rate, at some point in the whole heartsick process, my father took the case to court and finally won custody. He told a friend later it wasn't something he was proud of doing. I wouldn't see my mother again until I was in my 30s. Dad didn't talk much about it.

Les traveled out to Connecticut with my father to pick me up. According to Les, Evie "was a very, very nice woman—a good-looking woman—and she gave Sam up simply because, I'm sure, she knew Carl could afford to give him a good education." Evie later told a friend about what a very difficult situation it was. "You know, if I had two nickels to rub together to have caught a bus to go out there and get him, I would," she said. "But I didn't have any money. I couldn't afford it. I couldn't borrow it. And I tell you, it was the hardest thing in my life I ever did to not go and get him and have to relinquish custody of him."

Although this custody battle weighed on all our minds, occasionally something much bigger would put everyt hing in perspective. On December 7, 1941, my father uncharacteristically made an extensive personal note in his journal, which was mostly devoted to lab notes and thoughts about what he was reading. He began the entry like this: "This morning the Japanese bombed Pearl Harbor and Honolulu in the early hours of the day," then described the circumstances of the surprise attack. He concluded that "AT ANY RATE, America is united, as never before. The air is full of declarations of simple purpose. I'm interested to note how the *Star Spangled Banner* stirred me just now."

By 1942 and at the age of six, I was back for good. In February of that year, my father, too old for the draft or even to be accepted by the military as a volunteer, bought a 3.6-acre farm for $1500 out in the San Fernando Valley in Southern California. The "Reseda farm," as it was known, seemed to be out in the middle of nowhere. Dad and Cal were newlyweds now; they had officially tied the knot in Las Vegas, just after my sixth birthday. The three of us would go out to the farm during the weekends when it was being fitted out. At the crest of the Santa Monica Mountains, my father would shut off the car's engine to save gasoline and coast down into the valley as we listened to the Saturday morning radio programs.

My father hired a man named Sanchez to run the farm, but when the crops came in, we helped out with the harvesting. The scythe with the basket on the end of it weighed almost as much as I did, so Dad would swing that around on one side while I used a sickle to cut alfalfa tips on the other side. We would bring bed sheets with us to place the alfalfa in and then load the bundle into the back of the truck.

Once the alfalfa was on the truck, we drove back to the shop and my father began the long drying process. Sometimes Dad and I slept in the shop rather than driving back and forth to Cal's home in Windsor Hills. My father would unfold a cot and set up a little bed for me in the second office.

Sometimes at night, we would look at the stars with the small telescope we built together and set up outside the shop. Even in a big city like Los Angeles, the wartime blackout left the night sky glittering with stars. My father pointed out the planets and constellations. He explained how the sun is just another star around which the earth revolves, and how science had shown that all the billions of stars are composed of the same elements as our own sun and planet, as well as people, and even animals like my little cocker spaniel Sammie. "We are of the earth," he said, "and parts of the whole universe."

Now with me in his life, it seemed my father—who had a young spirit to begin with—had even more reason to indulge. During the constraints of wartime gas rationing, he had purchased a Whizzer, so he could stretch the limited gas coupons he and Cal received. The Whizzer was a motor that attached to a bicycle turning it into a quasi motorcycle. Once we attached the Whizzer to the bike, we would go everywhere—even to Aunt Sallie's home. Sallie and the rest of the Vaughn family were now living in a big two-story

Did You Know

… in 1943, the Nobel Prize in Physiology or Medicine was awarded to vitamin researchers Henrik Dam and Edward Doisy for their work on Vitamin K?

… in 1943, the B-Vitamin biotin was synthesized? Rats fed raw egg whites (which contain a biotin inhibitor) developed eczema and hair loss around their eyes that disappeared when biotin was added to the diet.

colonial near the beach in Santa Monica. Fuzzy was an executive at Socony Vacuum and worked at their downtown headquarters, while Sallie returned to nursing and was working at a local hospital. Their home was about 10 miles from Dad's factory. The whole trip, back and forth, barely tapped the tiny tank of gas as we coasted downhill, whizzed along the flats, and sometimes pedaled to assist the straining engine up the hills.

There was always something to do at the very small factory. Dad was often building or creating something, a camera or a microscope—you name it. And I got to help out. We built a microscope, and after we finished, we would look at pond water under its lenses. My father would point out all the tiny organisms that lived there. And while the steam engines puffed past across the street, my father helped me build my own train track that ran around the walls of the shop.

Once the alfalfa had been dried and ground and was ready for extracting, we would celebrate by driving down to a malt shop on Normandie. Sometimes Les would join us. It was a big treat for all of us. A hotdog was a nickel and a malted milk cost a dime, but it was worth the expense.

Dad continued with his more modest experiments. Looking for ways to bring in a little extra money, he made a batch of vitamin capsules "for pups," proposing the name K-9 capsules. My puppy was used as the guinea pig.

He also experimented with PABA (paraminobenzoic acid). In February 1943, he made 500 capsules containing the acid for personal use to determine its effect. In his notes for the formula, he drew a benzene ring with double bonds that struck him as attractive. It soon would become Nutrilite's logo. It was eventually learned that PABA, which helps folic acid to function, has an ability to absorb ultraviolet light. This led to its use as a component in sunscreen lotion.

One night, there was a fire at the shop. It may have started in the dryer, where something drifted down in contact with the flame, or it could have been due to an electrical short. However it happened, the wooden benches and dried concentrate were perfect tinder. The whole building quickly went up in smoke. Almost everything was lost. My father had never even thought to insure the valuable raw materials.

Dad and Cal immediately rebuilt, and from that point my father took the extra precaution of insuring the expensive and increasingly hard to get vitamins against burglary and fire, both at home and at the shop.

That fall of 1943, I started second grade at a boarding school, the Urban Military Academy, in Brentwood, just inland from Santa Monica. On weekends, Dad and Cal would pick me up and we would go out together to the farm. My father was a firm believer in education and wanted me to go to the best school. He felt that the Urban Military Academy would be a better choice than the neighborhood schools. The following year, I had some good news for him—I was able to skip third grade.

There were some problems on the home front, however. The relationship between my father and Cal seemed to be cooling. While they functioned effectively as business partners, the differences arising from the stress of working together tended to bleed over into their personal lives. The dual partnership was impossible to maintain, and it was the personal one that shattered first. Perhaps the relationship between the two had always been, at heart, a "virtual marriage," which couldn't survive the give-and-take of everyday reality. The knot that they had tied in Las Vegas in February 1942 had come unraveled by Christmas of 1944, and my father and I had to leave the comfortable new duplex near Westwood where we had been living. We moved back to the neighborhood near Nutrilite's headquarters, in a room close to the plant. Cal became Mrs. Calcote again and continued her property investment, settling back in Tulare County where she had been born and widowed, before she had met my father.

The hope for success was still out there for my father, of course, but it seemed as if it would position itself, as it had all along, still elusively "just around the corner."

CHAPTER TWELVE: THE BIRTH OF NUTRILITE

"Sometimes it is more important to discover what one cannot do, than what one can do."

—Lyn Yutang

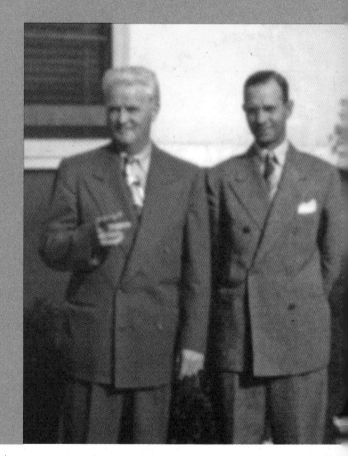

Lee Mytinger and William Casselberry, Ph.D., 1945.

Chapter 13 | The Salesman and the Educator

Over 10 years! As he began his new journal for 1945, my father could hardly believe the year would mark the 11th anniversary since he began his supplement business. At this point, the company was a survivor, but like a child suffering from an inadequate diet, it had failed to thrive. Outside its small niche market in Southern California, virtually no one had heard of it. Besides, my dad was still wearing too many hats; still manufacturing his product in his underequipped factory while trying to market it. The departure of Lela Calcote, along with her periodic cash infusions, revealed how thin the margin was. On January 10, 1945, the company legally became a sole proprietorship.

Once again my father was forced to reduce expenses. It was the only way for the company to remain solvent. He limited spending at home as well. One place he reluctantly cut was my tuition at private school. With Lela and her generous contributions to my schooling out of the picture, the cost of private school was an unaffordable luxury. I finished my fourth grade year at the neighborhood public school. It was a bit rough and tumble. Even though the school wasn't in the best area of town, it worked out fine and it really turned out to be a golden time for my father and me. It was just the two of us and we lived together in a little room near the factory.

During our time together, I helped my father at the factory and accompanied him on his sales rounds to customers—delivering bottles and collecting the used ones to be recycled. My job was to soak the bottles in a big aluminum tub filled with soapy water and put them on wooden pegs to dry. Dad called me his chief bottle washer. While at the factory, I also helped make the supplements; mixing up the mineral salts and pouring

The Nutrilite Story

in the raw materials and acids (with his supervision!) into big barrels. The combination would bubble and foam. For a 9-year-old boy, it was like magic.

When I wasn't at school, my father always seemed to be augmenting my education. In retrospect, I couldn't have asked for a better teacher. Every day I learned something new. He had an abiding love for the dictionary that he would share with me. He seemed to be always checking and double-checking the meaning of words. He loved words and loved to talk about them, what they meant and how to use them properly. As a young boy, he asked me to spell the longest word in the dictionary (antidisestablishmentarianism). I loved the challenge and would ask for tougher words. He never spoke down to me; he always spoke up to me and encouraged me to be the best that I could be and to do what I was good at—and keep at it.

While money was tight, we still enjoyed some special treats. When he lived on his own, he used to subsist for considerable periods of time on corn meal and raisins. However, with me at home, he used to make a tasty bread pudding that he baked in a tennis ball can. He would also splurge and we would go out for our weekly malt. While enjoying our ice cream, we talked about almost anything. I would tell him about school, my friends, and, of course, sports—I loved baseball. In fact, I carried my NUTRILITE™ Food Supplement in a little metal container in my pants pocket, which would clink and clank as I ran around the bases.

Dad shared with me what was happening at work. He would tell me of his dreams and how he hoped to help improve the health of people all over the world. I believed in him; to me, he was the smartest man I had ever met, and he was passionate about making his dream a reality. He said to me, "Son, one day this will be a million dollar company." I believed him.

The Educator

In the early 1940s my father started investigating the possibility of using radio as a means of expanding the market for his products and had enlisted the help of a local radio personality. He also appeared on radio himself as an authority on vitamins and nutrition and was delighted to find out that he had a knack for it.

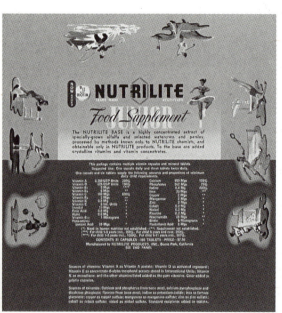

NUTRILITE JUNIOR Food Supplement label, October 1949. When I was young, my father used to give me NUTRILITE in half doses. However, in the late 1940s NUTRILITE JUNIOR Food Supplement was launched.

Journal Notes

"For the first time I went on air on KFAC, 'Man on the Street' 11:00 AM. The announcer interviewed me, and there must have been some 'oomph' in it because the leads finally counted up to over 260. I am delighted to learn I have a 'good' radio voice."
–Carl F. Rehnborg,
September 24, 1941

A broadcast on KFWB the next week was disappointing, though. "Poor program—1 lead."
–CFR, September 30, 1941

But another shot on KFAC, "bucking first game of 'World Series' between Brooklyn Dodgers and NY Giants," still brought in 75 leads.
–CFR, October 1, 1941

As he drove around the Los Angeles area on business and out to the farm, he would often catch the regular broadcasts of Dr. Bill Casselberry, the psychologist he had met earlier while taking the Dale Carnegie course. Dr. Casselberry's radio program offered psychological and vocational guidance. Perhaps Dr. Casselberry could help with his marketing dilemma?

Dad drove to Casselberry's office one day to talk to him about the problems he had been having trying to run both the sales and the manufacturing ends of a business.

Dr. Casselberry was a quiet and pensive man. He sat and listened. Education and training were his forte, although he also happened to have sales experience. As an undergraduate at the University of California, Berkeley, he had worked his way through school by selling kitchenware door-to-door. He served in the Army during World War I, then got involved in the real estate business and spent five years teaching Spanish, French, and English at a California public school.

By the time he was in his mid-30s, he had left teaching to pursue a degree in psychology. He chose to attend the graduate program at Stanford University where the psychology department was becoming noted for its work in intelligence testing. Professor Lewis Terman had published the Stanford-Binet intelligence test in 1916—which would become the standard IQ test in the United States.

At the age of 39, and at the peak of the Depression, Casselberry received his doctorate. So although he could eke out an existence, finding clients through his 15-minute weekly radio program, Casselberry was as desperately short of cash as my father and Les Lev.

In 1940, to augment his income, Casselberry started selling NUTRILITE food supplements. He had become interested in nutrition when he was 18 years old when his father became ill, hoping to find some way to improve his health. Nutrition, however, wasn't his big focus in life; although once he became a psychologist, his interest in nutrition was rekindled.

"I found soon after I started my practice," said Casselberry, "that in order to get best results I had to do something about the basic health of the people." The "sound mind in a sound body" approach was key to him. Recommending NUTRILITE food supplements was a natural fit and in sync with what he had learned while reading about nutrition.

By 1943, Casselberry added still another part-time job—working at Douglas Aircraft where he was hired as a personnel counselor.

The Salesman

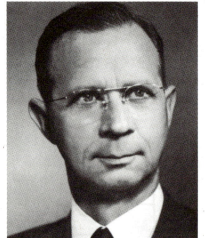

William Casselberry, Ph.D., circa 1952.

It was while Dr. Casselberry was at Douglas Aircraft that he met Lee Mytinger, a burly and flamboyant man with a full head of white hair, who in many ways resembled a classic salesman. Mytinger quit school after eighth grade to help support his widowed mother, first working as an office boy, then as a bank clerk and cost accountant. He served as a Marine during World War I, followed by a long history as a salesman selling tires, insurance, kitchen utensils, and burial plots from Maine to California. He eventually became the sales trainer, responsible for more than 100 salesmen at a mortuary service called Forest Lawn. Just before World War II, he was running a highly lucrative sales campaign for car tires, but that ended when wartime controls on rubber went into effect in 1942. This instantly put Mytinger on a different track.

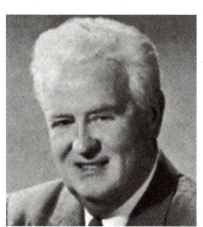

Lee Mytinger, circa 1952.

Mytinger, now working in the Personnel Department at Douglas Aircraft, met with Dr. Casselberry, who was giving various tests to help place employees in appropriate jobs. The blustery, husky Mytinger and the cerebral, skinny psychologist seemed to complement each other; both were interested in sales, but with two different approaches. They quickly became friends.

The two would often discuss the mechanics of sales. As Mytinger described it to Casselberry, most retail organizations had rules that, in effect, actually hurt their potential. What happened repeatedly was that the man in charge of a

Chapter Thirteen: The Salesman and the Educator

sales crew would search for, recruit, and train a salesman who, if he did a good job, was taken away
by the company and given a crew of his own. His old crew manager would lose both the man and the income he was getting from him, his cut of the man's sales. This limited the salesman's incentive to expand the business.

Casselberry, who was trained to listen and nod, nodded as Mytinger went on. "If ever I have my own deal someplace, I'll figure out a way so that you don't lose that [good salesman]—so [that] I keep the income from the people I develop," said Mytinger.

According to Mytinger, the J.C. Penney Company had found a way to motivate and keep good people. Penney offered the managers of the current stores the opportunity to open new stores as part owners. They would share in the profits from their original store while they sponsored and trained another manager for the new store. Their personal success was tied directly to the success of the company.

Casselberry told Mytinger of Nutrilite's business plan where distributors were able to recruit agents and get a kind of bonus on their agents' sales. These agents could also become distributors by recruiting their own agents. They would get up to a 40 percent discount.

As Mytinger and Casselberry talked, they eventually conceived what would be known as "The Plan." It differed from traditional door-to-door sales. If you worked for Avon or Fuller Brush, you were, for all practical purposes, an employee. You had a regular job. If you did well, you might become a district manager, but you never got much more than a salary or bonus.

The Plan, as it eventually developed, changed all that. It allowed industrious distributors to go far beyond the potential of a door-to-door salesman by allowing them to build their own distribution chain. It was a system bound by personal links and limited only by one's ability to forge them. And The Plan added a massive upside. It worked for couples who wanted to work together in a kind of mom-and-pop operation that came to people's doors. It took my father's 35 percent basic discount and added a range of performance discounts up to a total of 25 percent—offering a huge incentive for the most industrious to expand his or her sales and network of agents as quickly as possible.

Mytinger joked to Casselberry that if the first 10 agents each recruited two agents, there would be 20 more agents. And if they, in turn, each recruited two, there would be 40 more agents, and if they worked hard enough, everyone on earth would eventually be selling the product!

Casselberry had been selling NUTRILITE food supplements and knew it was a good product, one that people had been buying for more than 10 years now. The product generated significant repeat sales, the key to establishing a growing business. From conversations with my father, Casselberry knew that Dad's heart was in product development and manufacturing, not in sales. Casselberry described the sales plan he and Mytinger had bounced around and suggested my father give it a try.

Dad talked it over with his good friend Les Lev, who was now working at the Office of the City Attorney in Los Angeles. To Les, Mytinger and Casselberry were just another in a long line of distributors. "If they don't claim to talk big," Les said to my father, "they might work out."

At first, Dad brought Casselberry and Mytinger in as consultants. A special meeting was arranged with the distributors, who were in a minor mutiny over a number of concerns, including the desire to change the name of the product itself to NUTRILITE Food Supplement. The distributors identified with Casselberry and Mytinger immediately. Not only did they give the distributors a feeling that they were being listened to, they also made it seem that there would be an end to the status quo. They would finally have somebody helping them sell better.

Dr. Casselberry could assess their sales abilities and provide psychological guidance as well as effective promotional material, while Mytinger could assist and inspire them with hands-on sales training methods he had learned over the years. Both men spoke the unique language of sales: leads, prospects, calls, closes. They had experience not only selling door-to-door, but also through referrals and lecture methods. They knew what the Nutrilite distributors faced and how to handle it.

In June, Dad met with Mytinger and Casselberry to plan a joint venture. It looked like they would have a good working partnership. There were, however, a few differences of opinion. My father had the feeling that, no matter how many times he explained what he was trying to do, Mytinger and Casselberry weren't grasping the essential point. It seemed to him quite clear, as it had all along, that the goal was to supplement people's diets

Chapter Thirteen: The Salesman and the Educator

to provide a base for optimal health, not to cure them of anything. He knew his product would do that, and he believed the product would sell on its own merits.

But Mytinger and Casselberry kept driving the conversation toward what the product would cure; what powers could they claim for NUTRILITE food supplements that would help it stand out and justify its price or even its use in the first place. There was no question that the product itself didn't represent for Mytinger or Casselberry what it did for my father; the physical manifestation of years of painstaking research and deep personal belief.

My father was unquestionably an idealist. Mytinger and Casselberry were both purely practical men. But it was clear that Dad couldn't keep up the work of running both sales and manufacturing; it was wearing him out. Together, perhaps, they could accomplish things that none of them could accomplish on their own.

Mytinger and Casselberry established a partnership, which quickly became known as M&C. The partnership started simply, working out of Casselberry's office in downtown Los Angeles. On September 1, 1945, Dad signed an exclusive agreement with them that was drawn up in anticipation of rapid growth, addressing contingencies relating to size and volume. My father, who had been struggling for years trying to find someone to take the sales and distribution responsibilities off his shoulders, was satisfied to give M&C a free hand as long as results were good. For the time being, most business was still handled out of the factory on Slauson Avenue, but soon my father transferred his small number of distributors to M&C.

To an outsider, M&C may have looked and acted like the sales and marketing division of Nutrilite Products Inc., but it was in fact a separate company with independent ownership and decision-making. They wouldn't own any part of each other's company, but would work closely together. M&C would be NPI's only customer, and NPI would be M&C's only supplier. NPI was responsible for production and research; M&C, for marketing and distribution.

M&C developed a strong business plan, but realized that in order to make their plan work, they would also need a strong sales manual. In a system where the distributors would be largely self-educated as well as self-motivated, the manual would have to be the "compleat" handbook, persuading them beyond all doubt of the merits of NUTRILITE food supplements and giving them the facts, figures, and motivational materials to become successful marketers themselves. If Mytinger was the business-plan half of the team, the educational manual was right up Casselberry's alley. It was as if he had been born for this job. All his persuasiveness as a psychologist, his charisma as a radio talk show motivator, and his considerable layman's knowledge of nutrition, came together in this *pièce de résistance*.

His genius started right with the title. How to begin to tell people about the product? What sort of lead? He named it *How to Cheat Death*. That would be the touchstone bringing everything to bear around the crux: Our product enables your body to throw off disease as well as remain healthy.

Of course, this is the very claim that my father had been cautious about pushing—and for good reason. There's a thin line between a food supplement that helps the body maintain its natural rhythms at peak efficiency and a cure-all. My father had always stayed on the conservative side. And with the FDA's increasing efforts to crack down on hucksters and exaggerated claims for placebos—thanks to the passage of the 1938 Food, Drug, and Cosmetic Act—inspections were on the rise. Dad's factory and product labels had already been inspected several times, passing the scrutiny of the FDA each time.

But Casselberry knew full well that health maintenance didn't sell—at least not without the pizzazz of cure. Without ever exactly stepping over the line, his booklet pushed the edge as far as it could go. It started out with testimonials, mostly culled from customers and distributors themselves. These involved a variety of cures and recoveries, including everything from asthma and hay fever to bouncing back from death's door.

Moving into safer territory, it then went on to make the case that even in the apparent land of plenty, Americans were starving to death because of poor diet and depleted soil. Casselberry pulled out all the stops, every statistic he could find. He included statistics such as those from the Bureau of Education which reported that 50 percent of school children "need medical attention of some kind" and that "four million of the boys drafted for army service were rejected for physical defects and inability to serve." Both statements were true, but neither statistic in its original context mentioned malnutrition as a cause. Then the booklet introduced the cure for these deplorable and dangerous situations. With rather broad brush strokes, he painted the picture, although inaccurate, of a young man named Carl Rehnborg who graduated from an East Coast university with a degree in biochemistry who went to China to sell milk to Chinese mothers for their

Chapter Thirteen: The Salesman and the Educator

babies. He then introduced a story that he attributes to my father, but isn't confirmed by any of his known writings. The story mentions my father opening a demonstration clinic in the slums of China and feeding ailing infants canned milk. When initial results proved unsatisfactory, he went out and gathered quantities of green grass, alfalfa, and other fresh green plants, scrubbed them and carefully dried and ground them into a powder that he mixed into a thin gruel and fed to the babies along with their milk. Some of the babies showed improvement, but not all. According to the story, my father suspected it was because the plants were grown on depleted soil, so the plants grown on it could not supply the babies with all the nutrition they required. He then went on to grow his own alfalfa to create an alfalfa paste to provide the nutrition the babies needed. To make his point Casselberry wrote with excitement, italics, and capital letters: *"not ONE of the babies failed to IMPROVE!"* A drawing shows my young father wearing what looks like a pharmacist's outfit, standing by a worried Chinese mother holding her malnourished baby.

When sounding the disclaimer that NUTRILITE is a food supplement, whose purpose is simply to give Nature the tools needed to do her job, Casselberry couldn't resist sounding, one final time, the clarion call of healing and included a list of 49 symptoms or conditions that had been cured or greatly helped by the use of NUTRILITE food supplements. These conditions ranged from allergies, anemia, and asthma; to neuritis, night blindness, and migraines; to ulcers, being underweight, and worrying over small things. My father would have discouraged these statements, but since it wasn't part of the contract, he wasn't given the opportunity to review the pamphlet.

After 47 breathless pages, Casselberry ran out of steam. If he had done as good a job as he hoped, he had created the primary sales tool that representatives would use to build a national sales network. In terms of a marketing tool, it looked like a masterpiece.

Now, armed with a bold new distribution plan and a powerful sales and motivational tool, M&C was ready to set the world on fire.

If anyone knew what Mytinger and Casselberry's real goal was, they would have laughed out loud. Already their colleagues thought they were nuts. Total sales in August 1945 were just a few thousand dollars, out of which they would have to give their distributors a cut, pay themselves, and pay my father for the product. People joked about it and called them dreamers, so they never mentioned that their real goal was to double sales every six months for the next several years. They would simply let the results speak for themselves.

"We make a living by what we get, but we make a life by what we give."

—Winston Churchill

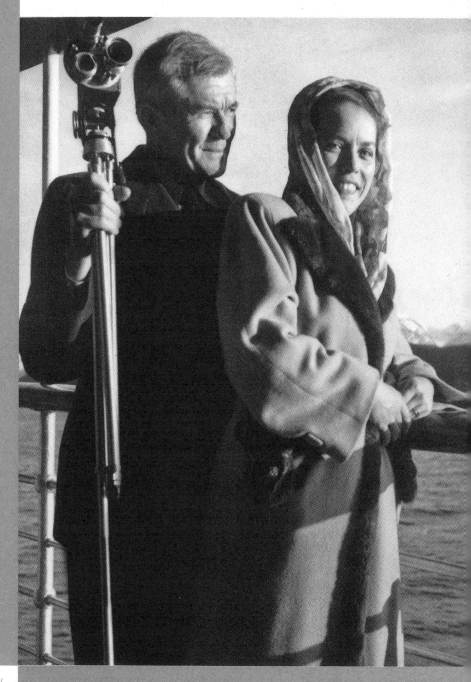

Carl and Edith Rehnborg on a boat in Alaska shortly after they were married, circa 1948-1949.

Chapter 14 | Jackpot!

The engine for growth started to build momentum slowly. At first, Mytinger and Casselberry had to recruit salespeople themselves. They would meet with new prospects every Monday at a restaurant on Normandie Avenue, close to Nutrilite's headquarters, paying 50 cents toward the breakfast of each person who listened to their pitch. In their dog-and-pony presentation, they outlined the business opportunity and showed how the distributorship system worked. They described the increasing performance discounts and bonuses salespeople would receive as they climbed the ladder, so to speak, selling product and sponsoring other salespeople in their organization.

They also described the sales kit. It contained all the material needed to get into the business: the sales manual, two copies of Casselberry's booklet, *"How to Cheat Death,"* a book called *The National Malnutrition*, and a 30-day supply of NUTRILITE™ Food Supplement. Also included were three sample bottles of concentrate, a big card listing the common ailments that may benefit from supplementation, five copies each of an eight-page and a four-page advertising folder, as well as order and delivery forms. It was a bargain. It retailed for $16.47 plus tax, which was less than what a customer would pay for a month's supply of the NUTRILITE product.

There was a certain inherent tension between recruiting distributors and selling products. The prospect found out at the meeting that the distributorship system was set up to discourage distributors from recruiting at all until they had established a strong customer base. Only after they had acquired 25 regular customers would they be considered experienced enough in sales to be able to become a sponsor and train others. This requirement had the dual effect of discouraging dabblers from signing up, while encouraging serious individuals to strive for the level where they would be able to enjoy a share of their recruits' sales.

Mytinger's son, Bob Mytinger, signed up early in the game and found he had a knack for this kind of sales. He quickly became the star. Sales had averaged about $2,000 a month before M&C's involvement. However, with the help of M&C, sales had doubled by the year's end, totaling $50,000 in retail in 1945.

Now instead of being awash with bills, Dad had some money in his bank account. He no longer had to choose between fixing a flat tire and buying a new pair of pants. He could afford indulgences grander than a malted milk at the end of the week. And one of those people who benefited from his growing riches was me. With education always a top priority, he was able to send me back to private school. In the beginning of 1946, when I was almost 10 years old, I attended California Preparatory School, a boarding school in Ojai, California, in the hills between Los Angeles and Santa Barbara. It had the dual effect of allowing me a better education while allowing my father more time so that he could focus on the business. During this time, Dad would send me weekly letters and I would come home once a month.

Every month that passed only further proved that Mytinger and Casselberry were more than just big talkers. Even Les Lev said, "You have to hand it to them!" People were signing up by the score, starting out in Southern California, but soon spreading out to the Midwest and East Coast. Dad's 40 distributors, collected over ten long years, quickly multiplied—in the early fall of 1946 about that many were signing up every month. There were so many new recruits that Les prepared a standard contract that M&C was using. No longer did my father have to find distributors one by one, now each new distributor had an incentive to find other distributors on their own. The more distributors they recruited, the more money they made.

It turned out that Mytinger and Casselberry had prepared their plan carefully—there was almost no way they could lose. Almost as soon as a shipment of NUTRILITE Food Supplement was delivered to M&C, Nutrilite Products, Inc. had money in the bank. It was like a chain-reaction all the way to the distributor. M&C was paid before boxes were shipped out to distributors. Distributors were paid before delivering the product to their

Chapter Fourteen: Jackpot!

customers. Everything was handled in cash, so that loans, even for operating expenses, weren't necessary. It was an early model of what came to be known as just-in-time inventory management; no receivables, and inventories turned as soon as they arrived.

The liquidity of the organization was tremendous. Once a week, when deliveries were made and payments received, Dad, Mytinger, and Casselberry knew instantly the status of their companies' cash accounts. They could see their accounts beginning to grow faster and faster as the months went by. By the end of 1946, the first full year with the new corporation, retail sales rocketed to $750,000.

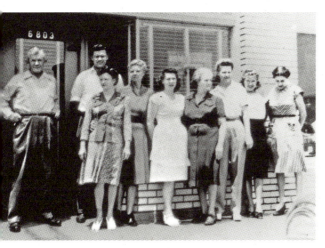

My father with staff members in front of his office at 6803 Hoover Street, Los Angeles, 1946.

Now with money coming in, Dad plowed the majority back into his company. NPI had outgrown the shop on Slauson Avenue. There wasn't enough room in the single storefront for the entire booming operation. To accommodate the growth, the extracting equipment and vats for making mineral salts were moved to a property on Grand Boulevard in Buena Park—a small farmtown just about 30 miles south, while the main office, vitamin compounding, packaging, and shipping and receiving was moved a short distance to 6803 Hoover Street in Los Angeles in October 1946.

Dad moved to Buena Park so that he could be available day and night during the lengthy drying process of the concentrates. Best of all, my father wasn't moving out there alone. He had found a new partner, Edith Louise Bruck, who would be with him for the rest of his life.

Edith had been an acquaintance of Dad's former wife, Lela Calcote. Edith and Lela had met at a real estate brokerage course at UCLA. The two would talk on the phone from time to time. When Lela wasn't there when Edith rang, Edith would chat with my father. The two seemed to have a lot in common and the conversations flowed remarkably easily for both of them. During the summer and early fall of 1945, those conversations flowed a lot more easily.

On October 3, 1945, just one month after Mytinger and Casselberry took over control of sales and distribution, Dad and Edith arranged to meet for the first time. My father had imagined Edith would be "small and dark, and perhaps like other women." However, when they met and Dad watched her come across the street toward him, he realized she wasn't

> "Now darling, I do not know absolutely that I was sure what was to happen. I am sure I did not love you lightly, or just look on you as a sweet adventure, but seven days is usually a very short time in which to progress from meeting to marriage… But I got married. Not because you asked or required it of me, but just as inevitably and naturally as I had fallen in love with you."
>
> —Carl F. Rehnborg,
> December 1946;
> in a letter to Edith

at all like other women. She was much larger than he imagined—not fat, but not petite—with long, black hair flowing down her back. She had an exotic look; she stood out in a crowd.

For my father, it was love at first sight. He asked Edith if she believed in love at first sight, thinking to himself "that wasn't very clever or adult." However, not since the passing of Mildred had he been so spontaneously, fully engaged.

Edith, like my father, was a several-times divorcee. She had come through a rugged history of difficult relationships, but there was a swashbuckling, ready-for-anything spirit to her. She took a bit longer than my father to warm to the new relationship, but by Christmas they were definitely a number. And soon, one year later on December 12, 1946, they were married. My 59-year-old father and his 44-year-old beloved seemed to balance each other perfectly—like yin and yang. The corner had been turned—business was booming and Dad now had his lifetime partner with whom he was not only deeply in love, but who also shared his passionate interest in his growing business.

Dad and Edith's first home sat on the site in Buena Park where the extracting equipment and vats for mineral salts were housed. It was the first home for my father since he had left China nearly 20 years before. My father still had his scraping-by mindset. Instead of building a fancy home, he and Edith lived in a Quonset hut. At that time, the market was flooded with these war-surplus, round-roofed, galvanized steel buildings. The one they chose was about 48 feet wide and 20 feet deep. Dad had one side of the curved roof chopped off to make a flat front. Although the quarters were a bit cramped and space was at a premium, Edith didn't seem to mind. At one point in her life, she had lived in a tent in a mining camp, so a Quonset hut was luxury in comparison. The hut not only housed Dad, Edith, and me—when I wasn't at school—

Chapter Fourteen: Jackpot!

but some of the growing operations. It essentially consisted of three parts—the living quarters on one end which was about 200 square feet and then the compounding (or tableting) area as well as the drying area on the other end.

As the money began to flow in, my father began building the equipment he had been dreaming about since his days on Balboa Island. He hired Wilcox Sheet and Metal Works to do it, and the actual fabrication fell to a pipe-smoking German named Al Liersch. Almost everything in the Quonset hut was made of stainless steel, using special welding techniques that very few people had mastered. Al set up the equipment in the Quonset hut and it was a sight to behold. Shiny tanks and vent pipes leading to a big exhaust duct suspended from the galvanized roof with gauges, thermometers, and putt-putting compressors seemingly attached to everything. It was quite a step up from the operation my father had set up earlier on Slauson Avenue.

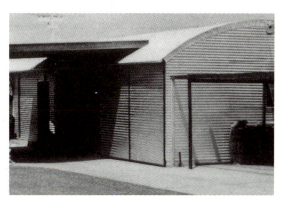

Pictured is the Quonset hut where my father, Edith, and I lived and part of the operation took place during the early years, circa 1945.

After a short period of time, Dad's finances were doing so well that it didn't make much sense to continue to live in the Quonset hut. My father and Edith decided to build an actual home close to the Quonset hut. Dad hired an architect and asked him to build something out of redwood. My father was able to supervise the construction simply by stepping out of the Quonset hut and walking about 20 feet. The house turned out to be quite nice. It had a modern design and a spacious feel with huge picture windows that faced Grand Boulevard. Even though everyone simply called it the "Redwood House," it had an impressive, modern design.

By this time, the farming operation had also moved from San Fernando Valley to Buena Park. Edith found herself getting up early in the morning to help my father harvest the alfalfa, taking over the tasks that Evie used to perform. When I was there, I'd help out, too. Now it was the three of us. It took some getting used to as a 10-year-old boy to have another de facto mother. But soon Edith became "Momedith" and then Mom. And when I wasn't at home,

The Nutrilite Story

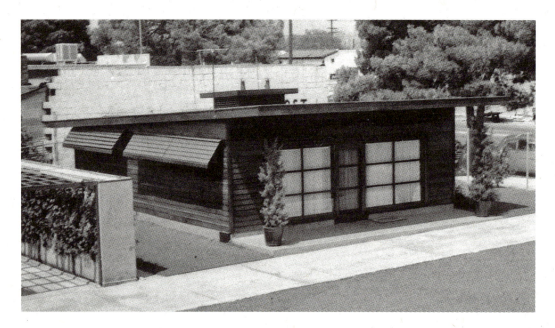

The Redwood House which was featured in the *Los Angeles Times Home Section*, undated photo. To the left of the house you can see the original "Strawberry Wall," where the most succulent strawberries were grown.

I would get weekly letters from her and my father with words of wisdom and encouragement to do my best at school.

Dad bought a little two-wheeled trailer with four-foot high sideboards to haul the cut alfalfa from the farm to the Grand Boulevard property for processing. As we arrived, Mom or I would hop out of the trailer to open the big gate to let Dad drive in. We would take the alfalfa to a small walk-in shed with the dehydrator and load it onto wooden trays with stainless-steel mesh on the bottom. The three-foot by seven-foot trays took two people to load onto the wooden racks. Inside the shed, it was like being in a tropical alfalfa garden that eventually turned into a dry sauna. Warm air was pumped into the room at the bottom; moisture-laden air was exhausted at the top. All day long, the racks had to be rotated to make sure that all the alfalfa dried evenly. At the end of the cycle, Dad would begin the leaching process.

The dried alfalfa was then ground up in an electric mill, kind of like a coffee grinder, in the Quonset hut. The flaky powder was poured into what my father still called "leach cans," but the system was more elaborate than it sounded. At each stage, the solvents were drained off into another can until the result was a beautiful, green extract. The Quonset

School Day Letters

"I hope you like your school, your school-mates, and your studies and that you are having a nice time on your rides. I will love to see you next week, and I love you very much. Edith said to give you a big kiss without any rouge, but I told her I couldn't lean that far, and to give this one to me and save another for you when you come next Friday. Lots of love, Daddy"
—Carl F. Rehnborg, January 25, 1946; in a letter to Sam

hut smelled like a distillery during the leaching process from all the alcohol being used and recycled. Dad had to have a special license from the liquor control board for its use.

After the extraction process, the remains of the alfalfa formed a brown mush completely drained of chlorophyll. Dad saved it to add to the compost for the farm. He would then put on a pair of big rubber gloves and mix the precious extract with powdered watercress and parsley on a big five-foot square table. The stuff was like dough when he put it into the foot-wide throat of a gigantic meat grinder, which extruded the results like hamburger. The grinder's rotating blade cut the extrusions into little pieces. He spread the black bits on to two-foot by four-foot wooden trays with stainless steel screens on the bottoms. The trays went into another dehydrator overnight. All night long, my parents would switch off rotating the trays. When the material was dry, Dad rubbed it through the screen to create little black granules. The concentrate was placed in five-gallon tins while the mineral powders were placed in cardboard drums and taken by truck up to the plant on Hoover Street in Los Angeles to be compounded and packaged.

Renovations had taken place at Hoover Street, too, now that my father could finally afford tableting machines. While those machines were chunking out mineral tablets, several ladies in white dresses and hairnets would fill vitamin capsules. They stood at narrow tables in front of machines with two aluminum rings that had little sockets to hold the tops and bottoms of the capsules. It was a bit more advanced than the process Leverne Parker had used back on Balboa Island. The ladies would spread the dark-green, almost black concentrate onto the bases with a spatula, just like Dad and Leverne had done, but now they could put the two rings into the machine where a vacuum sucked the cap onto the base. The capsules came out nice and clean, glinting reddish-pink in the lights of the factory. The mineral tablets and vitamin capsules were bottled, labeled and packaged and then transported down to M&C's office in Long Beach to be distributed.

By this time, Nutrilite Products, Inc. was growing so rapidly that my father couldn't run it like a mom-and-pop shop anymore. In June 1947, for the first time, Dad set up an accounts payable register. He also began to hire people to help him with both making the product and running the company. One man he hired he fondly called his "Number One Boy," like Hua had been back in China. Only this Number One Boy was Norwegian and named Otis Nord. Otis started out by doing landscaping at the Redwood House and gradually became an all-around helper.

Otis told his nephew, Dewane A. Bunting, about Nutrilite Products, Inc. and about the elaborate process my father devised to create concentrates out of plant material for use in a dietary food supplement. Dewane had always been interested in chemistry. NPI turned out to be smaller than Otis made it sound—with only a handful of people working there at the time and my father making all of the concentrates and mineral powders himself in the little Quonset hut behind the Redwood House. He applied for the job as a laboratory technician and was hired. The young man initialed all the documents: D.A.B. Dad started to call him Dab.

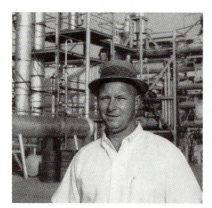

Dewane A. Bunting (Dab), June 1963.

To Dab, my father was some sort of genius who had designed all the equipment and the process. The stainless steel equipment glistened. Everything was spotless. It looked beautiful to Dab. At one point, my father asked Dab to handle an evening shift. One of his duties was to keep the condensers shiny and bright. He would polish them until they sparkled.

My father came through around 9 p.m. and noticed the sparkling condensers. "What are you hanging around for?" he asked Dab. Dab was a little surprised—he had only worked four or five hours, and my father was telling him he would be paid for eight. "That's the kind of man he was," Dab said later. "If you did your job, and you did it right, he'd reward you for it over and over again."

When I was home from school during the weekends, Dab would play catch with me. I know he was petrified that I would break one of the giant, plate-glass windows on the Redwood House ... I never did.

School Day Letters

"Perhaps the riding master has told you, but no one ever learns to ride really well unless there is some time spent riding barebacked. I mean the horses' backs, not yours. That way you learn to ride with your knees, which is the only way to ride, even when you are using a saddle. Perhaps I have told you that while I rode a lot when I was a boy, the very first time I used a saddle was when my dad gave me one for a present when I was fifteen. I did not even have a bridle for the horse, but only a halter without a bit, and I guided the horse with my knees and by pressing his neck. Sometimes when we were riding home and it was near dinner time, the horse would go faster and faster and I couldn't make him stop, and unless I jumped off when we got to the barnyard, he would scrape me off his back against the top of the barn door as he went charging in at full gallop to get his supper."
—Carl F. Rehnborg,
February 15, 1946;
in a letter to Sam

The company was growing quickly, and life was pretty casual at Nutrilite during those days. Dab thought of it as a kind of family. And in many ways it was. One of the people my father hired to help run the company was indeed family—his 29-year-old son and my step-brother Ned with whom he recently reconciled. Ned, who had run ordnance depots as an Army officer during the War, was hired as a vice president.

Ned had turned into a brilliant young man sharing many of our father's traits. His similar broad background allowed him to talk on diverse topics in the same fluid style as Dad's; he knew how to hold your attention. He had graduated from the Massachusetts Institute of Technology (M.I.T.) with a bachelor's and master's degree in aeronautical engineering, but before he got his Ph.D., he entered the Army.

On Dad's encouragement, Ned moved out to California with his young bride to start a Ph.D. program at the California Institute of Technology (Caltech). But after only two months, he dropped out, feeling the program didn't compare to M.I.T. Dad believed Ned had just been away from school too long while in the Army. It was too hard to get back into it after so many years away.

Dad was getting the family company he had dreamed of. He dissolved the old Nutrilite Products, Inc. on October 20, 1947, of which he was the sole owner, and reincorporated with Edith and Ned as co-owners. The three of them were directors, as well, along with Les Lev, who served as secretary. Dad was president; Edith, treasurer; and Ned, vice president. They held their first directors' meeting on October 28, 1947. At the same time, M&C's management structure changed from a partnership to a corporation. It was also in 1947 that NPI bought some land adjacent to Grand Avenue where a bigger plant could be built that would consolidate all the activity from Grand Avenue and Hoover Street. Construction of the new facility was slated to begin late in 1948 and, by 1949, all aspects of production for NPI would be together in Buena Park at 5600 Beach Boulevard (which the city had renamed from Grand Avenue).

By this time, my father was rich. It still took some getting used to, but it was true. The brilliance of Mytinger and Casselberry's sales plan and marketing strategy coupled with Dad's innovative product was a dynamite combination. Sales continued to grow at a spectacular rate, almost tripling in 1947 to over $2 million, bringing NPI itself around $500,000. Dad celebrated his 60th birthday knowing that the next year he would be a millionaire.

But it was never really about the money for my father. He had been affluent before, in China, and had lost everything. He had lived on little or nothing in the United States for decades. If he lost it all now, he could live on little or nothing again. It was the work that sustained him; the continuing adventure of nutrition, where there was always something new to learn, that had kept him going when times were tough and prevented him from getting a large ego now that he was a financial success. For Dad, it was immensely more satisfying to know he was making a difference in people's lives.

This point was driven home poignantly when he happened to meet an old friend from his days in China. Back in the good old days, my father had urged him to try his concoctions of green, leafy plant material and infusions of rusty nails for iron and powdered shells dusted on his food for calcium and phosphorus. His friend may have kidded him about it like so many others, but he certainly remembered what my father had taught him. The good times ended during World War II, when my father's friend had been held in a Japanese prison camp. Conditions in the prison camp were atrocious. The men were barely given enough food to survive. All the serious deficiency diseases that Dad had described to him began to appear in the men: beriberi, scurvy, pellagra. Remembering my father's earlier crude gruels and conversations about diet and nutrition over the Rehnborg dinner table, the friend created his own concoctions for himself and his men. Dad later described his friend's situation:

> *He made cider from apples and stored it in a closed stone crock under his bed, where it slowly became vinegar. He cadged oil from a friendly guard. Then he, and those who would follow his lead, picked all the dandelions and pig weed and other green things growing in the*

Did You Know

... sales of NUTRILITE Food Supplement grew almost exponentially from 1945 to 1947?

Year	Retail Sales
1945	$50,000
1946	$754,000
1947	$2,096,000

yard, and they had salad, and salad, and salad, every day. They made infusions of rusty nails. They pounded up shell and added them to their food.

He told my father that he and his men "were able to walk out of there a couple of years later reasonably fit. Many did not." This was exactly what my father would have predicted. To him, this was vindication of all his efforts, worth more than a million dollars.

Gradually, over the years, the purse strings loosened and Dad shed his bread-pudding mindset. He allowed himself his first toys: a little sailboat; a real car to replace the Whizzer bike that had been the standard means of transportation during those gas-rationed war years; a big new telescope to look up at the stars; a new home by the beach overlooking Newport Harbor. Over time, that sailboat became a yacht, and that car became a big, black Cadillac—in fact, a fleet of luxury cars including a Jaguar and a Mercedes. And yet, for all his success, my father would never forget how far he had come or the people who helped him get there.

One day, many years later, Ed Richardson, the boy who thought Dad was making rabbit pellets on Balboa Island back in the 1930s, was working in the office of the boatyard when what he described as a big, black limousine pulled up. The driver, Otis Nord, came into the office and asked if Mr. Richardson could come out and talk to the man in the car.

"If you mean my dad, he's a little hard of hearing," said Ed, "in fact he's deaf. But I can come out."

So he came outside and found my father sitting in the car. Dad apologized to Ed for skipping out on the rent 20 years back and was there to settle up.

> "I never sold vitamins and minerals. I sold the farm. And that's what I taught distributors: take your distributors, take your customers, and take them out to the farm…because I know that deep inside every human being there are farms."
>
> —Marty Loos, Nutrilite Distributor

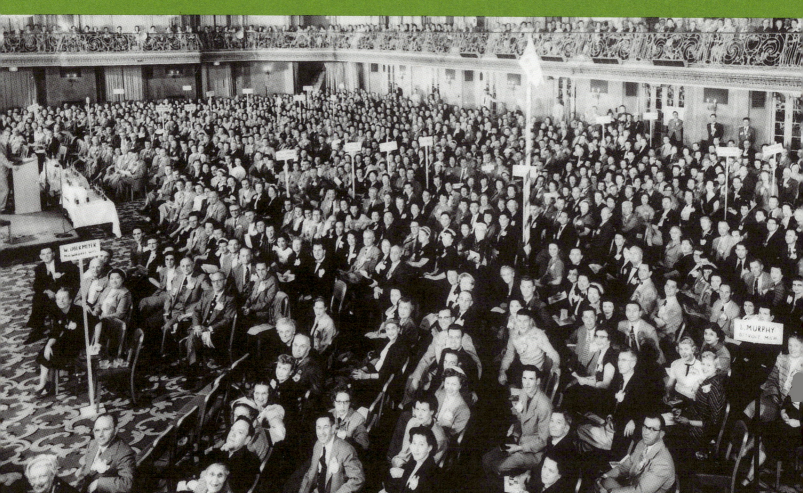

4th General Assembly of the Midwestern Nutrilite distributors at the Conrad Hilton Hotel, Chicago, Illinois, October 10, 1953. These conventions always seemed to draw a full crowd.

Chapter 15 | The Potentates

As Mytinger and Casselberry finished crafting their plan that summer of 1945, it occurred to Casselberry that one final touch was needed: how to give additional incentive, besides money, to those who were able to build their own distribution chain to the point where they received the maximum discount. They decided on a title that would honor that achievement: potentates. Just as a high-potency vitamin, they figured, is better than a low-potency one, a potentate salesman would be the best in the bunch. The potentates were also given a special 2 percent bonus if they sponsored another potentate, and some were even given the privilege of nurturing a closed territory if they moved to a different part of the United States. Little did they suspect that those final flourishes of the plan were a stroke of genius. As a matter of fact, the 2 percent potentate bonus is now considered by the Direct Selling Industry as the first instance of what today we refer to as multilevel selling.

Before long, a stableful of high-powered Nutrilite distributors would charge onto the field, changing forever the way marketing was done in the United States. Their passion, flair, and commitment were evident as they successfully built their sales networks in different parts of the country.

The "Revivalist"

One of the first recruits was Basil Fuller, who had returned from the war where he had served in the Navy as a radio operator. Before World War II, he had been studying chemistry. Now that the war was over, he thought he would work his way back into chemistry by finding a job in the field. Newly arrived in Los Angeles, he opened the Yellow Pages and began calling all the chemical supply companies starting with the first listing

THE NUTRILITE STORY

under A. By the time he got part way through the B's, he had landed a sales job with the Braun Corporation.

The office where he worked was across town from where he lived, so he would sometimes hitch a ride with a colleague who worked in the Purchasing Department. On one of these trips, Basil mentioned an ad he had seen in the paper for a sales course. His friend wasn't interested, but said, "If you're thinking about sales, you really ought to talk with my father-in-law. His name's Lee Mytinger and his new sales company has become the exclusive distributor of a vitamin product called NUTRILITE Food Supplement."

Basil was curious. He knew of the NUTRILITE™ brand name since Braun Corporation supplied Nutrilite Products, Inc. with some of their raw materials. He also knew the company was expanding, based on their growing orders. His curiosity urged him on. In February 1946, Basil followed his friend's advice and met with Lee Mytinger.

At the meeting, Mytinger told him how the sales system worked; how Lee's son Bob Mytinger could sponsor Basil, and Basil could sponsor his brother Warren, and Warren could sponsor somebody else, "on and on, ad infinitum."

Did You Know

… the bonus schedule was a milestone achievement? It was the first instance of multilevel marketing. For additional information, regarding the mechanics of M&C's Marketing Plan see Appendix 3: The Nutrilite Opportunity.

Chapter Fifteen: The Potentates

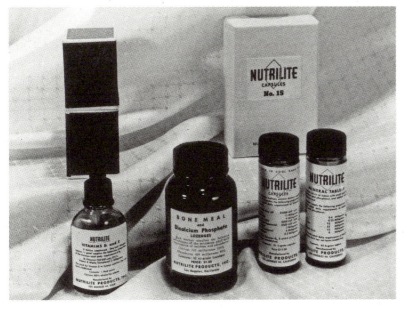

This group of NUTRILITE products is the forerunner of what would be known as NUTRILITE XX Food Supplement. Includes: Vitamin B1 and E (in liquid form), $3.50; Bone meal and dicalcium lozenges (32), $1.00; and No. 15 Vitamin Capsules (31) and Mineral Tablets (31), $15, mid-1940s.

Mytinger showed Basil the products that were available. The top unit, NUTRILITE Capsules No. 15 was sold in combination with a vitamin B and E liquid product and a big bottle of chewable calcium lozenges. The combination retailed for $19.50. They also had NUTRILITE No. 10, No. 7, and No. 5 that cost progressively less and were of decreasing potency. A total of four choices were available at the time.

The meeting went well enough that Mytinger invited Basil to join him at his partner Dr. Casselberry's office to take a preference test to find out what type of job Basil would be best suited for. It was the kind of test Casselberry had given in the Personnel Department at Douglas.

"Your score went off the chart!" said Casselberry after he reviewed the results.

"The way the test works," continued Mytinger, "is that you'd probably make a good preacher-revivalist."

Basil looked at the promotional material that Mytinger and Casselberry wanted him to pass out. He felt that the booklet that Casselberry created had a strong story; however, he was still somewhat skeptical. He wanted to meet the man behind Nutrilite Products, Inc.

So after work one day, Basil drove up to Nutrilite's headquarters on Slauson Avenue. He found the factory and wasn't too impressed; it was "just a little building about 25 feet long." Dad happened to be there.

Basil was invited in. My father sat on the corner of his desk and as the two men talked, Basil saw the sparkle in my father's eyes.

"Bob Mytinger's doing pretty well canvassing," said Basil, telling my father how much Bob was earning.

"We're doing about the same here," my father said, "but we're going to get ahead of him soon."

Dad talked about how the pay system got started. "Eighty-five percent of it," he said, "was Lee Mytinger." He told Basil that he had been previously paying a huge commission, 60 percent, to a few distributors under the theory that they would pay out a share of that to their distributors. Mytinger modified that system, giving a smaller percentage starting out and using bonuses as a motivational tool.

Basil walked away impressed. As he left, he thought to himself, "We're going to have to go out and sell a lot of NUTRILITE product so he can get a better looking building!" And that's exactly what he did.

Two months after Basil's initial introduction with the sales plan and the product, he started spending 30 days in the field working part-time with his sponsor, Bob Mytinger, and enjoyed every minute of it. He was the big star that month, celebrated in M&C's weekly newsletter, and proving to be a born salesman.

After that initial taste of success, Basil knew in his heart he was going to spend all of his time on it. His wife, Lena, became his active partner. The two worked beautifully together, taking advantage of each other's strengths. Lena wasn't a natural salesperson, so they worked out a plan.

Lena would go out on a Tuesday and lend copies of *How to Cheat Death* door-to-door. Basil would come back on Saturday to pick them up. Basil made some suggestions for when she dropped off the information.

"Keep it low-key," he said. "Go up to the door and knock on it, and when the lady comes up to the door, say 'Good morning. I'm lending these books that I have in my hand to everyone in this neighborhood. The booklet is about food deficiencies and how they affect our health. We're lending the book to everybody just as a matter of information. This is a way of advertising the product that we have. And we'd like to have you read the book if you have time to do so. My husband will be back in a few days to pick up the book, because it's not for sale. If you have any questions, he'd be glad to answer them. If you're not interested, if you have no questions, he won't bother you. He'll go on his way.'"

So, Lena went out and placed a dozen or so of these books on Tuesdays. On Saturdays, Basil went back to call on the people. He got at least one sale right off the bat, maybe two … that was the first week in May 1946.

Chapter Fifteen: The Potentates

On Memorial Day, he went out all day long and made at least a half a dozen sales. Nobody had ever done that before—go out all day and come back with six or seven sales in one day. Even his sponsor had never done that. Basil's last sale was at 9:30 p.m. He hurried home.

By 10:00 p.m., he was on the phone with Bob Mytinger to ask about a problem he had. "I hate to bother you this late at night," he said, "but I had half a dozen sales today."

"Boy," said Bob, "if you can do that, you can do anything. I don't care how late you call. It's okay!" He told Basil he could come right over and talk about it.

Bob poured him a drink, "and we had a good celebration right there that night," said Basil. "I guess that was my third day out," he continued, "so everyone was very happy."

Basil and Lena worked part-time that summer. Within a few weeks, Basil wanted to quit his job, but it was vacation time and he didn't want to leave his boss short-handed. He quit the first of September 1946. In the meantime, he looked up the Dun & Bradstreet report on NPI. There wasn't much, he found out; it said that Mr. Rehnborg refused to give them a statement. The estimated sales figures were small, but he expected that. He already knew that the first month of sales for M&C had been about $5,000.

It wasn't long before Basil and Lena found that the Southern California area was saturated with distributors, so they decided to strike out to develop a virgin territory. In March 1948, they headed out to Chicago, Illinois. Basil talked his brother, Warren Fuller, into joining him as a distributor.

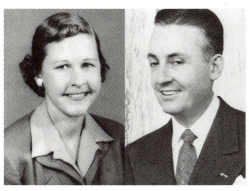

Lena and Basil Fuller, circa 1957.

Basil and Lena began with the same technique used in California: ringing doorbells and leaving a booklet behind. By now they had perfected the system. Basil's records showed that he rang 5,000 doorbells to make $10,000 in sales, or two dollars per door, even counting the ones where nobody answered!

One of Basil's early recruits, Neil Maaskant, started building his own organization in Michigan, which grew rapidly. He started a cousin, a Mrs. Van Andel, on the product. Soon enough, another group sprouted in Milwaukee, and one of Basil's recruits from Los Angeles moved to Cincinnati to start his own organization.

One of the things that Basil and his brother, Warren Fuller, created while in Chicago was the General Assembly of Nutrilite Distributors—a title that was inspired by the creation of the United Nations a few years earlier, but later simply called the "Pow Wow." It was an annual convention and one that turned out to be extraordinarily successful. In December 1950, two years after Basil and Lena had arrived in the Windy City, they had their first convention—inviting anyone within shouting distance to attend. Within the next few years, the number of people who attended grew enormously—and soon even the largest ballroom in the largest hotel in the world at the time, the Conrad Hilton in Chicago, couldn't hold everyone.

The crowd at the Pow Wows became so large that M&C hired a young audio-visual specialist named Barney Bailey to set up what may have been the first closed-circuit television event, to allow the overflow crowd in the two other ballrooms to see the proceedings. Basil and Lena turned out to be enormously successful, and within five years had 5,000 distributors in their organization.

As Basil, who scored so high on Casselberry's test that he could have been a preacher or revivalist, so aptly put it, "we did our revivaling in Nutrilite, rather than in religion!"

The Naturalist

Marty Loos and his wife Dottie moved to California from New Jersey. Marty felt the move would be good for his health.

The two packed everything they could into a trailer, hooked it to their car, and headed to San Diego. He found work in La Jolla.

However, Marty found that just moving to California wasn't good enough: the lab apron he wore as a dental technician always seemed to be full of handkerchiefs. His boss Ed Umsted, a Nutrilite distributor, noticed Marty's general discomfort and encouraged Marty to give his product a try. After a couple of months of taking, stopping, and then taking the product again, he eventually figured it must be helping to support his daily activities. He became a believer and signed up as a Nutrilite distributor in November 1947.

One day Ed said to Marty, "Hey, I want to take you to the Nutrilite farm."

"Farm? They have a farm?" asked Marty.

"Yeah," said Ed.

At that time, only a handful of distributors had ever visited the farm at Buena Park. My father happened to be there when they dropped by. Dad told Marty and Ed what he was trying to do with the farm, explaining it rather than selling it. Marty was intrigued with my father's message and was fascinated by his use of words.

Chapter Fifteen: The Potentates

"What I like is what Carl does," Marty said later. "I knew that Carl was doing things that nobody else was doing … He made the soil as perfect as possible, grows the most nutritious plants, is careful about the extracting, careful about exposure to light, heat, cold … gets the concentrate in there, protects it, adds to it, sells it. You can't do more than that."

Marty himself hated selling. He felt it was for people who couldn't do anything else. However, as soon as Marty saw the farm, he knew intuitively what he would say to potential customers.

"I knew what I was gonna tell people. I never sold vitamins and minerals. I sold the farm," said Marty. "And that's what I taught my distributors: take your distributors, take your customers, and take them out to the farm … Because I know that deep inside every human being there are farms. If you go back, all their ancestors had farms. Someway they had to eat. And basically that instinct is in there. I believe that. That's inside every person."

Marty would tell customers, "The quickest and easiest way that I can tell you about the Nutrilite philosophy is to take you on a trip to the farm." Then he would open a book with the pictures of the farm, and they would go through it step-by-step. He told his distributors, "Let them smell the compost." That soon became their business slogan.

Closing was very simple. After explaining to customers how the food supplements were made, the whole process, he would say, "Now do you think, in view of what I told you of how these things work, what they contain, and how they are made, the care that's taken, do you think it's possible that you could eat that kind of nutrition and have nothing good happen to you?"

"Oh, no, that's good."

"Do you think that if you eat this kind of nutrition steadily over a period of six months or a year, that it can help you?" Marty would continue.

"Oh, yes!"

"Well, when would you like to start?" Nothing mysterious about it. "We didn't talk about stuff we didn't understand. They knew what I was talking about the minute I took them to the farm. I knew what I was talking about—that instinct was there."

Marty was passionate about the farm. It might seem that passion like Marty's would be hard to resist, but for someone like him, who hated sales in the first place—unlike Basil—it was the only thing that kept him going at first.

The Nutrilite Story

Marty and Dottie started their Nutrilite business working in La Jolla, California—although they never made more than $25 a week working part-time. Four months later in March 1948, they were ready to move to "greener pastures," and they headed out east to St. Petersburg, Florida. If it worked in La Jolla, it should work even better, Marty figured, where many retirees lived.

Once they arrived, they rented a little one-story building. It was perfect; it had space in the front for an office and a big area in the back to hold meetings. In the front of the building in the display window, Marty placed NUTRILITE product, paraphernalia, and a sign. Anyone walking by was sure to notice.

He soon got a wholesale merchant's license. Marty joined the Chamber of Commerce and the Sales Club. He then placed ads in the paper inviting people to come learn about the product and the opportunity.

"Become a Distributor of NUTRILITE Food Supplement," the ad stated. "Earn $500 a month in six months, $1,000 a month in a year." The prevailing wage in St. Petersburg then was $140 per month.

Sure enough, people started coming.

When they came, they were immediately greeted by Dottie. Dottie was a partner in the business and she was in charge of doing the bookkeeping. The business looked official. Dottie was there as a receptionist to greet potential customers. There were typewriters, stacks of literature, and samples of the product on the shelves along the wall. Some of the folks signed up right away, others wanted to come to one of the sales meetings held in the back room. Marty and Dottie kept the chairs set up permanently.

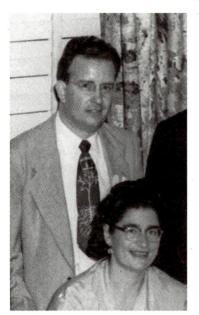

Martin and Dottie Loos, July 1957.

They had opened their shop in St. Petersburg on April Fool's Day in 1948. By June, they were Potentates!

Marty and Dottie became successful Nutrilite distributors largely by ignoring the Casselberry promotional material, especially the testimonials. As Marty would say, "I sold the farm … the alfalfa, the compost …."

The Showman

Rick Rickenbrode had successfully run a string of gas stations in the Pittsburgh area before the war. Flamboyant, young, and restless, with a passion for "statement" shoes

Chapter Fifteen: The Potentates

and flashy cars, he and his wife Jean wanted to travel. From their home in Erie, Pennsylvania, they traveled out to California, just for the thrill of it, but returned home not long after when they got word that Rick's mother was ill. After she recovered, they hit the road again, checking out New York and then heading down to Florida. Since Miami Beach was the only city they had heard of in Florida, that's where they went.

Jean, who had graduated from high school with shorthand skills, looked for work as a stenographer. It turned out that work as a waitress paid more. She didn't have any prior experience, but was quickly able to land the job.

After four or five months, Rick was able to lease a gas station. But business pretty much came to a standstill in the summer, and the young couple succumbed to the "on the road" passion and the lure of the West. They arrived in California, settled first in San Francisco, but found the cold and fog unbearable and headed into the heat of Sacramento.

There, Rick happened to see the headline of an ad in the paper, placed by a Nutrilite distributor: ARE YOU SATISFIED WITH YOUR PRESENT INCOME? No, he thought. Their present income was zero. There was a meeting that evening, which Rick attended. That night, he purchased a sales kit so he could review the business opportunity.

When he got home, Rick studied the material trying to calculate what would happen if every person he brought into the business was a crook, so that if there was a way they could cheat you, he would figure it out.

He worked it all out, all the sponsoring of people, bringing them in, percentages made, and all that, and he just worked it and worked it and worked it and finally gave up. Rick looked at Jean and said, "There's no way you can beat this."

He was so impressed that he drove over to Stockton to meet Bob Fields, the Nutrilite distributor who had placed the advertisement. They talked all day, and Rick signed up to be a distributor. After Rick left, Fields turned to his wife and said, "There goes either my first Potentate or the biggest flop ever."

Rick had a thing about shoes. His shoes always made a statement of some kind. Outside of Florida, most people couldn't understand the statement. His favorite pair at one time was light tan in color with a kind of paisley pattern in the leather, framing a cream-colored mesh underneath. Put on some pastel pants and a guayabara shirt and you had quite a look. But it wasn't a look people saw a lot in Sacramento. Jean wore casual Florida clothes as well, in bright colors, which she thought looked good with her dark tan and bleached blonde hair.

Rick drove her in their shiny gold Grand Prix convertible to Bob Fields' meeting to sign her up as a Nutrilite distributor. He felt that the Nutrilite business had potential and wanted to take advantage of that.

Jean had no sales experience, but she was interested in the nutritional aspect and read up on it. Nobody knew much about vitamins and minerals at the time. "It was an educational job to sell that product at that time," Jean said. She read about it and was sold on the idea.

"You know, this makes sense to me," she had told Fields, "I think I might be able to explain this to another housewife."

"Well, why don't you try it?"

So while Rick was going door-to-door in one area, making sale after sale, Jean tried her luck in another neighborhood. After four days, she still hadn't sold a single bottle. Rick got home that day and found her lying on the bed crying. It was the first time he had ever seen his wife cry.

"What's the matter?"

"You're selling every day and I'm not selling anything," she sobbed.

"Why don't you tell me what you're telling these people?"

She did, and Rick thought it was far better than what he was telling them.

"So what do you say after you say that?" he questioned.

"Well, I don't say anything. I just wait."

"What are you waiting for?" he asked. "Maybe you want them to take the NUTRILITE product away from you or something."

He asked her if she knew what a "close" was. She had no idea what he was talking about.

"I thought selling was you told them a story and they said, 'Hey, I gotta have that stuff.'"

Rick explained that the goal was to make a sale with one of the "closes" or special techniques that salesmen have developed over the years to get customers to sign on the bottom line. You had to project a start, middle, and finish in every sale, he told her. Once Jean knew a few closes, she would be able to watch for customers who were ready to buy and get them to commit to a purchase. He was right. Rick taught her two or three closes, and from that time on she started selling.

CHAPTER FIFTEEN: THE POTENTATES

He showed Jean how to turn M&C's yearly savings program into a close. The program was one in which a customer would pay full price for the product for 10 months, half price on the 11th month, and receive the product free on the 12th month. Each unit had a stamp in it, which the customer would put on a card at the end of each month. Rick told Jean how to turn that into a close: "You explain the program then you simply say, 'Isn't that a good program, Mrs. Smith?' And Mrs. Smith will say, 'Yes it is,' and you're in like Flynn."

The program worked out to 55 cents a day. That was another potential close. "Isn't good health worth 55 cents a day?"

To get customers to sign, Rick told Jean to hand them the book and the pen and say, "Press hard, it's three copies."

"All you have to do is tell them what to do," said Rick, "and they'll do what you tell them."

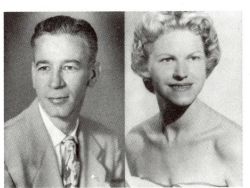

Rick and Jean Rickenbrode, circa 1957.

Jean started doing her own research on the topic of sales. She found that a successful salesman got the customer talking about something that was interesting to them to make them comfortable with the salesperson and then eventually with the product. Jean made her very first sale by talking with an elderly gentleman about the Golden Gate Bridge. He became a customer for life.

Although Rick and Jean were making sales, it wasn't happening as fast as Rick wanted. He was the type who walked fast, talked fast, and liked activity—lots of activity. Rick got an idea to help boost sales further, which he brought up to his sponsor.

He told Bob Fields, "Look, I've got an idea where instead of recruiting one person at a time you recruit a number of people, and I'll do the recruiting."

"What I want to do is find out whether my idea is any good," continued Rick. "You pay for the hotel room and the ad in the paper and so on." In return, all the distributors that Rick would recruit would go into Fields' chain, not Rick's.

At the first recruiting meeting, Fields introduced him as a kind of wild man from Florida. Rick stood there at the front of the room and noticed a box of sugar packets sitting on the table. He said, "I suppose after an introduction like that you're expecting me to pick up this sugar and throw it all over the room." And that's what he did. And then he went on to explain the Nutrilite opportunity.

Rick was a wild man, a showman, a dynamo. He knew how to work up the emotions; his clothes would soon be dripping wet. Everybody at the initial recruiting meeting—six or seven—signed up immediately. All the distributors, as promised, went to Bob Fields, who had spent his money to let Rick practice.

At subsequent recruiting sessions, Rick and Jean would tell the story of Nutrilite. "That's really what we did," said Jean years later. "How it came about and the fact that this was a food you added to your food, because the food you were buying in the grocery store was processed. It had to be … the farmers had to have a way to get the food to the tables in the urban centers. If they sent it fresh, it would spoil. So we got into canning … we got into freezing. And now we have radiation and so on. But each of these processes removes some of the food value from the food, and when you eat NUTRILITE Food Supplement—a product like NUTRILITE—it puts it back. And that's the way we sold it."

"We used to teach them to eat it," added Rick, "right along with their food. And you ate it, you didn't take it."

After couple of months running these recruiting sessions, Rick discovered that he was getting pretty good at it. He and Jean decided to move once again, this time to an unexploited territory where they could build their own organization. They chose Fresno, a city 180 miles south of Sacramento, California, in the heart of the San Joaquin Valley. Within six months, they had the largest per capita volume of any Nutrilite organization in the United States.

However, still yearning for more challenge and more money, Rick decided to pit himself against the untapped market in New York. He had always wanted to be able to retire by the time he was 30, and this could be the way to do it. Half a dozen distributors had tried to open up the New York market earlier with no luck. Jean wasn't convinced, although she finally succumbed to the decision.

When their local distributors heard about their decision, they came up to them at the meetings and said, "You've got it made here in Fresno. Everybody knows who you are. Everyone knows that this white Caddy belongs to Rick Rickenbrode, the Nutrilite salesperson here." But Rick had to prove that his system worked. He had certain sales goals to meet. There was no point hiding in Fresno. Los Angeles was too crowded. Basil Fuller had claimed the Chicago market. Marty was in Florida. The biggest market in the country was

Chapter Fifteen: The Potentates

in New York, worth a dozen Fresnos—two dozen!—and nobody had been able to make it work yet. They packed up and went to New York to start from scratch.

Rick and Jean arrived in New York in their big white Cadillac convertible and their flashy clothes and set out to make their mark. But this wasn't Fresno or Florida. They found an office, bought desks and chairs, and installed a phone that would ring both in the office and in their apartment, so they would be less likely to miss a call.

Then they contacted the *New York Times* to place one of their ads so Rick could put his system to work. Meanwhile, they were out ringing doorbells, and spreading the word in other ways, so the business was growing.

Their first ad was tiny, just a column inch, but the tiny ad was effective. After that meeting, the sales manager for a hosiery company, Selman Hauser, approached Rick and said, "That was the first time I've ever seen people give a standing ovation to someone who was trying to get them to go out and sell something door-to-door."

Sel and Rick became friends. After meeting for lunch one day, the two men went for a walk. Rick was pretending he wasn't going anywhere in particular. He had been previously thinking about buying some new suits. Rick said, "Oh, wait a minute, Sel, I saw a suit in the window. Gee, that's a good-looking suit. Let me see if they've got it in my size."

So they went in and he bought the suit, and said, "Look, while I'm here, why don't I buy another one?" So he did and then they bumped around another couple of corners and he said, "There's something I've always wanted." It was a place that made tailor-made shirts—expensive ones. Rick bought a dozen shirts. Sel's mouth was hanging open. He had never seen anyone spending money so casually. This Nutrilite thing must be a real opportunity.

Rick told Jean about it. "I no more than got back to the office than everybody in our organization in New York knew about it."

"You always were the crafty one," Jean said. He figured it gave him an edge.

The Merchandiser

Ned Ross was waiting outside the Piccadilly Hotel when some guy drove up in a flashy Cadillac the likes of which he had never seen. He parked the car right there in front of the hotel as if he owned the place. The guy was wearing some kind of sharp suit, and when he climbed out of the car, Ned could see he had the most amazing shoes. They were blue suede with white flames licking the heels. It was Rick Rickenbrode.

Ned happened to be at his wits end. Ned, himself, was already very successful. He was a salesman for the National Fisheries Corporation—a company that pressed fish livers and then refined the oil into vitamin A. The company was essentially a two-man show. It was run by Ned and his step-cousin who also happened to be his boss. In 1948, National had $18 million in sales—almost $140 million in today's dollars—all produced by the two men. Neither of them was married. They were two guys who lived for the business, working seven days a week, if necessary. It was assumed that one day the company would go to Ned once his boss retired.

Ned himself was a New York University graduate who had served in the Air Force during the War. He was bright and brimmed with energy. He never stopped thinking about the business, how to make it better, how to grow more sales. His focus made him a huge success and he was only 27. Soon, Ned, and then his boss, got married. What was once assumed was no longer true. Now that his boss had a son-in-law, there was a strong possibility of part of the business going to the son-in-law. Ned wasn't happy. He was one to control his fate.

At the Piccadilly Hotel, Ned watched Rick as he spoke to the crowd of about 40 people. By the end of it, Rick had taken off his jacket and rolled up his sleeves and his shirt was soaking wet. One thing that caught Ned's ear was when Rick said, "We don't want you to give up any job you have at present. We want you to keep your job until you're making at least as much in your Nutrilite business as you are in your regular job."

Once the presentation ended, Ned spoke to Rick. He said he was making between $10,000 to $12,000 a year (which would be worth around $100,000 today). Even Rick was impressed with the amount Ned was pulling in, but told him that his guidelines about not quitting his job until he was making as much in his Nutrilite business also applied to him.

"Okay," said Ned, "that's all I wanted to know." And Ned left. He came back next week like everyone else—and signed up.

Ned's approach to selling the product was to tell people, "Try the product, and I'll show you how to make some money."

"It's too simple," they would say.

Chapter Fifteen: The Potentates

"Some things are bound to work," he would reply. "Don't make it complicated. Why reinvent the wheel? It has generated millions of dollars ... I don't know why people don't see it the way I do."

Ned piggybacked on Rick's program. He never placed his own ads, but used his connections to find people who might be interested in selling NUTRILITE food supplements. Each month, he would have them come over to the Piccadilly for the meetings.

Ned would wait out front. There would be a crowd around Rick's car, because it was so unusual. "Isn't that some kind of car?" he would say. "Get in. Sit down."

"I can't do that!"

"No—get in, sit down. The car belongs to the guy you're going to hear tonight. He used to pump gas at a gas station!"

Ned received a letter from Mytinger and Casselberry on January 27, 1953, after he had made 25 sales at retail, "Congratulations! You are now a member of the special group of Nutrilite distributors who are qualified to sponsor other distributors." Three months later, he was making as much as he had at his old job.

In four years, he had $1.6 million in total volume—twice as much as Mytinger & Casselberry had brought in during their first full year. He had built his organization within their system. And he ran the whole thing off a card table in his apartment!

With the energy and passion of folks such as the Fullers, the Looses, the Rickenbrodes, the Rosses, and many, many others, Nutrilite soon had the country covered, coast-to-coast.

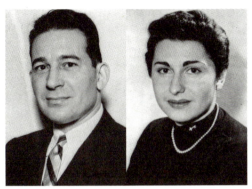

Ned and Doris Ross, January 1957.

"The basic idea at Nutrilite is that all of the factors required in nutrition are nearly always found in plant substances."

CARL F. REHNBORG

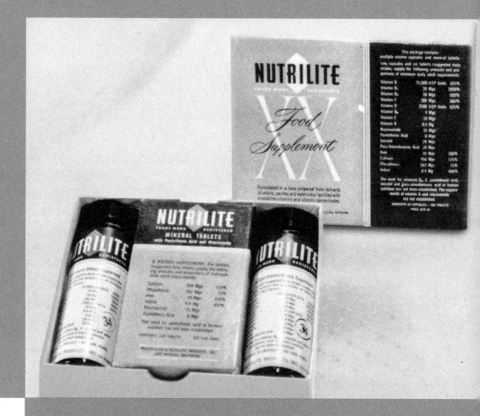

The launch of NUTRILITE XX Food Supplement (now DOUBLE X), 1948. The product, with two bottles containing red vitamin capsules and one small box with green mineral tablets, both with the exclusive NUTRILITE concentrate, would make the company famous.

Chapter 16 | DOUBLE X and Double Jeopardy

When folks such as Basil Fuller, Marty Loos, and Rick Rickenbrode began selling NUTRILITE™ products, it came in a motley assortment of bottles. My father had been looking for a way to simplify it and figured out how to do it. He consolidated the vitamins, minerals, and associated food factors into a single package he designed himself. Tucked inside the package were two glass bottles and one small box. The bottles held the red vitamin capsules; the small box, green mineral tablets. Both capsules and tablets contained the exclusive NUTRILITE concentrate from alfalfa, watercress, parsley, and yeast.

The price of the new product was the same as the former combination of products, $19.50 for one month's supply. Since the cost was close to $20, the product became known as NUTRILITE XX—meaning 20 in Roman numerals. In the spring of 1948, NUTRILITE XX Food Supplement was introduced, but would be better known as NUTRILITE DOUBLE X™ supplement.

Mytinger and Casselberry sent out an announcement to the field describing the advantages of the new packaging and formulation. It was more potent; it was less cumbersome; and it was packaged in a way to protect nutrient potency as well as the contents during transport. In the announcement, they also credited "Carl Rhenborg, President of Nutrilite Products, Inc. (NPI)" for being the leading force and scientific mind behind the product.

My father was probably amused by the misspelling of his surname and added it to a long list of other misspellings in his journal. But no matter how you spelled it, he had pulled off a major reinvention of the product.

Casselberry had also revised *How to Cheat Death* and retitled it to the less inflammatory *How to Get Well and Stay Well*. The changes were mostly minor, yet still close to the edge, a position

Journal Notes

My father kept a tally of the many different ways people spelled his last name:

Rehnbag, Rhemborg, Relinkey, Rehmborg, Rehborg, Rehnberg, Renborg, Rehnborh, Rhenbory, Remdort, Rhanborg, Remburg, Rhineburg, Bennborg, Reheborg, Wremborg, Renhebord, Rumbro, Bennborg, Rehnbong, Rehnly …

---

that always seemed to drive sales: NUTRILITE food supplements helped the body fight off disease and stay well. Also included was a stronger than ever emphasis on the power of plant concentrates to create and sustain health, emphasized by highly effective cartoon-like illustrations.

The results were amazing. Sales took off in what had already been a geometrically expanding market. In August and September of 1948, M&C sold as much NUTRILITE product as they had in all of 1947. It seemed that the Nutrilite steamroller was unstoppable.

Then the shoe dropped.

As sales grew and as the product was increasingly being distributed through interstate commerce, the federal Food and Drug Administration became wary. The FDA had been aware of my father and his company—almost from the start. In fact, the incorporation of California Vitamin Sales Company and the passage of the FDA's landmark legislation, the Federal Food, Drug, and Cosmetic Act of 1938, which granted the FDA sweeping powers to crack down on companies making dangerous products as well as those making fraudulent claims, occurred only three days apart.

My father continued to do all in his power to comply with this new law. Indeed, a copy of his promotional materials, going all the way back to the original mimeographed brochure *Stay Well* were in a file on the desk of the FDA's assistant commissioner, George Larrick.

The FDA kept increasingly close tabs on the company. By this time, the FDA had inspected Mytinger and Casselberry's offices in Long Beach—twice. The first routine inspection occurred in December 1946 and the second inspection one month later—at which time they requested copies of the literature used in connection with the sale of the product.

Five months later, on June 18, 1947, the FDA issued a warning of possible criminal actions against Mytinger and Casselberry. It came as a surprise and was the first time that my father's longtime friend and attorney, Les Lev, had ever recalled hearing from the agency. On Les's advice, an expert on food and drug regulation, Lee Myers, was placed on retainer to help in the matter.

On July 15, Les Lev and Lee Myers accompanied my father, Mytinger, and Casselberry to a hearing at the FDA's office in Los Angeles. At the hearing, the FDA officer expressed the agency's objections to certain discrepancies on the label of one of the food supplement products, which they contended had 40 percent less thiamin (vitamin B1) than what was claimed on the label. My father was surprised to hear this and asked, through his lawyers, if further tests of the FDA's sample could be done at an independent laboratory to see if there might be a mistake. In the meantime, the labels would be updated to comply with all the particulars of the Food, Drug, and Cosmetic Act.

The more serious objection, however, concerned the printed material used to promote and sell NUTRILITE products, particularly the Casselberry booklet. Although it was re-titled *How to Get Well and Stay Well*, the booklet still included the inflammatory passage about how to cheat death. The FDA considered this, along with some other items, completely misleading. Lee Myers promised them that M&C would destroy all copies of the current edition of the booklet and would revise it completely to comply with the FDA's concerns.

Confident that they had reassured the FDA, Myers consulted with another food and drug expert about the revision of the booklet. Meanwhile, the independent laboratory test on the FDA's sample product showed that the decline in potency was less than five percent, attributable to the age of the product between purchase and testing. The FDA was informed of the results and never raised the issue again.

Casselberry's red-flagged booklet, however, had caught the eye of federal regulatory agents. Stories began coming in from the field that employees of the FDA were interrogating Nutrilite distributors and customers.

On September 6, 1947, a second citation was issued; this one to Mytinger, Casselberry, and Carl Rehnborg as individuals and to NPI. In response to the citation, Myers included printers' proofs of the revised product labels and stated on behalf of Mytinger and Casselberry that they had promptly begun the rewrite of *How to Get Well and Stay Well*, and were working on it as rapidly as possible. He went on to mention that when it was complete, he was sure that none of the literature would be objectionable.

The revision was finished one month later, in November, at which time Myers notified the FDA that the objectionable booklet had been revised and that the previously distributed version had been discontinued. The updated version of *How to Get Well and Stay Well*, which became known as the 58-page edition, contained new language that referred to all diseases as a state of "nonhealth" brought about by "chemical imbalances." The direct curative claims were eliminated. Statements were added throughout the booklet reinforcing the idea that NUTRILITE food supplements were not a cure for anything, but a way to build up the body to optimize health. However, in his letter to the FDA, Myers failed to include a copy of the new booklet. The FDA, referring to it as "the alleged revised booklet" responded with a query to see proofs of the revised booklet and followed upon the query with a visit to Mytinger and Casselberry's offices a few days later. The inspector who visited found copies of the discontinued booklet in some of the sales kits. Casselberry, apparently resentful of the probe, refused to let the inspector look further into the files of the product shipments—behavior that the FDA agent viewed with suspicion.

By January 1948, Mytinger and Casselberry began using the new version of the booklet. Sales continued to flourish. Meanwhile, the FDA maintained a suspicious watch on the company's dramatically accelerating prosperity. Was this a legitimate operation or was this a get-rich-quick scheme of some kind? For my father, who became rich over a long period of time, this stepped-up regulatory attention was a novel experience.

In July 1948, the pressure from the FDA could be felt directly at NPI when the FDA conducted a routine factory inspection. My father told the inspector that Mytinger and Casselberry had responsibility for all the promotional material since September 1945. It was in the contract and allowed him to focus on R&D.

However, the visit may have gotten my father thinking. There were times when he wondered if the Mytinger and Casselberry sales and recruitment tail was wagging the NUTRILITE production dog. My father grew concerned enough to suggest unifying M&C and NPI. Mytinger and Casselberry, however, liked things the way they were. They completely owned their company, which not only got a markup on NUTRILITE food supplements, but they also had no manufacturing problems.

Chapter Sixteen: Double X and Double Jeopardy

On September 15, 1948, as a climax to what were considered years of "routine" FDA investigations, an indictment was returned in the Federal District Court in Los Angeles against Mytinger, Casselberry, and my father, charging two counts each of misbranding and fraud in connection with two interstate shipments of NUTRILITE product made in January 1947. The indictment was based on an earlier version of *How to Get Well and Stay Well* that had accompanied the interstate shipments of product.

The federal judge to whom this indictment was assigned for trial advised the parties that he considered the trial a waste of government money due to the discontinuance of the literature.

Undiscouraged, the FDA took their evidence to the county grand jury, which "returned a true bill indicting", M&C along with Lee Mytinger, Bill Casselberry, and my father as individuals for violations of the Federal Food, Drug and Cosmetic Act. They wanted an injunction to shut down distribution of NUTRILITE products. If they could shut down Mytinger and Casselberry's warehouse in Long Beach, they could halt the operation at its source and effectively quarantine the product. The FDA also recommended that the products be confiscated across the country.

On September 28, documents recommending that NUTRILITE products be seized nationally reached the desk of the FDA Associate Commissioner of Food and Drugs, Charles W. Crawford.

Crawford reviewed the documents sent to him, which included a *Finding of Fact* by a man named Dr. Robert Butz stating the literature used in conjunction with selling NUTRILITE products was misleading. Included was a copy of the 58-page version of *How to Get Well and Stay Well*. Crawford flipped thorough the booklet and read where it described my father's experience in China. He read about soils being inadequate, which in turn could lead to nutritionally inferior crops. He read about the effects of food processing on the nutrient content of food and how the average American diet lacked essential protective ingredients. He read the many pages of testimonials of people benefiting from use of NUTRILITE products. To Crawford, the booklet seemed, on balance, to be saying that people should buy NUTRILITE food supplements instead of going to the doctor. He concluded that there was probable cause to believe the booklet was misleading.

As Crawford put it, "The doctrine of *caveat emptor* [buyer beware] should not apply in the sale of commodities so vitally important as foods and drugs. Curbs were essential for those, in the industries, who abused their freedom."

Crawford recommended that a seizure case be instituted against a shipment of NUTRILITE food supplements found in Belleville, New Jersey. On September 30, 1948, he authorized multiple seizures of NUTRILITE food supplements in an *ex parte* decision—a decision made without all parties present—holding that the 58-page booklet is "misleading to the injury or damage of the purchaser or consumer" and that therefore the preparation was "misbranded" when introduced into interstate commerce.

On October 6, 1948, agents of the FDA seized the shipment of NUTRILITE products from a distributor in Belleville. The distributor called M&C in panic. Nobody had warned him of an impending seizure. Nobody had warned my father, Mytinger, or Casselberry, either. It took almost a week for Lee Myers to obtain a copy of the FDA complaint, which referred specifically to pages 37 to 58 of *How to Get Well and Stay Well* and excerpts from another pamphlet called *Nutrilife*.

That same day Myers wired all key agents, the new title for potentates, instructing them to:

> *Inform all agents and distributors in your group immediately that pending court ruling pages 37 to 58 inclusive of customer book, and Nutrilite circulars number 1 and 3 must not be used in selling NUTRILITE [products]. Remove pages 37 to 58 by cutting along fold with sharp knife. Wrap, seal and place disputed material in third party's hands to be held pending final ruling. Books and circulars in hands of prospects, junior distributors and customers to be treated same way. Full explanation will appear with Nutrilite News, but follow above instructions at once.*

Myers also sent a letter to the FDA advising that the disputed pages had been discontinued. The pages that remained described the discovery of NUTRILITE food supplements, pointed to the dangers and prevalence of illness, and recommended the booklet to those who wanted to get well and stay well. According to his letter:

The Food and Drug Administration seizes NUTRILITE product shipments throughout the U.S. on the basis that claims in the booklet, *How to Get Well and Stay Well*, by Bill Casselberry two years earlier, are misleading.

Chapter Sixteen: Double X and Double Jeopardy

> *... I want to say the filing of this libel in New Jersey was the first intimation that we had received that any of the literature we are using at present was objectionable to your office. In the future I will appreciate it if you will advise me if you find anything in our literature that you take exception to.*
>
> *... I need not point out that the offense of misbranding is not a well defined one in the light of present day scientific knowledge, and it is very easy for a firm in the nutritional supplement field to make statements in the best of faith which do not 'square' with the views of your office. In this case a letter from your agency pointing out your objections would bring about a correction without the necessity of court action.*
>
> *NUTRILITE is an excellent food supplement, and thousands of persons have benefitted from using it. With mutual cooperation, I believe that much trouble and expense can be saved for all parties concerned.*

John P. Harvey, who received Myers' letter at the FDA, summarized the agency's position:

> *Myers is an astute attorney, specialist in F&D [Food and Drug] cases. He is thoroughly aware of our procedure ... He really doesn't say anything in his 10-12-48 letter that requires an answer. Our failure to answer cannot prejudice any finding or future action. The letter may be filed without answer with this memo.*

By the time Harvey got around to not answering Myers' letter, the FDA had already initiated a slew of seizures around the country. Seeking to minimize the seizures, Mytinger and Casselberry wanted to consolidate all seizure actions in their home district in Los Angeles. The two of them, along with Les Lev, flew to Washington, D.C. to talk with the decision makers personally. As it now stood, they would have to hire local attorneys to defend them in every locality where product was confiscated.

While Les was busy lining up lawyers to help fight the seizure cases, he remembered an attorney he knew, who practiced constitutional law in Washington, D.C. Although Charlie Rhyne was only 36 at the time, he had already argued several cases before the Supreme Court and was one of the American Bar Association's rising stars. He was the personal attorney for the New York mayor Fiorella LaGuardia, and General

Counsel for the National Institute of Municipal Law Officers, representing thousands of city attorneys around the country. This was a man who knew his way around Washington.

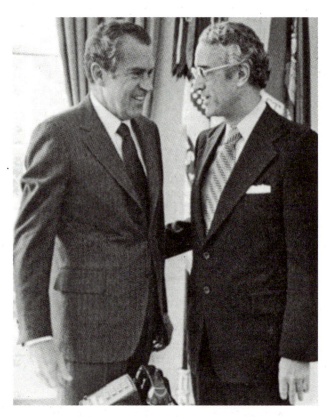

Richard Nixon and Charles Rhyne, undated photo.

But Charlie also understood the challenging lives of men like my father and Mytinger and Casselberry. Working his way through Duke Law School as a carpenter, he had seriously injured his right hand. Multiple operations to repair damage from the infection kept him in the infirmary for most of the year. Out of the entire highly competitive class, only one student came to visit him there, bringing his daily homework and discussing case studies with him. That student, Richard Nixon, had now become a congressman from California, representing my father's old town of Montebello and the district just north of Buena Park.

Les called Charlie and explained the situation: the FDA was seizing product and doing so not only in violation of the federal statute, but also in violation of the Constitution. He explained that the agency was harassing them and making seizures to run them out of business before Mytinger and Casselberry had a chance to revise their educational materials in good faith. Charlie didn't know anything about NUTRILITE food supplements, but he thought it unfair for the FDA to be playing so rough against a product that even they had admitted wasn't harmful. Charlie offered to help by getting a restraining order.

Meanwhile the seizures continued. On December 1, NUTRILITE food supplements were seized in Hastings, Nebraska. The FDA swooped down on Belleville again on December 15, and then two days before Christmas, seized more product in Spokane. On January 3, 1949, a shipment was seized in Chicago and then another in St. Petersburg the following day.

Stories continued to filter in from the field that FDA agents were questioning Nutrilite salespeople and customers as well as confiscating product.

Chapter Sixteen: Double X and Double Jeopardy

"They seized my product in Chicago," said Basil Fuller. "I went over to the Federal Building to see a federal attorney in Chicago to discuss the situation."

"I certainly didn't say anything about any of this going on to any of my distributors," Basil recalled later. "As far as I'm aware, most of my distributors didn't know this was going on for quite a while, and I wasn't about to tell them. I do recall that somewhere, early in the game, I had a distributor that heard about it, and he came in and said, 'Well, that's the end of Nutrilite. You'll never make it. When the FDA attacks you, you're through.'"

Marty Loos had everything in his storefront shop in St. Petersburg, Florida seized. "I made it convenient for the FDA to come in and seize my stock, which they did ... but that didn't bother me. I called up Mytinger and Casselberry and said, 'Ship me some more—they got it!'"

It was a stressful time for my father who had been working for decades to develop a product to help people balance their diet, only to see the FDA try to prevent its distribution. But that wasn't the only stressful thing happening. During this time, when the FDA was making life extremely difficult, my father lost a key ally. In January 1949, my father's youngest sister, Sallie, whom he had taken under his wing when she was younger and who had returned the favor years later by keeping an eye out for Evie and me while he spent long hours in the factory, died from leukemia. She was only 49, and the loss took its toll on all those around her. Fuzzy's hair turned white within two weeks of her death.

As so often is the case in life, as one door closes another door opens. Sallie was gone, but Charlie had now walked into my father's life. He was there to offer support, guidance, and expert advice. Sharp as a whip and extremely knowledgeable in the law, he succeeded in obtaining a temporary injunction, which put a stop to the seizures. M&C then sued the Federal Security Administrator, the head of the parent organization of the FDA, in order to obtain permanent relief. The case made its way to the District of Columbia Court of Appeals.

The mysterious Dr. Robert Butz who set the whole regulatory ball rolling in the first place with his *Findings of Fact* had disappeared to Texas. The FDA was reluctant to have him testify because he had received his medical degree from a correspondence school. The case, which dragged on for months, was tried before a panel of three federal judges. Charlie found a doctor who had studied nutrition independently for years, who testified in a convincing fashion that vitamins played an enormous role in health and that there were such things as subclinical deficiencies that could be alleviated by the use of vitamin supplements.

The FDA presented a series of doctors with a long list of credentials. They seemed to be unfamiliar with nutrition's role in health and proved to be less than effective witnesses. The FDA attorneys longed to get my father on the stand, so they could attack his credibility and lack of formal scientific or medical credentials. Charlie kept my father off the stand, not because he didn't think that my father wouldn't present himself well, but because he was afraid they would try to smear him personally. He had also encouraged my father to avoid speaking to groups in the belief that anything he said might be monitored by the FDA and quoted out of context. Nevertheless, since Dr. Butz was never presented as a witness, the FDA never made its case that the seizures were justified—even under the agency's own rules. In the end, the judges decided in Mytinger and Casselberry's favor: the FDA had no right to approve multiple seizures without a hearing in advance. It was a violation of Mytinger and Casselberry's constitutional rights.

The FDA, however, appealed the decision to the Supreme Court, where the justices, in a split decision, overturned the Lower Court's verdict. The court sent the case back for retrial, and in October 1950, the FDA filed with the District Court in Los Angeles an amended complaint for injunction asking that M&C refund everything that customers had paid for NUTRILITE products.

Charlie felt it was a "cheap publicity stunt." Depositions were taken in preparation for the trial. However, before the case could go to trial, the Federal Security Administrator, Oscar Ewing, overseer of the FDA, stepped in and ordered the agency to settle.

The settlement talks were long and exhaustive. The lawyers from the government and those representing NPI and M&C met in the Los Angeles County Courthouse where they eventually hammered out a consent decree on April 5, 1951. It was the first official governmental policy on what claims a company could make for dietary supplements.

During the settlement talks, Charlie took the vitamins and minerals, one by one, and wrung allowable claims out of the FDA. The consent decree listed 54 claims that anyone could make about vitamins and minerals. The claims generally reflected the same information that my father had disseminated before M&C's involvement: scientifically

Did You Know

... that the consent decree issued in 1951 listed a slew of vitamins and minerals for which the need in nutrition had not been established? This included vitamin E, folic acid, pantothenic acid, biotin, and vitamin B12, and the minerals manganese and zinc —all of which were in NUTRILITE products, and all of which were eventually proven to be necessary.

proven facts or claims justified by a preponderance of evidence.

It was finally over. For four long years from 1947 to 1951, the FDA case hung over NPI like a big cloud. Finally, the cloud had lifted and sunshine returned.

A question still remained, though. Even if you were to accept the worst-case scenario of M&C trying to imply in their booklet, without actually stating it, that the product was a cure-all, you have to wonder why the FDA took such a harsh line targeting NUTRILITE food supplements. Their own investigators commented repeatedly— and with some surprise—that distributors hadn't made claims that it was a cure-all or that it could cure anything, and the customers they interviewed didn't believe they were buying a cure-all. The FDA itself admitted that they had received no complaints about the product or the labeling. So why did the FDA turn their full force against NUTRILITE food supplements?

One reason that the FDA acted in such an adamant manner is that they, along with the American Medical Association (AMA), felt that there was no need for vitamin and mineral supplements. They felt the American diet was perfect or could be perfect if Americans learned to choose more wisely from the available food choices.

The FDA also felt the obligation to protect the American public. The big fear was that people would take supplements rather than see a doctor. And it was difficult to distinguish between something intangible like a dietary supplement and the pie-in-the-sky cure-all claims made by hucksters and others.

But why was the FDA so unwilling to accept the benefits of vitamins? The scientific evidence on vitamins was readily available, and the efficacy of the product, when taken as directed, was documented chapter and verse.

The real reason may well lie in the existence of two different conceptions of nutrition. On the one hand, the FDA and AMA believed that vitamins were, in fact, very much like drugs. If you had scurvy, you would be treated with vitamin C. If you had beriberi, you would be treated with thiamin (vitamin B1). Only a doctor should prescribe drugs. So a salesman who used to pump gas suggesting that a customer should take vitamins was usurping the doctor's role. What did a gas station attendant know about drugs? It could be very dangerous, especially if

someone with a serious illness relied on vitamins instead of getting a checkup from their doctor.

On the other hand, my father believed—with good, sound science behind him—that scurvy, beriberi, and other vitamin deficiency diseases were preventable. With a balanced diet, those ailments would never appear. But not every diet provides all the vitamins, minerals, and associated food factors that the body needs.

The FDA believed that nutrients needed to be tested like drugs before you could learn of their effectiveness, one at a time, isolated from every other nutrient, so you could also discover their side-effects and find ways to counter these effects.

My father believed that nutrients all worked together in some unknown way that was difficult or impossible to test. The Royal Navy didn't need double-blind studies to conclude that feeding lime juice to sailors would prevent scurvy. Whether nutrients come from a lime or a food supplement, the body would pick and choose which ones it needed and discard the rest, but you could be sure that you were getting what you needed by including a full spectrum of nutrients in your diet every day. The human body had been doing this for millions of years, long before scientists and doctors and drugs. It didn't matter whether you got your nutrients from a medical doctor or a farmer or even a gas station attendant, as long as you had the balance of nutrients.

My father constantly spoke of the linkages between man and nature and understood the body as part of a system. Nobody knew exactly how much the body needed of this or that nutrient, but it was becoming increasingly clear that they worked in combination, not alone. That was the beauty of the NUTRILITE concentrates which contained vitamins, minerals, and associated food factors. In this systems theory approach, my father was at least 60 years ahead of his time—in 2002, the Journal of the American Medical Association recommended that all adults should take a multivitamin every day.

"*Diet must conform to the universal physical laws which control man's being, and enough is known to make this course of action feasible… If habit cannot produce the patterns of diet which satisfy the requirements of man's physical body, science must. It is the essence of science for someone to produce for the use of human beings a supplement which will to some degree compensate for the inadequacies which habit, with respect to their diet, allows to exist. One such product, the one we sell and the one we believe in is NUTRILITE Food Supplement.*"

—Carl F. Rehnborg, 1958

> "Quality is a blend of many ingredients. At NPI, quality is a composite of carefully selected raw materials, precise scientific compounding, dependable stability, and reliable performance, plus an unseen, priceless ingredient known as honor and integrity."
>
> —Carl F. Rehnborg

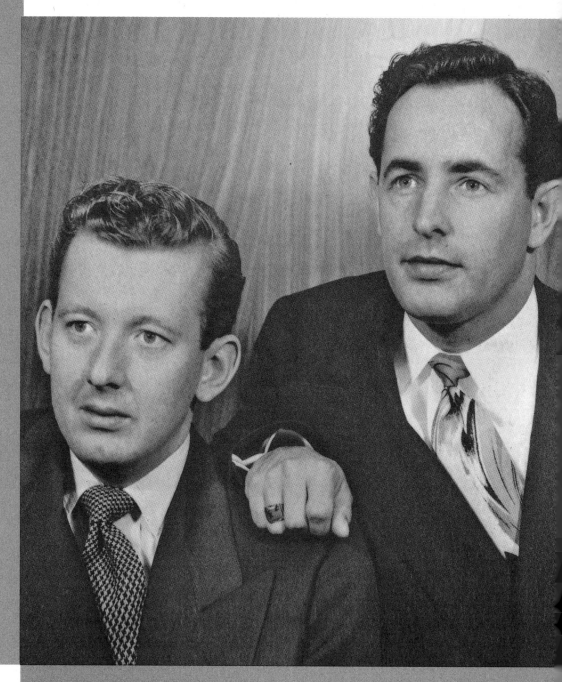

Jay Van Andel and Rich DeVos, 1945.

Chapter 17 | BEST OF NATURE, BEST OF SCIENCE

"We're still alive!" thought Basil Fuller after he plowed through the consent decree. It was true, Nutrilite had been dinged, but managed to survive. The "cheap publicity stunt," as Charlie Rhyne referred to it, that the FDA had tried in October 1950 had almost succeeded in achieving what years of legal wrestling had failed to achieve: putting sales growth on hold. Annual sales had leveled off after more than doubling in 1950.

But the FDA had underestimated the entrepreneurial genius, not to mention the "potency" of the sales force. It didn't take long for most of the key agents to turn lemons into lemonade. Soon distributors were using the consent decree as a sales tool, pointing to each and every one of the 54 claims that the FDA agreed could be made about vitamins and minerals.

During this time, Basil was keeping an eye on two young distributors from Michigan, Jay Van Andel and Rich DeVos, already enough of a team to be known as Ja-Ri Corp. They had been among the earliest recruits, signing up in his organization in 1949 under Neil Maaskant.

The two young men had wanted to go into business together ever since high school. After World War II, they had started an aviation business. Neither knew how to fly, but figured they could hire people to do that. They purchased a two-seater Piper Cub for a down payment of $700 and paid pilots by the hour. Calling their business Wolverine Air Service, they offered flying instruction, but also passenger rides, group transportation, and sales and rentals of airplanes. To increase revenue, they opened a restaurant on-site called the Riverside Drive-Inn. Their aviation business was so successful that after two years they had 12 airplanes and 15 pilots.

After three years of successfully running their aviation business, they thought it would be fun to take an adventure while they were still young. They had read a story about a yachtsman who bought a sailboat and sailed to the Caribbean. They liked the idea so much that they sold their business and bought a boat—a 38-foot schooner named *Elizabeth*. Neither of them had been on a sailboat before. According to Jay and Rich, "We got stuck, we got lost, we got to Florida and sank off Cuba. That was the end of that story."

After their sailboat adventure, they trekked around South America, discussing what kind of business they would like to get into when they returned home. Shortly after their return, Jay's second cousin Neil Maaskant spoke to Jay about NUTRILITE™ products. It sounded interesting to Jay (and a good addition to another new business of importing Haitian mahogany woodenware), so Jay bought a sales kit and two boxes of NUTRILITE Food Supplement with the implicit instruction that if Rich didn't like the idea, he could return the merchandise. Jay explained the program to Rich and shortly thereafter both men had signed up to be Nutrilite distributors.

Basil Fuller felt these young and energetic guys were clearly the ones to watch. However, unlike most other distributors, Jay and Rich felt the consent decree was a huge setback, and NUTRILITE food supplements were not necessarily an easy sell. But this reservation didn't seem to dampen either their enthusiasm or their effectiveness.

After years tussling with the FDA, Nutrilite was soon back in the saddle. Sales started to boom again, rising 20 percent in 1952 and another 30 percent the following year to $16.3 million.

Meanwhile, Mytinger and Casselberry continued to do what they did best, promoting and distributing NUTRILITE products. They had begun a national advertising campaign, which included the sponsorship of the *Dennis Day Show* on prime-time radio on Sunday afternoons. After the consent decree was finalized, the *Facts Folder* was published,

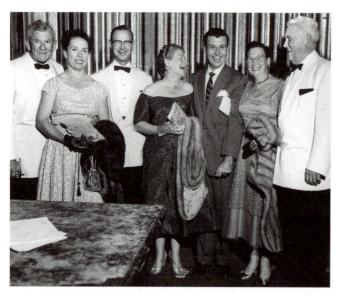

From left to right: My father and mother along with Dr. and Mrs. William Casselberry, Dennis Day, and Mr. and Mrs. Lee Mytinger at a social event, circa 1950. M&C's national advertising campaign included sponsorship of the *Dennis Day Show* on prime-time radio.

Did You Know

... between the years 1948 to 1954, sales of NUTRILITE Food Supplement continued to increase? This was due to the high rate of recruiting and the favorable result from the litigation with the FDA.

Year	Retail Sales
1948	$4,584,000
1949	$5,968,000
1950	$9,740,000
1951	$10,567,000
1952	$12,425,000
1953	$16,319,000
1954	$25,222,000

to replace the previous sales booklet. It too was a powerful educational tool.

As sales continued to grow, amounting to over $25 million in 1954, it became apparent that M&C needed more professional management than a consulting psychologist and a salesman could provide.

Casselberry hired his son-in-law, Dug Duggan, to be the first business manager of the company. Dug had graduated early from Pomona College and had gone into the Army. After mustering out, he took classes in personnel and business administration. Dug was only 26, but all in all seemed to be a good choice and balanced Casselberry's fear that the two Mytingers, Lee and his son, Bob, would somehow take over the company. His fear was not only assuaged, but now with Dug and Bob, who was firmly ensconced among senior management, there was a second generation of "M&C" leadership in place.

Growing the Farm

Meanwhile, back at the farm, my father was extremely glad to have the FDA case behind him. With the marketing aspect of the operation succeeding brilliantly, he now had all the time and money he needed to devote himself to his greatest love:

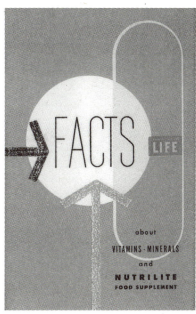

FACTS, 1951. Created after the consent decree, *FACTS* provided up-to-date information on vitamins, minerals, and food supplements. The preface states: "Health, like freedom and peace, endures as long as we exert ourselves to maintain it ... and that is why intelligent people everywhere are seeking knowledge regarding proper nutrition as well as the other factors like exercise, rest, proper sleep, fresh air and freedom from accidents and disease ...."

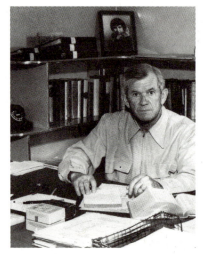

My father in his office at Buena Park, circa 1950. In the background is a photo of Edith taken as a young woman during the 1930s.

building the business into the very best, scientifically grounded, respectable vitamin company in the world.

In this he had a good strong role model in his friend George Merck, Jr., who in 1933 had vowed that his company, which made not only vitamins, but also pharmaceuticals and specialty chemicals, would "play the part of a true partner with medicine," by establishing a rigorous research organization staffed by leading scientists. Merck had been one of my father's suppliers almost from the start. Dad had engaged in in-depth discussions with Merck's chemists on ways to improve the quality of his products. Eventually, George Merck himself would come out west to visit with him. Like my dad, his father George Sr. had crossed the ocean to build a branch office for his company, only in this case, he had left Germany and come to America. During World War I, the American branch had been severed from its 300-year-old parent company, and become a huge operation in its own right, headquartered in Rahway, New Jersey.

George Merck became an ally, a close friend, and mentor to my father. He had appeared on the cover of *Time* Magazine, and his approach to the intelligent merging of pure and applied research would later be featured in *Built to Last*, a study of highly successful companies. For my father, a self-trained scientist, Merck's research organization was a prototype for what he hoped to build at Nutrilite.

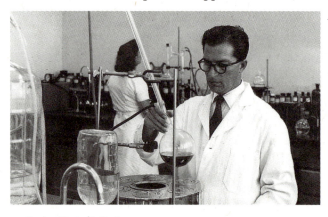

Stefan Tenkoff, Ph.D., in the laboratory, May 16, 1952. Dr. Tenkoff would play a key role at NPI.

Implementing that vision received a huge and unexpected step forward with the sudden arrival of Dr. Stefan Tenkoff. Dr. Tenkoff had joined NPI as a considerably overqualified laboratory assistant in the spring of 1950. He was bright and energetic. He spoke Bulgarian, German, Russian, French, and English fluently and had received his doctorate degree in industrial chemistry from the Berlin Institute of Technology during World War II. Dr. Tenkoff was from Bulgaria. His father was Bulgarian; his mother, German. It was while Tenkoff was living in Germany that the Russians occupied Bulgaria as well as his sector of Berlin and ordered all expatriate Bulgarians to return home. Instead of returning home, Tenkoff

Chapter Seventeen: Best of Nature, Best of Science

and his wife fled to the United States and wound up at his uncle's place in the farm town of Fullerton, just up the road from Buena Park.

Once he arrived in the United States, Dr. Tenkoff was eager to find work. He happened to notice the brand new NPI headquarters on Beach Boulevard. He walked in and filled out a job application. He was directed to the general manager, Les Lev.

In his thick accent, Tenkoff told Les that he had an advanced degree, but was willing to do anything. Les said there was no official laboratory, but they did have a quality assurance department. Unfortunately, there were no openings. Les didn't want to put him back in the plant.

"I'll do anything back in the plant," said Dr. Tenkoff. He wanted work. He kept coming back, and eventually found that they had decided to start a lab after all. He was hired on June 1, 1950, as a laboratory assistant.

As sales of NUTRILITE food supplements kept growing, it soon became apparent that more farm land was needed—the farm in Buena Park was no longer sufficient. In March 1951, a 100-acre parcel of land in Hemet was purchased and farming operations were moved there. Old buildings were razed and fields were prepared for growing alfalfa, watercress, and parsley. It was about a 90-minute drive from Buena Park. Located in the San Jacinto Valley, my father thought that it was an ideal place for the new farming operations. It combined the three basic requirements he had been seeking for superior plant growth: rich soils, a warm climate with a long growing season, and deep aquifers for an ample water supply.

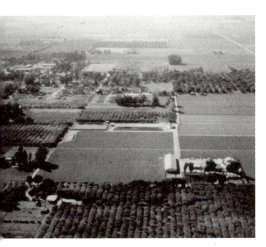

Hemet Farm, 1950s. The fertile soil and ample water supply of Southern California's San Jacinto Valley made it the ideal location for growing alfalfa, watercress, and parsley used in NUTRILITE concentrate.

By that time, Dr. Tenkoff was in charge of technology at the farm and had become director of R&D in 1951. Tenkoff was 34 and had been in the United States for barely a year.

Dr. T, as he had fondly become known, was the first one my father really trusted as an equal in the scientific aspect of the business. My father learned tremendously from the world-class processes that Tenkoff brought to the table that complemented Dad's brilliant seat-of-the-pants instincts.

On the managerial side, my father tried out a variety of general and sales managers, such as Ned, Les Lev, my father's younger brother Kay, and even Fuzzy Vaughn. But the real manager and co-partner was my stepmother Edith.

According to Les, my father "thought the sun rose and set on her," and while she had an office upstairs and a title no one could remember, her real title was Mrs. Rehnborg. As Les reminisced years later about Edith, "I forget what her title was, but she was much more than the title. Carl thought he ran the company, but in many ways Edith was in charge. He was crazy about her …."

Meanwhile, back at the farm, my father continued his research on growing the healthiest crops for use in NUTRILITE food supplements. He believed that conventional farming methods depleted the soil and negatively impacted the environment. Way back in his days in China, when he had various plants analyzed for their nutrient content, he knew that plants grown in deficient soils would fail to synthesize normal amounts of nutrients. He commented that "we must learn to feed our soil if we expect our soil to adequately feed us."

My father's philosophy on how plants should be grown for NUTRILITE food supplements became known as Nutrilite Farming Practices—the heart of which involves keeping a "balanced" environment in order to nourish and protect crops. He achieved this by soil and crop management,

Did You Know

… Nutrilite Farming Practices are based on nourishing and protecting the crops? This is accomplished by soil and crop management.

Soil Management involves building and maintaining long-term farming practices to create healthy, fertile, biologically active soils. This includes using composting to add nutrients back into the earth and earthworms to aerate and fertilize the soil, prevent soil compaction, hold water, and allow oxygen to enter. It also includes using cover crops that loosen and improve the soil's texture and when turned back into the soil adds natural humus (the organic portion of soil).

Crop Management involves keeping crops healthy by controlling pests and weeds and keeping their environment healthy. Such methods used include relying on naturally occurring predator insects, such as lady bugs and praying mantises, to control insect pests. Keeping plants healthy helps them naturally resist harmful insects, while plants under stress attract harmful insects. Proper habitats are provided for beneficial insects so they can continue protecting the crops.

Chapter Seventeen: Best of Nature, Best of Science

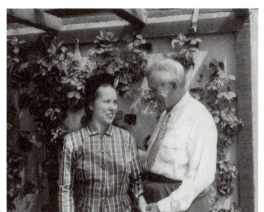

My father and Edith standing in front of the "Strawberry Wall," undated photo. In the late 1950s, the Hemet Farm was the location of an experimental hydroponic farming operation.

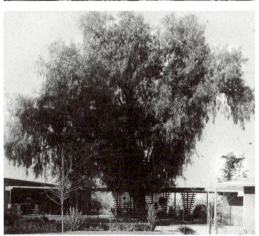

The pepper tree at Hemet Farm, circa 1965.

which not only maintained healthy soils, but also healthy plants that are able to resist pests and disease.

In the course of his reading, he came across the concept of hydroponics, growing plants without soil. My father thought this might be a method where he would know exactly what was going in and how it affected the grown plant. He built a concrete-block wall eight feet high with the blocks laid on their sides. He planted strawberries in the holes using his own mixtures of fertilizers, noting which strawberry plant in which hole had what mixture. He also set up separate hydroponic beds.

My father read about a special kind of earthworm called an "Egyptian earthworm." They are small reddish worms that are "active as heck," according to Dab Bunting, who was working at the Hemet facility in the 1950s. "They really go through the soil." Known for their ability to go very deep in the soil, my father thought that they might help aerate the soil at the farm, improve soil saturation, and work as a fertilizer as they left behind their casings.

With the Hemet farm up and running, distributors could come and take a tour of the facility. Basil Fuller happened to be visiting the Hemet farm when a board meeting was taking place. He recalled Edith calling out to my father, "Come on inside. We're having a meeting. We need you!" But to Basil, my father seemed to be more comfortable talking with distributors than attending those meetings.

Years later, my father wrote about a similar encounter in *NPI News and Views* when he introduced a new column for the newsletter entitled *The Pepper Tree Talk*:

Some years ago a Senior Key Distributor came to the Hemet Farm with a group of distributors. He found by inquiring at the office that I was in the farm house, and decided he and his group would visit with me.

As it happened, I was napping. But don't think that small fact stopped him. Making the round of the house and peeking in the windows, he located me sleeping soundly. So he

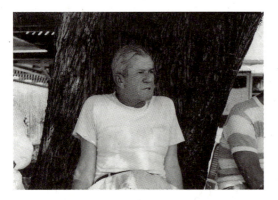

My father sitting under the Pepper Tree at NPI Hemet Farm, circa 1965. This was on a different occasion than when dressed in his robe!

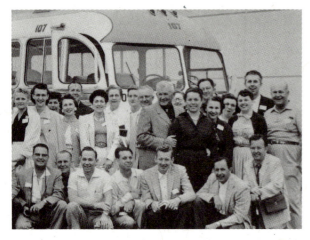

Rich and Jay (bottom row, second and third from right, respectively) and their group of senior key agents pose with Dad and Edith in front of their tour bus, 1956. A bus tour of M&C's offices in Long Beach and the NPI farm in Hemet preceded their yearly conference in Yosemite National Park.

waked me, and I, thinking it was just one distributor, pulled on a bathrobe and went to the door to let him in. But as you know and I then found out, opening the door was simply walking into a group of distributors collected under the big pepper tree in the court, and my nap became permanently unfinished business. The group greeted me warmly and we all shook hands.

The court under the big tree is paved with cement, there is a curved bench built around the trunk of the tree, and there are chairs and benches and a low parapet wall with a flat top, so we all settled down like a bunch of magpies (one of us in a bathrobe), and had a long talk that lasted a couple of hours and ranged over nearly every subject under the blue sky, with very special attention to product and to sales.

It was a wonderful session. Since then whenever those people and I have met, we always say, "Do you remember our pepper tree talk?" and the name has come to mean a treasured, long, informal exchange of ideas and thoughts about the enterprise which concerns us all.

So it seems to me that if I preempt a small space in NPI News and Views *now and then, on no fixed schedule, to write something having meaning to us as companions and fellow workers, it can be an informal way to communicate on one aspect or another of the things and thoughts that concern us mutually. So the "column" will be Pepper Tree Talk…*

One day, a competitor turned up on a tour. "You couldn't hardly get Mr. Rehnborg angry in any sense," recalled Dab Bunting, "but this guy got his ire up by saying, 'I don't believe you have a process. That's a bunk of junk. I just don't believe it.'"

According to Dab, my father took the person in for a quick tour through extraction and the man's "eyeballs just lit up." There he saw "several rooms full of big equipment. So the guy had to eat his words."

Others would visit as well. By this time, Marty and Dottie Loos had moved back to California following their stint in Florida and enjoyed taking people out to the farm. There was no better place to learn about the product.

"As soon as I saw what was being done on that farm," said Marty, "I knew why the product worked. Because of the way they were doing it … first of all, in their fertilization

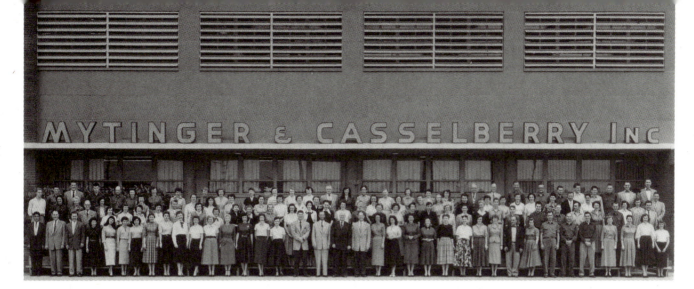

M&C employees in front of M&C's building next to their office at 1702 Santa Fe Avenue in Long Beach, California, April 1954. The two-story, block-long building was built in September 1951 to house the growing staff.

of the ground and the way they treated the soil. And then they had the compost piles that took six months to create…. And this compost pile, they would turn it and turn it and turn it. And then they had a big sump, covered, and I'd look down in there and see this black, tarry juice that ran off all these compost piles … and I knew that stuff was full of nutrition."

According to Marty, as they approached the farm, they "passed lots of other farms that were growing alfalfa, too. But you could tell the alfalfa where the Nutrilite farm was, because it was a deeper, richer green than any of these other farms had. You could see it."

Jay Van Andel and Rich DeVos also brought a busload of people all the way from Michigan. Their first trip to the Hemet farm was around 1951, after which they would drive out once or twice a year. They would pack as many distributors as they could into a car. They would share the driving and drive straight through, not stopping at a hotel since they didn't have money for rooms. When they arrived, they would go out to the farm and then visit M&C's offices in Long Beach.

By this time, Lee Mytinger and Bill Casselberry had opened a beautiful new facility in Long Beach. Distributors could visit it and talk to M&C's sales managers. Sometimes distributors would catch a glimpse of Mytinger and Casselberry themselves, who were always very gracious and helpful.

NPI and M&C had indeed recovered from so many years of FDA investigations. Things were looking up.

"One generation plants the trees and another gets the shade."

—Chinese Proverb

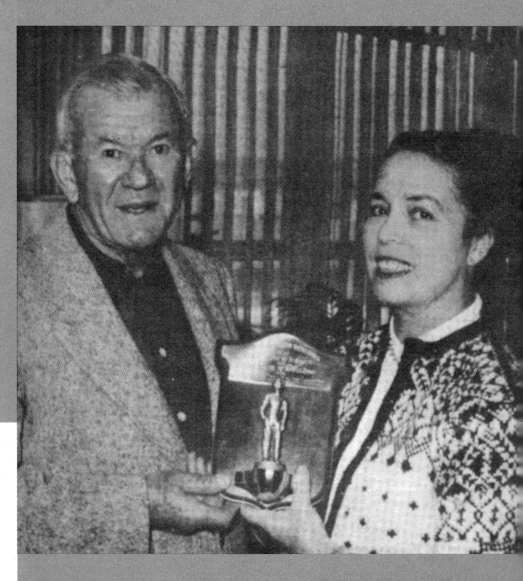

Carl and Edith Rehnborg, 1961. My father and mother are recognized for their outstanding contributions to the youth of the local community through their creation of an organization that would later become the Boys & Girls Club of Buena Park.

Chapter 18 | Global Citizen

In 1952, Dad turned 65—"retirement age" for most executives, when a man is able to lift his nose from the grindstone and look at the world in new and broader ways. For 25 years, my father had kept his nose very close to the grindstone; his brilliant mind and strong will focused on the task of developing a food supplement and finding a way to distribute it. But now that those jobs were brilliantly accomplished, there was finally time to broaden his horizons and create a legacy that would be far more than just vitamins.

A consultant who worked for the company once did an IQ test on my father and discovered that his score was 200—genius level. Dad always played this down, but the genius aspect certainly was evident in the way he was able to absorb knowledge and synthesize it. These traits were certainly given free reign again as he moved into the next chapter of his life.

The first step in this newer, expanded vision was a leisurely trip around the world with Edith. They left in 1953, just after my father's 66th birthday. For more than four months, they worked their way around the world, using the newly expanding international air travel, combining business and pleasure. They started in England and traveled through Europe, making a stop in Germany to visit the Merck plant. They visited the Middle East and its Holy Lands, including the newly created state of Israel, which had long fascinated my father. They also traveled in Asia, visiting Bangkok and Hong Kong, before heading home. My father kept careful notes, as ever, and wrote home to friends and associates.

His letters were generally packed with details of his trip and nuggets of his philosophy of life and living—such as the letters he sent me while visiting Greece and Pakistan. By this time, I was too big to be Sammie, so he addressed them with his latest nickname for me:

Athens, September 26, 1953

Dear Sambo:

When you and I come next to Greece, with Edith's permission you and I alone will visit the monastery at Mt. Athos, in the north of Greece, where women are not permitted to enter. Your mother says that any organization of males so superior they rule out women is doomed to failure, and for proof points out that Mt. Athos has not grown, but stood still, in all centuries since it was founded.

We came here from Israel on the 24th. That first evening we went to a performance of Hippolytus by Euripides, done in the ancient manner. I had never seen it done so, and it was interesting to watch, but the dialogue was all Greek to me. Enclosed is my seat check. How would you like to find your way by directions written like that?

Yesterday we 'did' the Acropolis, and today we went to ancient Corinth. They are, of course, complete ruins (man-made). I gather the two greatest calamities ever to visit Greece were Maminius, the Roman Consul who destroyed Corinth in 146 BC, and Lord Elgin, who despoiled the Pantheon and the Acropolis. What is left goes all the way back to perhaps 5,000 BC (the Greek to 1,000 BC), and stirs the imagination, but whatever is spoiled was spoiled by men, from the Christians who defaced the statuary to the Turks who made lime from all the marble which could be shattered and removed. They even tried to get the gold out of the tiles by making a furnace of the stone Byzantine Chapel Dofini, near Athens, but only ruined most of the mosaics. Under the soot, one was left in the undersurface of the dome, a magnificent portrait of Jesus as a black-eyed, black-haired, black-bearded Jew.

Nothing certain of Jesus and his times of 2,000 years ago was left in Israel except the scenery, but I soaked myself in that for background, and took very many pictures. All this land from Israel to Greece and all around the Mediterranean is more desert than Southern California, made so by the stupid humans who have lived here and removed the forests utterly. They all admit the lands were once forested, and seem to think nothing was lost but the trees. Instead they lost rainfall, rivers, climate, and fertility, and now are on the edge of starvation. The Jews, alone, have started to reforest on a grand scale.

We will have much to talk of. Tomorrow we go back to Rome, and on the 1st start flying

Chapter Eighteen: Global Citizen

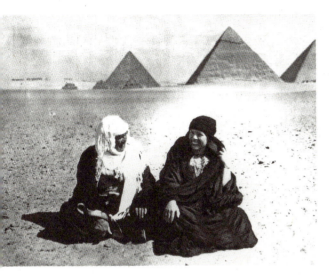

Dad and Edith in Egypt with the pyramids in the background, 1953. The black chador fit Mom's appearance well, making her look more exotic than usual.

east to come home. We love you very, very much.

—Dad

Karachi, Pakistan—October 3, 1953

Dear Sambo:

When we got back to Rome from Egypt, Pakistan, and Greece, we found not a single letter at the American Express except one from Virginia and only one letter from the Brucks at the Hotel Flora—nothing from the office, or Mrs. Cooper, or the Blades, or you. But the letter from Virginia was dated September 17th, and the letter from the Brucks the 22nd.

This left us in the middle of a guessing game. Our letter from Rome to the office had taken two weeks to get home by air mail, but the letters from Virginia and the Brucks had made the return trip in 5 days or so. Therefore, either nobody else had sent a letter, or else all the other letters were delayed.

But even if you wrote us after returning home, you still are not off scot-free. You sent two postcards from Oslo. Thereafter you were in Scotland, England, France, and Gibraltar, and a week or more on the steamer, and in New York, without sending us any further word, when only a postcard would have been sufficient—and your mother was most grievously disappointed. So here is your lecture, which please read carefully.

One of the penalties—if it is to be regarded as a penalty and not a reward—of living in a group larger than a prehistoric family in a cave, is that in the larger group, with stable government, civilized comforts, free communication, and dependence on the literature and arts and commerce, every one of which is the result of community cooperative effort, it is absolutely impossible for a man to live entirely for himself, except by retiring to an island or a monastery or a cave. There he can evade—but not escape—his inescapable social and cultural obligations, because these are an integrated element of the whole complex.

The intelligent man, as compared to the boor or the dolt, not only meets his implied obligations as a member of the human group, but also considers—because it is true—that they add grace and true pleasure to the business of living.

The wisest teachers have reduced it to a simple rule—you must love men. Love in this sense has extensive implications, and one of its forms is the Golden Rule. You know what to expect of other people, and they know what to expect of you. Perhaps I have told you *the Japanese word for "rude" means literally "other-than-expected," which puts it in a nutshell. And this love for other men must be selfless—not expressed for any other reward than itself—because it is the truth and not a sarcasm to say "Virtue is its own reward." It should be. And doing as you should extends to such apparent trivialities as writing a bread and butter letter to a house where you have been a guest.*

Let's put it another way: Doing what you should do as a member of the human group is "selfish" to the extent that it actually benefits you more than anyone else, but it is also the basis of all the cooperative efforts that makes whatever human progress there may be. The more nearly all men achieve it as individuals, the more nearly we shall approach the ideal human society.

Perhaps the highest expression of selfless love in humans is the love we sentimentally etherealize as "mother love." A woman who "mothers" a man gives more than any other human, and gives it selflessly. And Edith is your mother. I would expect it to be normal that a young man of your approximate upbringing, age, and disposition, would give a fair share of his waking thoughts to considering what form he can give his expression of appreciation, and then act on it, even if it is only to recall what interval has elapsed since he sent a message, and what there is to report, and then to send a postcard reading "Hi, old gal, I'm fine. Lots of love. Sam."

I love you, too.
—DAD

While my father analyzed the character and culture of these ancient places that were brand-new to him, he couldn't help but view things through his own particular lens—nutrition. He saw those barely recovering from the devastation of World War II. He wrote that food supplements could benefit many in Europe, particularly the English due to their poor diet, but felt that it would be years before there would be disposable income for this to happen.

My father was captivated by the energy of the newly created state of Israel and much admired their active land-reclamation and intense farming activities. And above all, in Egypt, India and other parts of Asia, he saw people starving, and the devastating effects of rigid caste systems, famine, and nutritional deficiencies.

Dad returned home from this world tour with two great inspirations. One was to find ways to eliminate the poverty he had seen throughout the Middle East and Asia. The

Chapter Eighteen: Global Citizen

other was how to promulgate his views on how the world could work better together to make this a better place to live.

The first was easier to address. Although the term "third world" would not be coined for another decade, it was these countries that most concerned him. The poverty he had seen throughout the belt from North Africa through India and into Southeast Asia, combined with the growing population, convinced my father that something had to be done to feed all these people. The sight of people with scabs on their eyes from lack of vitamin A and the crooked bones of rickets caused from a lack of vitamin D reminded him of the malnutrition he had seen so many years earlier in China. But these people were suffering not only from a lack of vitamins, but also from an inadequate intake of protein. They filled their bellies up with carbohydrates from rice, which failed to give them everything they needed to live.

Perhaps the memories of his trips to China across the North Pacific, where plankton blooms glowed in the dark seas at night, gave him the idea for a solution. By the fall of 1954, he decided to find a way to harvest plankton straight from the sea and use it to make a protein supplement.

Why plankton? More bang for the buck, he figured, or more protein by the pound to be more accurate. Sure, one pound of plankton might be roughly equivalent to a pound of fish, but a lot of food value was lost between the plankton and the big fish that humans ate. As he put it in a later memo, 10 pounds of microscopic zooplankton might have to be eaten to make a pound of larger plankton. Ten pounds of the larger plankton went into one pound of sardines or herring. Ten pounds of the small fish would be eaten to produce one pound of tuna or other food fish. So "fishing" for plankton would be much more productive than trawling for tuna.

The trick was to find a way to catch the plankton. A fishing line, even with microscopic hooks, wouldn't be much good, and the tiny creatures would slip right through a regular fishnet. Whales did it all the time, though. Baleen whales could glide through the water with their gargantuan mouths open, scooping up tons of plankton and filtering it from seawater with giant comb-like structures in their throats. My father thought that if a device could be created to emulate the siphoning function of a whale—an artificial whale of sorts—he might have success at harvesting plankton cheaply enough so that he could distribute inexpensive protein powder to the poverty-stricken people in the sun-beaten countries girdling the equator.

He shared this idea with his friend George Merck who was entranced by it and introduced him to a set of other prominently positioned scientists who were also intrigued, including the famous biochemist Dr. Thomas Jukes. My father had admired Jukes from a distance for several years, since reading his groundbreaking work on the B-complex vitamins. Merck also introduced my father to another of his colleagues, the director of the newly founded Institute for Oceanographic Research at Woods Hole, near Cape Cod, of which NPI would become an early corporate sponsor.

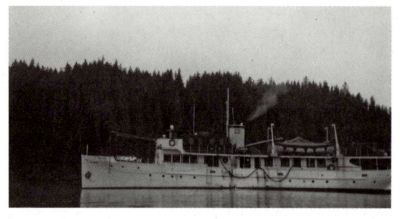

The *Acania* (above) was purchased in the 1950s and equipped as a research vessel to explore the feasibility of harvesting plankton as a source of protein for the world's malnourished people.

My father was able to develop the plans, procure funding, and find a boat, the *Acania*. The *Acania* was one of the biggest yachts in the country. It was a luxury vessel built in 1929 for a Wall Street banker who later gave it to silent-film star Constance Bennett. It seemed perfect. My father bought it and had it refitted for plankton hunting. By the summer of 1956, the *Acania* set sail, bound for the waters off Alaska.

I was able to join the crew that summer, during my summer break from Stanford University where I had completed my sophomore year studying chemical engineering. Everybody in the labs at NPI wanted to go. Even my father and Dr. Tenkoff spent some time aboard.

From the *Acania*, we would send these big coned-shaped nets (which were designed by Dr. T) down 100 feet in water to scoop up the protein-rich plankton. We would follow the plankton on sonar. We could see the fluorescent plankton rise up at night with the dwindling sun, when we could get close enough to harvest it. We would bring it onboard via big pumps that sucked the plankton out of the water and into the bowels of the boat, where it was spray-dried with relatively little treatment. Every night, we would catch 100 pounds. It produced a very high quality material that was 85 percent protein.

Chapter Eighteen: Global Citizen

The trip was a success, proving that plankton could indeed be harvested and a healthful protein supplement easily made from it. However, the operation wasn't successful economically. Harvesting plankton was simply too costly at the time to be viable, particularly as a supplement whose primary market would be the world's most poverty-stricken areas. Nevertheless, the adventure certainly got the attention of the scientific community and placed NPI on the map as a company, like Merck, whose interests weren't only in manufacturing, but also in long-range, philanthropic R&D.

Without a scientific mission, Nutrilite used the *Acania* for company outings while trying to figure out what to do with it. The *Acania* was eventually sold to the Stanford Research Institute and eventually became the property of the Naval Postgraduate School in Monterey.

Prior to the world tour, my father had developed the Nutrilite Foundation, which was initially concerned with philanthropic activities. He believed whole-heartedly that people had an obligation to give back to their community—in whatever means they could, whether it was financially or with service.

One of the first projects of the foundation was the establishment of an organization in 1949 called *Buena Park Kids*. The purpose of the organization was to provide a location and services for children of the community, who could come together and grow as individuals—socially, intellectually, and physically. It was originally intended for both boys and girls, but when parents didn't want them to mingle, it became a place only for boys and was renamed the *Boys' Club of Buena Park*. The funding was shared with the Andersen Trust, an endowment program for Boys Clubs in the Southern California area. My parents donated the Club's first building in Buena Park on Whitaker Avenue, as well as its present location on Knott Avenue, which was dedicated in 1961.

Dad's interest in sharing his thoughts on ways for the world to get along better was addressed in what was probably considered one of his most unusual and ambitious projects.

My father had had a philosophic bent right from the start. Even in college, he had been drawn to comparative religions. In China, he had read a book likening Jesus and Lao-tze, which vastly exploded the horizons of his thoughts.

Over the decades, my father had read voraciously on the subject of religion. His personal library was a virtual comparative religion department with more than 200 books on religion alone. He also helped fund research on the Dead Sea Scrolls, which had recently

"… It is as much a public responsibility to give direction to the development of boys in their activities outside of school, as it is to organize their school activities and to instruct and train them at home, and the nature of this wise control and direction is just as truly a charge on the whole community and the whole nation, as our schools and home training. This is increasingly true as society becomes more complex.

The answer is a natural one—boys' clubs. Every spontaneous formation of a neighborhood group—something boys have always done on their own volition—is a boy's club. The difference is, that if the community organizes the club for all the boys of the community, the boys can have their own club facilities, rather than some packing cases or a tree house or a cave dug in a bank, and they can have scientific organization of their natural curiosity and energy under direction of a trained youth worker. The activities also, rather than games of "cops and robbers" and of mischief, like breaking windows in any abandoned building, can comprise not only organized games, but constructive activities such as working assignments and field trips—and the quite wonderful experience, for a boy, of well-equipped premises of their own games and work and social life quite separated from parents and parental fault-finding…"

—Carl F. Rehnborg,
  August 3, 1960

Chapter Eighteen: Global Citizen

been discovered, to help further understand Jesus's true purpose and mission. On his trip to Israel, walking the shores of the Sea of Galilee where Jesus taught, he was even more drawn to the presence of this powerful teacher.

My father started a publishing company with Les Blades, a psychotherapist who had been hired to assess the staff at NPI. He then began to write on his own. His thoughts, investigations, and meditations were compiled into a book—written and rewritten over a period of 40 years—that was privately circulated in 1955. The result of his collected essays was *Jesus and the New Age of Faith*. The book reflects both his passion for and depth of learning.

While my father may have not been able to implement Jesus's sweeping visions for making the world better, he could at least begin with a smaller version closer to home. He began developing a program at Nutrilite called profit-sharing and began studying the possibility of turning the entire company over to its employees after his and Edith's deaths. There were tuition grants for the children of the employees and grants to colleges. Dad was proud that fringe benefits for employees amounted to 57 percent of their yearly pay. This was perhaps a small step toward the radically changed human community he envisioned. But it was a step in the right direction.

Dad's desire to make the world a better place included efforts to help the environment. One thing that my father began looking into more seriously when he returned home from his world tour was a way to protect the old-growth forests of America. He had been impressed with the active land-reclamation activities he noted taking place in Israel, which reinforced what he had learned in his conversations with George Merck, who led efforts to preserve the remaining forests of New England.

Many years ago, when he had first traveled by train across North America, he had noticed evidence of deforestation. My father observed the denuded hills of Wisconsin and the clear cuts in the Pacific Northwest. In China, he saw the results of centuries of deforestation, in the massive floods, in the silt-filled rivers, and in the near-desert conditions of the surrounding lands. The pages of *National Geographic*, which he read as a boy, contained articles deploring the devastating effects of forest mismanagement.

Now that he had money, he looked at ways in which he could do something about the problem. In 1951, influenced by *Our Plundered Planet*, a book by Fairfield Osborne that introduced the term "ecology" to the public consciousness, my father wrote a letter to the

The Nutrilite Story

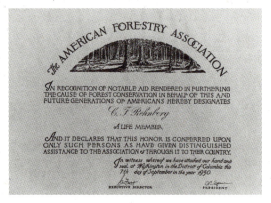

Certificate in recognition of work in furthering the cause of forestry conservation. My father was made a Life Member of the American Forestry Association in 1950.

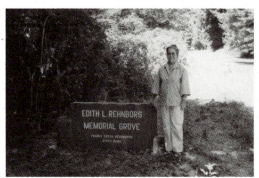

Edith standing by plaque bearing her name. The plaque commemorates the donation of a 40 acre tract of giant redwoods as part of the Prairie Creek Redwoods State Park in northern California.

author describing his intentions. "My interest is in the sub-problem of watersheds," he wrote. "This is specifically forestry and includes protection of the regional climate."

Dad had already been a supporter of the American Forestry Association, which awarded him a life membership in 1950, but felt that a more practical organization was needed as well, "with a hard core of men dedicated to his objectives."

My father had given a great deal of thought to the issue and was working on a proposal for an organization he created. By this time, he was calling it the Foundation for American Resource Management, or FARM for short. He wanted to focus on small areas that could be considered "ecologically autonomous," such as the giant redwood groves stretching from Ukiah to Eureka near the Northern California coast.

He wrote a complete proposal around 1954 that explained the rationale in more detail. "We take it," he wrote "that the meaning of the word conservation should in this connection signify management of natural resources in such a manner as to make these resources continuing entities for the use and benefit of the human population." One extreme tends toward the destruction of the resources, while the other wants "everything in nature to remain in its 'natural' state. As usual, the middle ground is the golden mean." Special areas should be preserved, but otherwise the resources "should be used, but never destroyed."

FARM would provide "intelligent management [and increase] of America's remaining renewable resources." The foundation would begin by sponsoring research that would have immediate economic value both to industries and the general

Did You Know

... acerola is one of the world's richest sources of vitamin C? One eight-ounce glass of acerola juice contains as much vitamin C as eight quarts of orange juice or 27 pounds of cabbage.

public. The objective was to establish "natural balances," starting with reforestation in a small part of California as a prototype.

He proposed that the foundation be dedicated "to full protection of the basic resources of a specified area, but directly engaged in forestry of redwoods and firs." He wasn't opposed to harvesting lumber, but he was utterly opposed to the mindless devastation of forests. He believed that by the truly wise use of the land, including reforesting previously denuded areas and using sustainable harvest techniques on second-growth forests, much land could still be spared for wilderness areas and public parks. There would be wood for building and forests for forest lovers. And most importantly, the watershed would be preserved.

Meanwhile, Dad led the company to expand its horizons. About three years after the Hemet farm was purchased, even more acreage was needed to grow alfalfa to keep up with product demand. In 1954, the Lakeview farm was purchased—which initially consisted of 630 fertile acres (and later more) in the San Jacinto Valley in Southern California. Under the direction of Dr. Tenkoff, who was now Vice President of Production, the extraction and concentration facilities were moved from Hemet to Lakeview in 1955, and the Hemet property was sold because it wasn't big enough and was too close to downtown Hemet.

That same year, 500 acres in Hawaii were purchased in order to grow acerola for use in a vitamin C supplement. The acerola, which looks like a small green cherry, is one of the richest sources of vitamin C. Nutrilite was one of the early investigators of the nutritive value of this succulent fruit. In cooperation with the University of Hawaii, Nutrilite supported and carried out research on this valuable plant. Acerola cherries were cultivated and propagated on Nutrilite's Hawaiian plantation under controlled conditions.

The green cherries were harvested at their peak for vitamin C; the juice was quickly extracted, concentrated, frozen, and delivered to the Lakeview processing facilities.

It is of interest that the University of Hawaii, College of Tropical Agriculture named a superior strain of acerola cherries "The Carl Rehnborg Variety," in honor of my father's efforts.

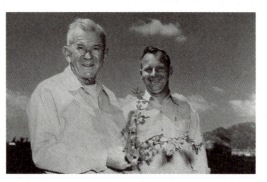

Carl Rehnborg and Dewane A. Bunting in a field of alfalfa at Lakeview, 1958. Lakeview is located on a prehistoric lake bed, which accumulated nutrient-rich sediment, contributing to the fertile top soil.

While Dad was globetrotting and exploring the world of religion and ecology, Nutrilite continued to expand in the nation's consciousness. On April 26, 1954, a NUTRILITE™ ad was featured in the biggest selling magazine of them all, *LIFE*. M&C reprinted the ad by the scores and sold the reprints to distributors.

That same year, Dad and Les Lev traveled to Europe to investigate the possibility of selling NUTRILITE food supplements in Germany, Belgium, Scandinavia, and Switzerland. Two years later, he took a trip to the South Pacific where another opportunity presented itself.

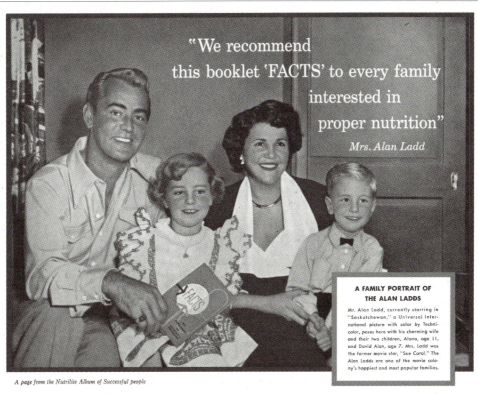

"We recommend this booklet 'FACTS' to every family interested in proper nutrition"

Mrs. Alan Ladd

A FAMILY PORTRAIT OF THE ALAN LADDS

Mr. Alan Ladd, currently starring in "Saskatchewan," a Universal International picture with color by Technicolor, poses here with his charming wife and their two children, Alana, age 11, and David Alan, age 7. Mrs. Ladd was the former movie star, "Sue Carol." The Alan Ladds are one of the movie colony's happiest and most popular families.

A page from the Nutrilite Album of Successful people

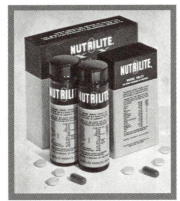

NUTRILITE Food Supplement advertisement, 1954. This advertisement was released by Mytinger & Casselberry, Inc. for the April 26, 1954 issue of *Life Magazine*.

It's wonderful to feel that you are a successful wife and mother! To maintain this feeling, women are constantly seeking and absorbing new ideas in many fields of homemaking. Not the least among these fields is family nutrition.

Today, women are not satisfied with the vague compliment, "She sets a good table"...instead, they strive to make sure their families receive every benefit available through the discoveries of modern nutritional science. This is the reason many wives and mothers make certain the diet of the family is supplemented with additional amounts of vitamins and minerals *every day!* Because of this, Nutrilite Food Supplement has received greater and greater acceptance in homes across the nation.

Perhaps—after reading the authoritative booklet, "FACTS...about vitamins, minerals, and Nutrilite Food Supplement"—you, too, will realize the extreme importance of the essential vitamins and minerals in relation to the well-being of yourself and your family.

Your neighborhood authorized Nutrilite Distributor will make this booklet available to you without cost or obligation. Look in the Yellow Classified Telephone Directory under the heading "VITAMINS" or "FOOD SUPPLEMENTS" for the Distributor nearest you, or write Mytinger & Casselberry, Inc., 1702 Santa Fe Ave., Long Beach, Calif.

Nutrilite is sold or offered for sale as a food supplement to supplement or fortify the diet.

NUTRILITE *A distinguished product among food supplements*

Copyright 1954, Mytinger & Casselberry, Inc.

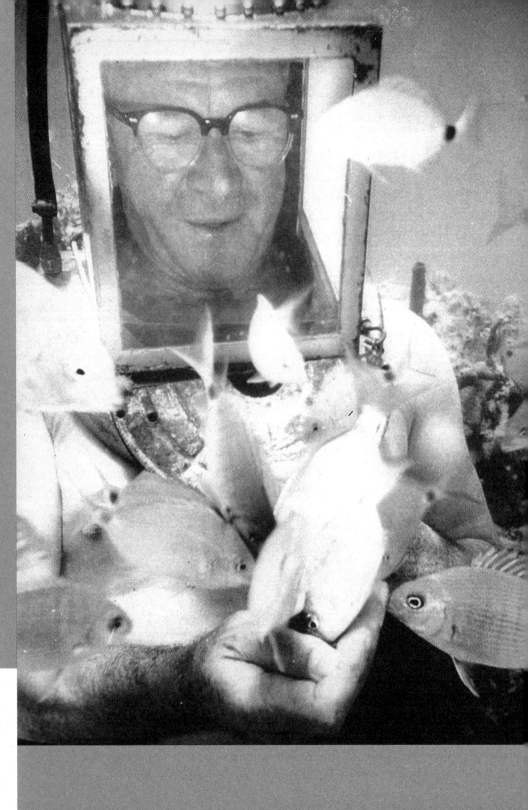

*"Wherever you go,
go with all
your heart."*

—Confucius

My father finds the fish as interested in him as he is in them, 1950s. My father was passionately interested in a variety of fields—from the stars to the deep sea.

Chapter 19 | South Seas Adventure

As a young man, my father had dreamed of seeing the South Seas. He had read many books on the topic. A copy of Zane Grey's *Tales of Tahitian Waters*, which he read while landlocked in dusty Trona, sat on one of his library shelves. Other books could be found in his library as well, such as Margaret Mead's study *Coming of Age in Samoa*, Bengt Danielsson's *Love in the South Seas* about Polynesian sexuality, and Thor Heyerdahl's *Kon-Tiki* describing the theory that Polynesia was populated by settlers floating in reed rafts from South America.

In the summer of 1956, with the business fabulously successful, my parents were able to travel to the South Pacific for the first time. I was able to join them for part of their trip, at least while they enjoyed their layover in Hawaii.

My life had taken on a new dimension. I had just gotten married. I had met my wife, Gay Armstrong, while I was home in Corona del Mar during spring break from Stanford University. She was a friend of a friend. I would have to say that I was pretty much smitten with her from the start. She was a high school junior and a local beauty queen. I had taken her to a Stanford football game and her arrival brought most of the Stanford men's rooting section to its feet. She was gorgeous—a California beach girl with a heart of gold. We were young; I was 20 and Gay was 17 when we got married. I knew my parents weren't enamored over the idea. Dad was concerned that I would get sidetracked and not finish my schooling.

Gay and I spent our honeymoon in Hawaii—where we met up with my parents for a short time before they continued on their way to the South Pacific. Their plane first touched down in Fiji's Laucala Bay. Here, a car was waiting to take them to the elegant Grand Pacific Hotel that sat on the waterfront of the beautiful city of Suva.

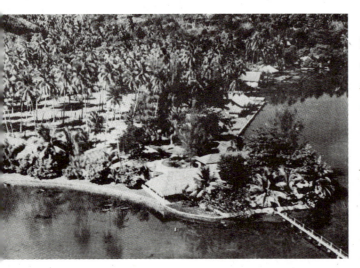

Les Tropiques resort, Tahiti, circa 1961.

The next day they embarked for Western Samoa, a four-hour flight, setting down in a crystal lagoon on the north side of the island of Upolu. They were taken 20 miles along the coast to the capital, Apia, where they were met by the legendary Aggie Grey—who was the model of James Mitchener's "Bloody Mary" in *Tales of the South Pacific*—at her rambling seaside hotel.

Prior to the trip, my father had been thinking of purchasing a home in Tahiti where he could stay for months at a time, relaxing and listening to the surf and watching the bright stars in the sky. But once arriving and seeing the Grand Pacific Hotel and Aggie Grey's Hotel, he got lost in the magic of the place and started imagining what it would be like to own a hotel there himself.

The South Pacific would be a major tourist destination—my father was sure of it. A new water and sewer system had already been built in Tahiti's capital city Papeete, and the main road around the island had been paved. New schools and bridges were springing up along the road. There was even talk of an airport in Tahiti. Flying boats—boats which take off and land on water—and soon jets would be bringing swarms of tourists.

To my father, the beauty of the islands and of the people was irresistible. He joyfully immersed himself in the culture of the native South Pacific Islanders. He was intrigued with what he saw and the people he met.

During my parents' stay in the South Pacific, they checked out the hotels that were available for sale in Tahiti. The pickings were slim. Most had fallen on hard times. Of the hotels they checked out, Les Tropiques seemed to be the best of the bunch. To the west, it had an amazing view of the island of Moorea; to the north, the panorama of Papeete. Hundreds of coconut palms soared into the air around its 14 cottages. The main hotel building stood on a point of land that poked into the shore reef, giving the impression from the open-air dance floor that you were in the lagoon itself. The combers broke over the outer reef less than a mile away, splashing into a calm and crystalline lagoon. A plank path set on concrete piers led from the hotel property to an artificial island in the lagoon. It was paradise, although the hotel and cottages, like all the others they had seen, were in poor repair.

CHAPTER NINETEEN: SOUTH SEAS ADVENTURE

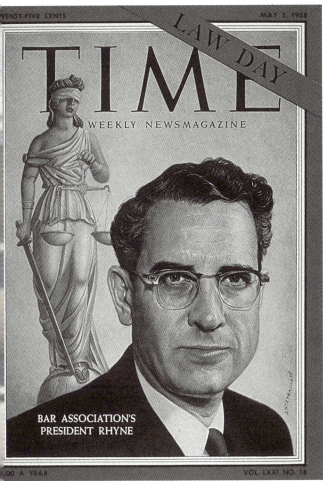

Charles Rhyne featured on the cover of *Time* Magazine, May 5, 1958. Charlie Rhyne was a close friend of my father and helped NPI in various legal matters. [Reprinted through the courtesy of the Editors of TIME Magazine © 2009 Time Inc.]

The man who owned the lease on Les Tropiques was a character named Donn Beach. He had a clause in the contract giving him the option to buy. Beach was living in Honolulu at the time. On my parent's trip home, they stopped in Hawaii and met with him to discuss the hotel.

My father couldn't have found a more experienced person to help navigate the waters in the hotel business than Donn Beach. Beach had invented, along with his own name, the whole concept of Polynesian cocktail lounges and had started the trend of the Tiki lounge in Honolulu. Like my father, Beach was an inventor of a kind, only his specialty was rum; he had devised over 75 rum drinks since his bootlegging days at the end of Prohibition, including the Zombie and the Mai-Tai. In his flamboyant manner, he had a way with women, bowing to every beauty that walked into his place and offering her a pearl from his pocket.

Both Donn Beach and my father saw the possibilities of Tahiti as a vacation destination and were willing to put money into it. Their backgrounds were different, but they both had the ability to dream—and to dream big.

Beach helped my father purchase Les Tropiques. It was a complicated deal. Only a French company could own property in Tahiti. Even then, transferring the deeds was like slogging through a swamp. To expedite the situation, my father purchased the company that actually owned the hotel—Societe Hoteliere de Tahiti.

Charlie Rhyne handled the incorporation of the parent company. Charlie had been elected President of the American Bar Association in 1957, so he lent some prestige to the project. People were beginning to recognize him—especially after landing on the cover of *Time* magazine.

After having made several trips to Hawaii, Tahiti, and other Polynesian islands in the South Seas, my father started to envision a large-scale hotel project throughout the area. Such a project could encourage the development of the economy by bringing in tourists to this beautiful but remote part of the world.

My father acquired some acreage with a white sand beach on the island of Moorea, 10 miles from Tahiti, as a second possible hotel site. The prized land belonged to Princess Pomarè of the Tahitian royal family. My father sought additional investment capital to develop his idea further. In his various drafts for the prospectus—a document used to describe the scope and details of the project for prospective investors—he kept coming back to his goal of developing the economy of the islands in a way that protected the local cultures. He had seen the changes that had come to Hawaii since his first stop in 1915 on his way to China, where the native people seemed relegated to picking pineapples on their own land or serving overbearing foreigners from the mainland. My father wanted things to be different under the aegis of a subsidiary corporation he called South Seas Enterprises, Ltd.

"The South Seas," concluded the prospectus for the project, "constitutes a tremendous attraction for visitors, and has philosophical impact of a living object lesson in more natural attitudes toward life and living, and in the relation between people as individuals. It is the last great area of native culture, of absorbing interest alike to the anthropologist and to the tourist. If it is changed it will be lost forever. The governments of these peoples do not want it changed, and if we help in the ways we can to prevent change, the area will remain for a very long time a refuge from stress and artificiality into a simpler concept of living, and a very much greater joy in living."

The project was shaping up to be an integrated chain of accommodations from Fiji through Samoa to Tahiti, including service from a competent travel agency and even flying boat service and "outpost" facilities to the more isolated and inaccessible locations—places where visitors, if they wished, could live like the natives. Native fishermen were recruited to take visitors deep sea fishing. A floating hotel, sailing yachts, motor boats, and equipment for skin and aqualung diving were lined up. It was all part of an integrated network that visitors could plug into at any point, packaged in any way they wanted.

The South Seas Enterprises concept had even grown to include a coconut processing component. The idea was to get more value out of the coconut by using everything—the husk, the fur, the meat, the milk, and the oil—and to do it with fresh coconuts right from the islands. My father negotiated with Crown Prince Tungi of Tonga for the nuts to be

Chapter Nineteen: South Seas Adventure

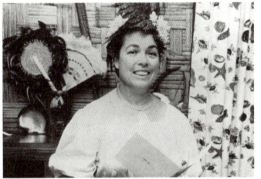

Edith is wearing a special headdress woven of fronds and flowers, undated photo. My parents took great pleasure in furnishing their home with native arts and crafts, and loved the Tahitian relaxed lifestyle.

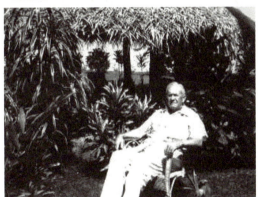

My father sits outside the lanai which is open to the South Sea breezes, enjoying the balmy climate.

grown in Tonga and then shipped to a processing plant in Western Samoa. Tahiti, however, wasn't involved because the French required that all the dried "meat" of the coconut, the copra, be shipped to France for processing. My father had a complete analysis done of the market for coconut products. Would bakers prefer coconut flour? Would they want to use coconut oil? Did it matter if it had a flavor? The list of topics to be analyzed covered dozens of pages.

My parents also built a vacation home on land they purchased at Punaauia, Tahiti. It had a wonderful view of the ocean and the island of Moorea across the strait. They enjoyed their time there.

My father continued his studies—immersing himself in his surroundings. Just as he had while in China, he learned the language. While in his 70s, he learned French to help in his efforts to launch South Seas Enterprises. Meanwhile, he continued to document what he observed in the island paradise:

I have always had a romantic interest in the South Seas—particularly in the area covering Tahiti, Samoa and Fiji—and in the past couple of years Mrs. Rehnborg and I have had the chance, after 40 years of wishing to do so, to visit the area, and to acquire some firsthand information, as well as to develop a very sincere admiration for, and interest in, the area and its people.

The area we have grown to know better stretches from French Polynesia in the east to the beginnings of Micronesia in Fiji and New Caledonia—a distance of over 3,000 miles. There are literally hundreds of islands in this expanse of the Pacific Ocean, of which the total land area is extremely small when compared to the tremendous expanse of the ocean surrounding them. Always, on these islands, one gets the effect of terrific isolation. ...

The range of temperatures in these islands is almost steadily between the low 70s and the high 80s. The air itself is like a caress. There is a crystal clearness and plenty of sunshine, and on the high islands, copious rainfall in the hills, and plenty of water…

And the people themselves are incredibly beautiful—the men of magnificent physique and the women beautiful by any standard. It is very probable that in the isolated areas, where the terms of living had balanced themselves out, that these people, living on a natural and adequate diet, and superbly healthy, did not have a single ailment of the kinds that plague the western world. No contagious or infectious diseases, not even the common cold. Dental caries was an unknown thing. Very old people wore their teeth down on rough food, but nobody lost any teeth. …

These were the people, outstandingly attractive as human beings, living lives of love and laughter and song, with vigorous dances and vigorous warfare, and a tremendous lust for living, who were found by the first of the intruders. …

For very small payments, usually in the form of booze, the traders persuaded the chiefs to let them denude the high islands of their camphorwood and sandalwood. With the backing of their own governments, they moved into the lagoons of the atolls and mined the pearl shell and pearls. Among natural mineral resources, gold and manganese were discovered in Fiji, and a potash deposit near Tahiti, and these have been taken away also. The copra trade was organized and developed for the benefit of the interlopers, not the natives. …

Nothing was brought to the natives that they needed; much was taken away that they should have now … What we have given them of western progress—if it is indeed progress—does not fit them, and they did not need it. The whole effort, now, should be to preserve what is left.

One day while I was at Stanford, I happened to be watching television with some friends. A clip about Tahiti came on. The newsreel showed some scenic shots of the island and then focused on a traditional Tahitian celebration with hula-dancing women and fire-juggling men, but the camera crew seemed more interested in what they described as peculiar activities of the tourists. The camera zoomed in on one man in particular, wearing a wild Tahitian shirt and a floppy straw hat, who was cranking away on his camera. You might have guessed. It was none other than Dad.

Thanks to his extraordinary range and depth of knowledge and his lifelong passion for learning, my father was able to encourage and inform me at every level of my

Chapter Nineteen: South Seas Adventure

education. It was during this time while my father was increasingly involved with South Seas Enterprises that I happened to be taking a tough physics course at Stanford and was struggling with some basic concepts of time and space. My father wrote me a letter that provided some insight into my predicament—about the idea of time as a fourth dimension:

> *I assume that matter and energy are considered to be different aspects of one ultimate 'reality,' and that this matter/energy can be regarded as electromagnetic fields of force, although its 'final' nature is unknown. If, however, time is in fact a spatial dimension, as indicated by its use mathematically, then just as a point has no dimension in space, and a moving point creates a plane in two dimensions, and a moving plane creates a solid in three dimensions, so in turn a 'moving' solid in the time dimension creates an event.*

This was a long way from an interested father helping his son with his homework. It also was something deeper than a very smart father showing off his stuff. In some ways, it was a bridge of knowledge that would, as it had in the beginning, link me more and more with his world and business. In the letter he continued:

> *It seems to be generally understood and accepted that the final nature of 'reality' may never be deciphered. Nevertheless, there are and have been successive steps toward such understanding. The concepts of relativity and quantum physics substantially invalidated the classic view of the physical universe which had prevailed up to that time.*

He continued to impress me and my friends with his knowledge. Prior to my marriage to Gay, he had paid a visit to my fraternity where I lived briefly during my sophomore year. The Fiji House was a rowdy and eclectic conglomeration of free spirits. One of my fraternity brothers, Tony Serra, who would later become a nationally famous criminal defense attorney, had a room that was painted all black, including the windows, in homage to Plato's Parable of the Cave. In his room, he had a headstone from a grave, inscribed in Chinese. My father, in his soft-spoken yet friendly way was very much at ease in what was in many ways a bizarre atmosphere, stunned my fraternity brothers by examining the headstone, and translating it.

During the late 1950s and early 1960s, my father was spending more and more time attending to business in Tahiti and the South Pacific. He felt he could since the business back home was in good hands. Dr. Stefan Tenkoff was doing a great job with R&D and was

Papeete, April 29, 1961

Sweetest darling—

It is mail day, and mail days slip up on me unexpectedly. I was just reminded when I heard the blast of a steamer in the harbor. I did not know one was due, and I do not know which one it is. I need you with me just to feel organized and in step with events.

There is so much to get onto my discs that I do not get the time to dictate it. There are enough hours in the day but not enough system to my use of time. I need to manicure my nails, but I did get my hair cut. If you were here both would have been done days ago.

Today is typically crowded. It is 9:00 a.m., so I have taken too long to dress. I dash next to Les Tropiques, where I have an appointment. Then I'll get off a few more discs. Then at 3:00 p.m. I go to see a princess, the aged daughter of Pomare V, and then with Simone to outline what has to be done at Punaauia to get it in condition by June. It has been sadly neglected, but Simone will hire the gardener or gardeners and get it done, and keep supervision of their work. I gather this is being done for you, sight unseen.

More and more, it seems to me, I realize how much I adore you, and how smooth and rational life is when we are together. I go my own way alone, and some of my events might not occur if you were along, but it is like the kid who is coursing through the neighborhood until Mama calls him home to wash behind his ears and get ready for dinner and homework. Both are fun, but home is more orderly, and much more satisfying.

I love you hugely and absorbingly, and I am lonesome.
Millions of kisses and a long hug.

—Your adoring Carl [in letter to Edith]

CHAPTER NINETEEN: SOUTH SEAS ADVENTURE

taking on more responsibility, relieving many of the business pressures weighing on my father, and two professional managers were hired to run the business.

Luther Hester, who had been brought in to oversee FARM, the forest resource management project, was running the show as President of Nutrilite Products, Inc. (NPI). Fletcher Kettle, another professional manager, who had been brought in to oversee the Nutrilite Foundation, the philanthropic arm of the company, had become the titular President of South Seas Enterprises. While my father remained Chairman of the Board and Edith retained certain responsibilities at NPI, the two managers, who always seemed to be referred to collectively as Hester and Kettle, were in essence running the company.

By 1957, at the age of 70, my father's status had advanced to that of an industrial statesman. As a favor to Charlie Rhyne, whose term as President of the American Bar Association was drawing to an end, my father hosted the dinner before the inaugural session of the American Bar Association. The dinner took place at the luxurious Ambassador Hotel in Los Angeles.

Dad's lifelong interest in China and his newly passionate concerns for the people and the economy of the South Pacific intermingled in this eventful evening. The guests began arriving at the function to find the room decorated as if it were a feast in Tahiti. Handwoven baskets and other gifts from Tahiti were given as gifts to each of the guests. This was the kind of trade my father was trying to encourage to help make the islands self-sufficient.

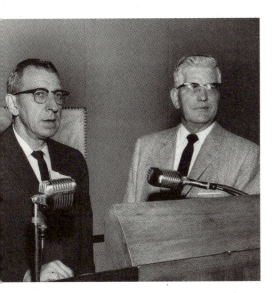

From left to right: Luther Hester and Fletcher Kettle standing in front of a podium, circa 1950s. Hester was the president of NPI and Kettle the president of South Seas Enterprises during the 1950s.

The guests attending the function, who had traveled from all over the world, had never attended anything like it before. Almost all the members of the Supreme Court were there. Solicitor General Lee Rankin was there, along with future Watergate special prosecutor Archie Cox. Charlie Rhyne had also invited Madame Chiang Kai-shek. My father was especially eager to meet her. None of them had ever met my father. Charlie was busy rushing around making sure everything was running smoothly, so he barely had time to check in on my father. He was amazed to find him chatting amiably with these national and world leaders as if he had known them all his life.

Dad had his chance to spend some private time speaking with Madame Chiang Kai-shek, who professed herself profoundly impressed with my father's deep knowledge of

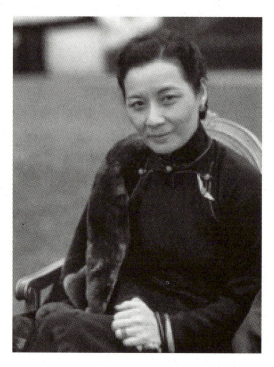

Madame Chiang Kai-shek, 1943.

Chinese culture and fluent command of Mandarin. She later told Charlie that my father was the most fantastic person she had ever encountered.

Meanwhile, other exciting things were happening for the company—one such event was the repackaging of NUTRILITE™ DOUBLE X™ Food Supplement. Hired for the job was Raymond Loewy—the same creative mind responsible for Studebaker's futuristic Avanti sports car and the redesign of the Coke bottle. The butterfly-shaped plastic green package with its two compartments that Loewy designed held the vitamin capsules in one compartment and the mineral tablets in the other and helped to separate Nutrilite further from the competition.

However, during this time while Dad was pursuing his interest in helping to develop the economy of the South Seas and I was at Stanford University, retail sales for NUTRILITE Food Supplement seemed to be slipping. Compared to their peak in 1956, sales were down 20 percent in 1957. The money that my father had anticipated to help build the South Seas projects was beginning to dry up. Something had to be done.

CHAPTER NINETEEN: SOUTH SEAS ADVENTURE

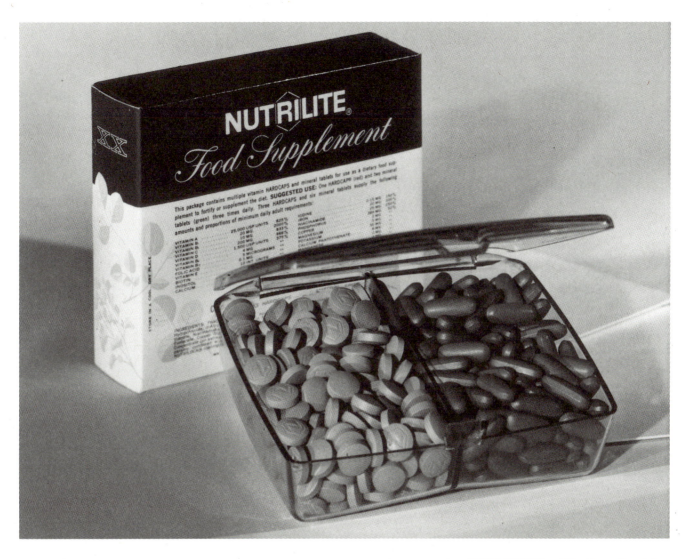

NUTRILITE XX Food Supplement container designed in 1957 by Raymond Loewy. Loewy was the same creative mind behind the redesign of the Coke bottle and Studebaker's futuristic Avanti sports car. The butterfly-shaped, plastic green package with its two compartments to hold the vitamin capsules and mineral tablets helped separate Nutrilite further from the pack of competitors.

> "As one sees a reflection in a polished mirror, so can one know the present by studying the ancient times."
>
> —Chinese Proverb

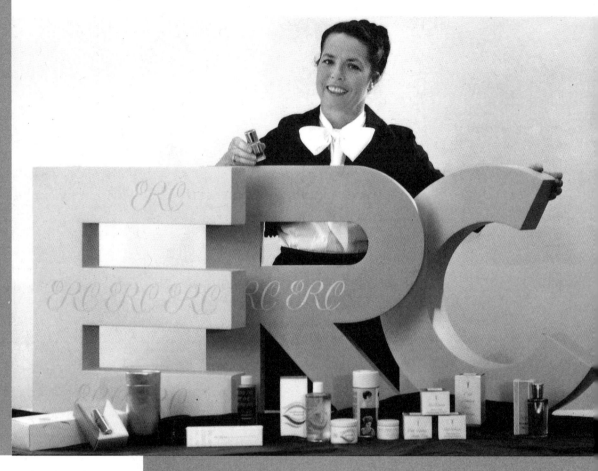

Edith Rehnborg and part of the Edith Rehnborg line of cosmetics, 1958. Facial creams, lotions, shampoos and conditioners, make-up, and perfumes were all part of the Edith Rehnborg Cosmetics line. Introduced in 1958, Edith Rehnborg Cosmetics were formulated blending the finest ingredients from nature and science to produce the most luxurious beauty aids.

Chapter 20 | The Clash over Cosmetics

Basil Fuller was the first distributor to notice it. One year after the unprecedented success of 1956 when sales skyrocketed to well over $28 million, the volume in 1957 didn't seem to be rising so quickly. Something was off and something had to be done immediately to keep sales growing. Lee Mytinger and Bill Casselberry called a Senior Key Conference at the spectacular Fontainebleau Hotel in Miami in 1957 to address the problem.

Basil's suspicions were correct: "Everyone was singing the blues." It became evident that the wrangle with the FDA, although it had ended in victory, had left stress fractures in the organization that were now beginning to open up. Some distributors thought the consent decree with its very specific listing of what claims could be made cramped their style and deprived them of their most powerful sales material: the testimonials. Others thought the prices were too high. There was also a general sense that the sales material from M&C was outdated and no longer appropriate for the situation.

But the real solution to the problem was not just new promotional materials; what was really needed, my father thought, was an additional product line. For some time, he had been preparing lotions and creams based on natural plant concentrates for my mother. A line of such cosmetics, he figured, could capitalize on years of existing research and development and be a logical extension of the nutrition items. And, since cosmetics didn't qualify as food or drugs, they were outside the purview of the FDA. In the spring of 1956, my father informed Lee Mytinger and Bill Casselberry that NPI was planning to develop a line of naturally based cosmetics. The cosmetics would be named (naturally!) after Edith and would be priced competitively.

Mytinger and Casselberry were initially conflicted over the idea of whether to sell cosmetics. Lee Mytinger, the gung-ho salesman, thought it made sense to have a product extension that the salesman on his monthly delivery route could mention to customers. Bill Casselberry, however, was adamantly opposed to the idea, feeling that there should be no dilution of the established NUTRILITE™ fever. Casselberry, however, was eventually brought around to the idea with a bit of persuasion from his son-in-law, Dug Duggan, who pointed out that M&C was like a one-legged stool. "It's alright if we're milking the same cow all the time sitting here," Dug said, "but when we have to keep moving, we've got to have four, three, maybe two spokes down there. We want to have another leg or two." Once convinced, Casselberry decided to get into the act—but rather than supporting the proposed NPI cosmetic line, M&C would create their own.

This decision would have far-reaching implications. As the two companies raced to get their products to market, neither company had any incentive to help the other—or so they thought.

M&C worked with a Detroit consulting firm on a skincare product called Magicare. It would sell for $20. Casselberry was convinced that there was magic to the $20-per-unit formula that made the economics of the distributor chain work.

My father had his own opinions on how to develop the cosmetics. He took a global view of the project. Rather than just come up with yet another set of beauty products, he proposed that NPI scientists begin with extensive research on the history of cosmetics going back to ancient civilizations. He felt that by studying the use of cosmetics over an extended period of time, they would unearth some fundamental ideas which, on examination, would be found to be entirely scientific.

NPI set up a cosmetic division in March 1957. Pete Hazell was hired away from Avon to develop a sales and marketing plan for the distribution of the cosmetics. Maurice Lernoux was lured from Max Factor to develop the cosmetics themselves, and Raymond Loewy, who had contributed the unique butterfly tray for NUTRILITE DOUBLE X™ supplement, signed on to design the packaging.

As the two companies, once inextricably linked, rushed to get out their competing product lines, it naturally created confusion and conflict. What did that exclusivity agreement really mean?

> "When we set out to develop the Edith Rehnborg line of cosmetics we were also developing an idea. First, we were sure cosmetics would open doors for distributors and add to their incomes. Second, was the matching of inner care with food supplements to outer care with cosmetics."
>
> —Carl F. Rehnborg

Would NPI have to sell its cosmetics through M&C? Did M&C have to distribute whatever products NPI came up with? Could NPI sell their cosmetics through their own sales plan? The two engines driving sales—production and marketing—which had worked so beautifully in tandem in the sale of food supplements, now seemed to be pulling in diametrically opposite directions.

M&C felt that NPI couldn't sell Edith Rehnborg Cosmetics. The disagreement, in fact, got so heated that Charlie Rhyne went to court, and in a successful argument in a case before the Federal Trade Commission, argued that distributors should retain the right to sell whatever product they want—otherwise they would be considered employees. The upshot was that it cleared the way for NPI to sell its cosmetics through a separate sales force.

Meanwhile, supplement sales continued to slip. Dug Duggan, from M&C, hired Clair Knox, a retail consultant from Toledo, Ohio to help develop new sales material. Knox was convinced that with the proper tools, NUTRILITE food supplements were not a tough sell. He felt a more positive approach to sales was needed. Knox's project eventually culminated into a new pamphlet called *Food and Your Family* and a very effective set of graphics used to recruit distributors. The material even had the FDA's approval.

Knox also had some other suggestions to make. As he worked on his project to revitalize M&C's sales material, he had quickly noticed a far more serious underlying problem in the management structure: Lee Mytinger and Bill Casselberry were no longer talking with each other. They were communicating through messages carried by their respective secretaries. The face-to-face operations were being carried on by the younger generation of M&C: Bob Mytinger and Dug Duggan. Once having observed this, Knox had some organizational suggestions to make—such as the obvious: if Lee Mytinger and Bill Casselberry were no longer a functional team, why didn't one buy the other out?

NPI's organization didn't have the obvious problems that were handicapping M&C, but still there were obstacles. My father was gone much of the time tending to his dreams for the South Pacific and trying to set up a European and Japanese distribution system. Meanwhile, the two men that he had entrusted to run the company were not necessarily the right ones for the job. Luther Hester had come out of the foundation world, a slower-paced and more predictable environment than that of a fast-growing company. Fletcher Kettle was a strong-willed businessman who seemed to rub people the wrong way.

As sales continued to slip and as the launch dates for the new cosmetic lines drew closer, my father realized he was going to need to position himself more prominently in marketing and renew the personal links with the sales force. In the past decade, he had drifted away from this. After all, his first love was research and manufacturing, and M&C were spectacularly successful at the marketing end. He was also given specific legal advice to do so. The earlier FDA case had been against M&C; NPI was not technically implicated. But legally, Charlie Rhyne felt, it was important to maintain a clear line of demarcation between the organizations.

My father, however, felt the need to re-establish direct links with the distributors. Charlie was skeptical. The FDA would be in the audience taping my father's speech and analyzing it to see if it conformed to the letter of the consent decree. Charlie, however, finally relented and gave Dad his okay. My father was thrilled—he had won over his friend's calculating mind. It was arranged for him to give the keynote address at the upcoming Fiesta de Oro sales rally on May 3, 1958.

When the big day came, my father put on his white dinner jacket and black bow-tie and drove to the Ambassador Hotel in Los Angeles—the same hotel in which he had hosted the American Bar Association dinner only nine months earlier.

Thousands of people came to hear him speak. The crowd filled the immense room that held the function. A series of speakers addressed the crowd that night—Lee Mytinger joked about how sales could grow into the billions and the audience laughed. However, everyone anticipated the moment when my father, the mysterious founder of NPI, would finally stand at the microphone.

At last, he was introduced. As he began, he had trouble making himself heard over the applause filling the room.

Chapter Twenty: The Clash over Cosmetics

"I am rather moved," he said. At emotional moments like this he would often tear up a bit. "It has been a very long time since I have had a chance to talk to a group of Nutrilite distributors. And, as a family man should, I am telling you that I have missed you very much."

The energy in the room was electric as he spoke of his beliefs:

> *"I think what I have missed most is the feeling of warmth between us, because this is not just a group of people thumping the tub to appear enthusiastic, but a group of devoted believers rekindling the fire of conviction and purpose. What we are all doing together, in our distribution of NUTRILITE Food Supplement, is nothing less than a sustained drive to convince every human being who lives, beginning with the persons next to us each day, that health and well-being are not things merely to be regained when lost, but rather gifts to be maintained with all our power, on a regular and constant basis."*

He told the crowd they were:

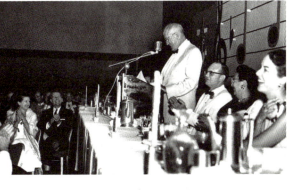

> *"The most beautiful bunch of grocery salesmen in the whole world."*
>
> *NUTRILITE Food Supplement isn't just a "package weighing a few ounces—it is a physical manifestation of a powerful ideal, the conviction that it is truly and really and actually the means by which any person may make his or her adjustment to the conditions of living. It is the instrument by which a person may overcome the nutritional handicaps unwittingly caused by man himself in his choice and use of foods—the substances which, when added to his foods, may provide the things quite possibly missing from his ordinary diet."*

He went on to mention that:

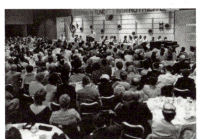

My father speaking at the Fiesta de Oro banquet, May 3, 1958.

> *"Ideals are the only dependable and trustworthy drives for human effort. They are the motive power for all the advances of the human spirit, whether in what are called moral values, or in the arts and sciences, or in government, or in the rearing of our families, or in business!"*
>
> *"I can best drive home the thought that your product is the expression of an ideal,"* he continued. *"I'll try to re-state it in a few words. The reason for our effort is our product, and the reason for our product is the ideal on which it is built. This ideal is of good to the human race ... So let us determine our course and dedicate ourselves to take this message to the world ... let's tell everyone!"*

And take the message to the world, the salesmen did. When it came to the cosmetic line, by the end of 1958, the tally was in—in the form of sales—and Edith Rehnborg Cosmetics was outselling Magicare ... hands down.

However, the existence of two separate cosmetic lines, the rift between NPI and M&C, and the lack of strong, clear direction created morale problems among the distributors. Like children being faced with the likelihood of their parents' divorce, all felt uncomfortable being forced to choose between the two cosmetic lines. Some distributors, like Jay Van Andel and Rich DeVos, chose both.

Whether because of the stress of the business or some other factor, my father had a stroke two months after the Fiesta de Oro Sales Rally, while on a return flight from Hawaii. He had fallen asleep with his head on his shoulder. When he woke up, he couldn't move and had to be carried off the plane. He experienced a slight slurring of speech, which quickly corrected itself. There was no serious impairment, just a slight shuffle when he walked, which was not so unusual for a man in his early 70s. Most people wouldn't even notice it, but it was an intimation of mortality in an active man whose last serious illness had been 40 years earlier during the influenza epidemic of 1918.

For the people charged with looking after NPI, particularly Luther Hester and Fletcher Kettle, my father's stroke, combined with his absence while traveling and his various intellectual and entrepreneurial pursuits, presented them with an unsettling combination of insecurity and opportunity. Were the Founder and Chairman of NPI to die suddenly or be permanently disabled, what would happen to the direction of the company? Would NPI without its inventor, the embodiment of the organization, wither away or be swallowed up by another company such as M&C, taking jobs like Hester's and Kettle's with it?

Neither Luther Hester nor Fletcher Kettle had any sort of personal history with Lee Mytinger or Bill Casselberry. To them, M&C was mainly a paper organization taking an extremely large share of income for distributing NUTRILITE food supplements and now competing with Edith Rehnborg Cosmetics.

Hester and Kettle felt that NPI could get along fine without M&C. As they saw it, there were difficulties with M&C—such as the problems that had developed with the Sales Plan. The biggest one, which hadn't escaped the notice of the Federal Trade Commission, was that the company had thousands of distributors. And, once they signed up, distributors

Chapter Twenty: The Clash over Cosmetics

retained their status for life—regardless of performance. To measure performance and increase revenue, M&C decided to institute a 50-cent charge for every new customer. The new policy proved to be a disaster. Distributors threatened to revolt, which further intensified the existing disagreement between Mytinger and Casselberry.

NPI had already developed its own roster of distributors to sell the Edith Rehnborg Cosmetic line, which was independent of the previous M&C contract. Why not take it a step further, bringing the food supplements and cosmetics under the same umbrella?

So Hester and Kettle, feeling that they were now in charge of NPI's future, decided to make their own "declaration of independence." On March 23, 1959, they placed a full-page ad in *The Wall Street Journal* announcing that M&C was no longer the distributor of NUTRILITE Food Supplement. Anyone wanting to sell the vitamin products, let alone the cosmetics, would have to sign up with NPI. Like the original, this "declaration of independence" was also a declaration of war.

M&C obtained a restraining order and the ad never ran again, but the damage was done. The damage to the sales force was unprecedented, but the real verdict was in the bottom line. By 1959, sales for food supplements had dropped by more than half compared to their peak in 1956.

Earlier, at the 1958 Senior Key Conference on Mackinac Island, the Study Group had elected Jay Van Andel as chairman. He spent a lot of time at NPI, apparently at my father's request, trying to find ways to promote the products and settle disagreements between NPI and M&C. My father liked Jay's energy and had offered him the position of general manager. Jay turned him down, partly because it didn't come with control of the company and partly because it didn't include his partner Rich DeVos. Jay preferred to go back to Michigan and take his chances with another plan that was beginning to form in the back of his mind.

Total Retail Sales of NPI's Products

Year	NFS	ERC
1955	$27,241,000	NA
1956	$28,563,000	NA
1957	$22,848,000	NA
1958	$23,414,000	$1,566,000
1959	$11,893,000	$6,638,000

NPI denotes Nutrilite Products, Inc.; NFS, NUTRILITE Food Supplement; ERC, Edith Rehnborg Cosmetics; and NA, not applicable.

"I believe that one of the most powerful forces in the world today is the will of people who believe in themselves, who dare to aim high, to go confidently after the things that they want from life."

—Rich DeVos

Chapter 21 | Amway

Jay Van Andel and Rich DeVos had been finding it difficult to keep up their momentum. NUTRILITE™ Food Supplement had never been an easy sell for them—they figured each initial sale required a one-hour presentation. Besides, it was costly, and much of their management time was devoted to thinking up new ways to justify the price. My father had agreed with their position and liked the momentum and energy of this young team. But his hands were tied.

In fact, everybody's hands were tied. Following the skirmish over cosmetics, things seemed to settle into a siege mentality. Lee Mytinger and Bill Casselberry held each other at a standoff. Mytinger & Casselberry, Inc. held Nutrilite Products, Inc. at a standoff. Nobody seemed to be able to move. Sales continued to plummet. Clearly, something or someone would have to give. But who would crack first?

As the stalemate dragged on and Jay's summer of attempted mediation between my father, Mytinger, and Casselberry came to nothing, Jay became concerned about the supply of product. By this time, Jay and his partner Rich had built the Ja-Ri Corporation into one of the largest distributor organizations in the country—selling and distributing NUTRILITE products. As heads of their own company with their own distributors to supply and support, they would have a lot to lose should M&C and NPI go belly-up. Jay realized that he would have to break his own way out of the stalemate.

From the start, Jay had been one of those arguing for the need of a more diverse product line that was more competitively priced. Now, an opportunity had arisen with the stalemate between the companies. Jay and Rich developed a plan to keep up sales momentum for their organization. As early as a 1957 Key Distributors Conference, Jay informed Chicago Key Agent Basil Fuller that he and Rich had put out word to their top sellers to find a suitable product to sell on their own—and they would do it through a new company. The key criteria for the new product was that it had to be one that just about anyone would be familiar with and could sell.

Soon a product was found that they thought might drive sales: a concentrated liquid soap called *Frisk* that contained no phosphates and was biodegradable. There was an aspect to the product, which would be later renamed L.O.C.™, or Liquid Organic Cleaner, that was intriguing: its lack of impact on the environment. In recent years, those strolling along lakesides and seashores had noticed the white foam or "head" that seemed to linger on some beaches, a bubbly froth that many experts attributed to the widespread use of household detergents. As ecological awareness began to grow in the late 1950s, Jay and Rich figured *Frisk* might just catch on. And, like NUTRILITE Food Supplement, it was "concentrated."

One month after the infamous ad in *The Wall Street Journal* stating that M&C would no longer distribute NUTRILITE Food Supplement, the new sales venture called "the American Way Association" and later named Amway began in Jay's basement.

Jay and Rich had kept the other key agents in the Study Group informed. Most of the key agents were skeptical. NUTRILITE Food Supplement wasn't only a product, but a regimen, to which customers committed themselves as a safeguard to their personal health and well-being. The incentive for regular use and repeat purchase was built into the product. But who would commit themselves to faithful use of a particular kind of household soap? Many of the key agents were dubious. "Good luck, boys," Rick Rickenbrode said. He didn't believe they could make it happen.

The tension was palpable as the various players assembled for the Senior Key Study Group held in 1959 at stunning Lake Louise in the Canadian Rockies. The hotel looked out on a mirror-like lake that reflected the snow-capped mountains and thick glacier at the other end of a small valley. It was a restful setting, but not restful enough to disperse the anxiety in the air.

For one thing, the question of who should distribute Edith Rehnborg Cosmetics or even NUTRILITE food supplements had not been resolved. For another thing, the strain between Mytinger and Casselberry was so great that people were beginning to speculate which of the partners would be the first to quit.

Chapter Twenty One: Amway

This year, for the first time, the meeting had been extended to include others outside of the core study group—people like Neil Maaskant, Jay and Rich's sponsor. Lee Mytinger and Bill Casselberry were both there, along with Dug Duggan and Bob Mytinger from the M&C team. Luther Hester and Fletcher Kettle were there from the NPI team, along with Pete Hazell, the marketing consultant for the Edith Rehnborg Cosmetics line, who would unveil NPI's new sales plan.

Marty Loos was one of the key agents at the meeting as well. He was happy to have a free trip up to Lake Louise with Dottie. He knew that Rich DeVos and Jay Van Andel were selling other products. However, he had an inkling that something else was up when they pulled him and Dottie aside. He was right. One or two of Marty's successful distributors had forced their way into the Ja-Ri organization and were now selling the new soap product. Legally, Jay or Rich couldn't get them out. Marty was furious. He never wanted to talk to them again.

At the meeting later in the day, Basil Fuller noticed Bill Casselberry writing a note on the back of an envelope and handing it to Lee Mytinger. Mytinger shoved it in his pocket to read later. When he did, he told Basil that Casselberry had offered to be bought out. The distributors were stopped in their tracks. What would happen next?

With the question electric in the room, Pete Hazell proceeded to outline NPI's new sales plan. The chief difference in it had to do with the bonus plan. It was significantly different than that used by M&C—with the top of the new plan calling for only $2,500 as opposed to $7,500 in bonuses.

The NPI management team at the meeting thought the plan was wonderful because it prevented top leaders from profiting on the work of their downlines without actually having to sell the product themselves. However, a cloud began to form over the distributors the way a vicious weather front suddenly could move in over the Rockies. You didn't want to be out blazing new trails in weather like that.

As the plan unfolded, Luther Hester asked for questions. At first, distributors were quiet, cautious, and polite. Except for the members of the Study Group, the other distributors weren't used to giving feedback in the meetings. Rick Rickenbrode broke the silence: "I don't think much of it." One by one, the senior key distributors all joined in, their comments becoming bolder and more critical. Even gracious Basil said, "It's a lousy program you're offering us." When the time came for Jay to give his response, he said, "Well, if that's what you're going to do, you can forget about us. We're through!"

Jay and Rich tried to be as gentle and fair as possible. They continued to sell NUTRILITE Food Supplement, and they vowed not to recruit distributors from outside their own line, but conflicts inevitably arose, causing a serious breach between themselves and NPI. Even without some poaching, NPI had lost more than half of its Midwestern sales force.

Jay and Rich were able to utilize what had worked well in M&C's sales plan and eliminate what didn't. They tweaked it to include a system of annual renewal and instituted a service charge on orders. The Amway Plan was more efficient economically. By taking onboard what was effective and scuttling what was not, Amway began to grow dramatically, adding new products and new distributors, continually re-energizing the business.

Jay and Rich had also learned from the mistakes of the past. They had seen firsthand the dangers that could arise if a conflict would occur between them. As smart businessmen, they found a way to prevent themselves from taking the stress out on each other or on their families. It was in the form of Clair Knox—the man who had helped orchestrate the new sales materials for M&C, and the same man who had made management recommendations to M&C.

Knox was a man, they realized, who would be able to stand up to them no matter how hard they fought back, no matter how much they disagreed with each other on a particular day. Jay and Rich didn't want there to come a day when they would communicate to each other only through notes from their secretaries. Knox's job would be to keep that from ever happening.

With energy, a strong new product line, and a tight partnership, Amway took off. In 1960, Amway's total sales would reach $7 million, about half of the total sales of NUTRILITE Food Supplement and Edith Rehnborg Cosmetics combined. As Amway continued to expand their product line with items that were easier to sell than food supplements and cosmetics, more and more Nutrilite distributors would abandon the mother firm for the upstart.

CHAPTER TWENTY ONE: AMWAY

> "We are just now as a company in a tough bind, but this is strictly an invitation to grow and not an occasion for despair or fear."
>
> —Carl F. Rehnborg

Chapter 22 | Weathering the Storm

Back at Nutrilite, the events of that Lake Louise conference precipitated a crisis that plunged the company into its darkest years. In one blow, the Mytinger & Casselberry empire had caved in. Even under the best of circumstances, the demise of a 15-year-old, phenomenally successful marketing flank would take some delicate transition as the new players got used to each other. This was a far cry from the best of circumstances; in fact, it was just about the worst: M&C was in collapse, the distributors were confused, and there was an aggressive new competitor in the field.

My father had been caught off guard. Preoccupied with his other, more globally and philanthropically oriented projects and serenely confident that NPI would keep growing at its phenomenal rate, he had turned too much of the managerial operations over to Luther Hester and Fletcher Kettle, who had told him what he wanted to hear. Now their managerial ineptitude had betrayed itself: first in the gaffe of *The Wall Street Journal* ad, and then with the new sales plan, which had badly alienated both M&C and the distributor force. The distributors, even the loyal ones, were badly shaken. The whole organization needed to be rebuilt, almost from the ground up.

It couldn't have come at a worse time for Nutrilite. The company was in the midst of a rapid expansion of the facilities in preparation for a project that was the fulfillment of one of my father's deepest dreams: to build a world-class nutrition laboratory at NPI.

During 1958 and 1959, while the battle lines were tightening between NPI and M&C, my father had been involved in a series of exchanges with Dr. Thomas Jukes, the distinguished biochemist he had met four years earlier through George Merck and the plankton project. In a flurry of visits and correspondence, it appeared that Dr. Jukes could be lured away from academia to head up a vastly expanded research laboratory.

Dr. Jukes was the chairman of the Committee on Fellows of the American Institute of Nutrition. The fellows program had recently been established, and awards were given to members of the institute over 65 years of age who had distinguished careers in nutrition.

The founding batch of fellows included such dignitaries as Elmer McCollum (who discovered vitamin A), Roger Williams (who coined the word "nutrilites"), and Casimir Funk (who coined the word "vitamine"). Jukes led the group that picked them, so it was an enormous vote of confidence in the legitimacy of my father's dream for Jukes to want to join the NPI team.

Together, Dad and Dr. Jukes worked out the specifics for the research laboratory. Dr. Jukes had suggested a budget of $700,000—approximately 7 percent of NPI's projected sales for 1959. They figured the research laboratory would include a staff of 35 to 40 people, including a stable of the brightest researchers heading up studies in animal nutrition, microbiology, physiology, experimental pathology, organic chemistry, biochemistry, enzyme chemistry, pharmacology, and toxicology. The new laboratory would be cutting edge not only in equipment, but also in design. No longer would applied research be carried out exclusively within academia, but rather in the field itself. There would be immediate possibilities for the implementation of discoveries made. The research lab would be home to a group of scientists who would follow a less formal, more free-ranging, and more fundamental approach to new knowledge. It was an idea my father had seen modeled by his friend and mentor George Merck. Merck's unexpected death in 1957 left my father more resolved than ever to develop the model.

There was a second profound benefit for my father in the research lab as well: scientific legitimacy for both himself and his product, and an additional anchor to windward against his old foes in the FDA who still doubted the legitimacy of his product and the validity of the research on the associated food factors that supported it.

For Dr. Jukes, it was a big move to leave the safety net of academia to try his lot with a daring vitamin company. The appeal to him, aside from the personal respect between himself and my father, was the freedom to design and run a state-of-the-art laboratory facility with both intellectual freedom and adequate funding. He checked and queried several times: "Can we safely assume that the increase in sales in 1959 and 1960 will be

Did You Know

... Dr. Jukes discovered that two B-vitamins, riboflavin and pantothenic acid, promoted the growth of chicks? He also helped develop a method for the synthesis of pantothenic acid that was used by manufacturers.

sufficient to support a research program of the size I propose?" Luther Hester, NPI's president, assured him that it would.

A tentative organizational chart for the department and a wish list for the first three department heads were put together. The men who were recruited were real powerhouses in the nutritional field. Dr. Jukes had no names to suggest for the rest of the departments other than the type of scientist he was looking for: young, creative, original thinkers.

Dr. Jukes arrived at NPI in June 1959, just shortly after the unruly Lake Louise meeting. Two weeks after his arrival, he gave a press conference and spoke about a new technology that NPI was working on to create a biological pest control that worked without developing resistance in insects in ways such chemicals as DDT did.

Things looked bright for the company—at least from the outside. A writer from *Medical Economics*, a magazine from the publisher of the esteemed *Physicians' Desk Reference*, met my father for an interview in the summer of 1959.

Lois Chevalier had done her research and knew about NPI and its struggles with the FDA, and was primed to expect the worst: fast-talking, hard-sell salesman pushing something people didn't need. She met my father and was immediately struck by his eyes. "Bright-eyed," was how she described him, "a vibrantly healthy man of advanced years." She had no idea that he had suffered a stroke the year before.

She was impressed by NPI's $300,000 research program, sophisticated scientific equipment, and "a staff of Ph.D. chemists doing experiments in the spotless laboratory." The photographer that accompanied her took a picture of one of the scientists standing by the expensive new spectrophotometer. The scientist told Chevalier about the research taking place—research attempting

Did You Know

… NPI developed the first biological pest control in the marketplace? The first version of BIOTROL was registered for use in 1960.

In the late 1950s, the Mexican spotted aphid had begun rampaging through the alfalfa fields. My father knew that chemical insecticides could not be used, that they would contaminate the alfalfa concentrates and possibly be harmful to humans. He had his researchers at NPI contact scientists at the University of California, Riverside to help find a solution to the dilemma.

The scientists combed the fields in search of dead aphids. Dad described their efforts. "It is very much like looking for a needle in a haystack, but they found dead aphids which had curled up their toes and quit for unknown reasons."

The scientists dried and powdered the dead insects, and scattered the powder onto petri dishes, one insect to a dish. They tested the resulting cultures on living insects. One earlier aphid had been covered with fuzz from mold. The test insects that were exposed to the powder from this earlier aphid died very quickly and were covered by the same mold. The researchers thought that the spores from the mold might be an effective solution to their aphid problem, so they brewed up hundreds of pounds of the fungus material and sprayed it onto fields infested with spotted aphids. It took longer than chemicals to kill the aphids, but they all died, and they didn't come back. The aphids also did not develop a tolerance for the fungal control either, as they often did for chemical insecticides. In addition to that, it was totally harmless. My dad was intrigued with this and recognized there might be a commercial product in this method of insect control. He quickly realized that the fungal material had no economic potential out in the marketplace, as the spotted aphid wasn't that big of an insect pest, but on further discussions with the scientists at the University of California, they recommended that he investigate a way to produce commercially a bacteria called *Bacillus thuringiensis* that was a very effective control of caterpillars of various kinds that were infesting vegetable crops all over the state of California. When chemicals were used, it often led to a buildup of chemical insecticides on the crops, which could be harmful to people.

My father hired entomologists, biologists, and fermentation experts to figure out the best way to produce a commercial product from this material. It took a long time and more than a million dollars to prove that it worked and that it was safe for humans. NPI ended up with the first pesticide petition for a natural insect control agent, *Bacillus thuringiensis*. The commercial name was BIOTROL.

Chapter Twenty Two: Weathering the Storm

to establish that the NUTRILITE™ concentrate increased an organism's resistance to stress.

My father told Chevalier about the alfalfa, watercress, parsley, and yeast that went into the concentrate. She tried to get him to tell her more about the concentrate, but he said that it was a trade secret. He told her that he had started out making it by hand almost 30 years earlier. "That was about the time they had just begun to make vitamins in crystalline form," he said.

Chevalier asked about the problems with distributors making false claims about curing diseases, causing problems with the FDA. "We're totally in favor of what the FDA stands for," he told her. "The distributors are forbidden to make such claims. We don't want them to be amateur doctors. They're supposed to be grocery salesmen." He gave her a copy of the sales manual, so she could see how they were trained to sell food supplements. She flipped through it and noted that it had a counter for "every possible form of sales resistance—without naming a single disease." It didn't seem unreasonable to her that distributors were able to tell customers what government publications said about nutrition in general, or to explain the importance of specific vitamins.

As the trio toured the facility, the photographer wanted to get a shot that captured my father's spirit. When he showed them his pride and joy, a gull-winged Mercedes, the

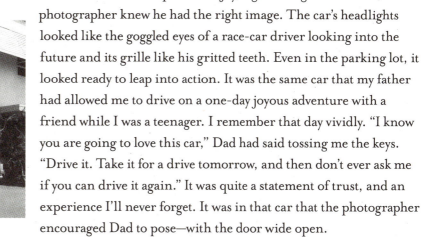

Dad posing by his Mercedes, 1959.

photographer knew he had the right image. The car's headlights looked like the goggled eyes of a race-car driver looking into the future and its grille like his gritted teeth. Even in the parking lot, it looked ready to leap into action. It was the same car that my father had allowed me to drive on a one-day joyous adventure with a friend while I was a teenager. I remember that day vividly. "I know you are going to love this car," Dad had said tossing me the keys. "Drive it. Take it for a drive tomorrow, and then don't ever ask me if you can drive it again." It was quite a statement of trust, and an experience I'll never forget. It was in that car that the photographer encouraged Dad to pose—with the door wide open.

While they were chatting, he explained that although he had developed the original concentration process, he wasn't a scientist so much as a "self-educated chemist." He also explained some of the new things that were exciting him. Chevalier wrote in her notes about his "hotel chain in the South Sea Islands," and his "new process for extracting coconut oil that he hopes will bring prosperity to Tahiti."

While things looked bright for NPI, the company continued to struggle. The feud between NPI and M&C over cosmetics had left distributors feeling confused, and the new sales plan that NPI introduced had alienated many of them. The conflict was eating away at the sales field. Meanwhile, Rich DeVos and Jay Van Andel were busy growing Amway, and distributors in their organization felt isolated from the discord between NPI and M&C while simultaneously offering a product that was easier to sell.

Also unsettling were some of the dynamics occurring within NPI, forcing my father to step in and take control. While my father was pursuing interests abroad, he had put too much faith in the hands of Luther Hester and Fletcher Kettle only to find that the men were planning to take over NPI. By using their influence with the Nutrilite Foundation Board, the two had hoped to vote my father out of the company. When my father got word of this in August 1959, he fired both of the men.

Dr. Thomas Jukes also left within the month. The collapse in sales cut the ground out from under his plans. He also had some fundamental disagreements with my father—questioning the use of natural plant concentrates and the associated food factors found within. According to a memo written by my father to Dr. Jukes on August 5, 1959:

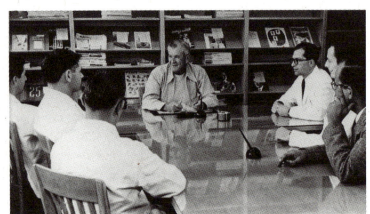

My father with researchers in NPI's library. Staff research and development meetings were held frequently in the company's library, which was considered one of the finest technical libraries in the area.

> *You are proposing that we say that the vitamins that can be synthesized in the laboratory are all there are; and, finally and definitely, they are all that mean anything in nutrition. Whether I am scientific or not, I do not believe this, and neither do our customers, and neither does the world; and I do not think that we are in any way required to make such an idea the exclusive basis for what we offer for sale.*

Dr. Jukes returned quietly and seamlessly back to academia. A colleague Dr. Jukes had brought with him summed it up: "Tom Jukes and I [were] catastrophic in California!"

CHAPTER TWENTY TWO: WEATHERING THE STORM

It was a bitter blow for my father. He had lost a set of eminent research scientists, a huge number of distributors, and over half the company's sales in a slide that appeared to have no end. The rift with M&C and the white-knuckle drama of the past year had taken its toll on him as well. About one year after the shakeup in executive staff, he had suffered a second stroke. While he recovered nearly fully once again, it was a reminder that his time to accomplish his dreams was finite. So was his energy.

This stressful time for my father also turned out to be a rather difficult time for me. After three years together, Gay and I decided that our marriage couldn't last. We were just too young. However, we were intent to remain friends. This was especially important because during our time together we had a beautiful baby daughter named Lisa and neither of us wanted Lisa to suffer from our decision.

By this time, I had received my bachelor's degree from Stanford University in chemical engineering. Although my father was under severe business pressure and could have used my help, he encouraged me to stay in school and persist in acquiring the full academic credential he lacked. I had toyed with the idea of going to business school or even into the Underwater Demolition Team (the precursor to the current Navy SEALS). My father's advice to me was, "Son, go on and get your doctorate, go and get your advanced degree in science, that will be the thing that will be the greatest help to us in the future." And so in the fall of 1958, I entered Stanford's graduate program in biochemistry.

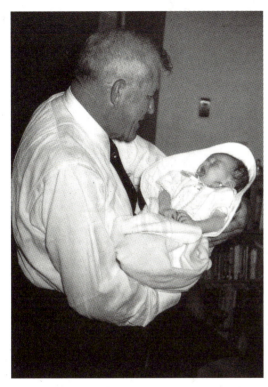

My father and two-week-old granddaughter Lisa, 1957. Throughout his life, he would augment her education.

Emergency Measures

When the dust had cleared from the purge of 1959, Dr. Stefan Tenkoff was left at the helm of NPI. As it turned out, there probably couldn't have been a better person. Steady, experienced, and deeply loyal to my father, he steered the only course possible to carry Nutrilite through a storm that might otherwise have sunk it.

Once Hester and Kettle were gone, the extent of the problems became clear. It was worse than anyone had imagined. Dr. Tenkoff discovered that NPI had no cash to pay its suppliers. Even after convincing the suppliers to accept payment after 90 days, he had no idea how to cover payroll. He thought the research expenses were too high for a company that couldn't even pay its employees. The company was geared up for success, pumping out products that weren't being sold. Inventories were piling up. The farm was expensive to operate and the new, improved soft-gel capsules were melting in the trunks of distributors' cars in the August heat. In addition, NPI was borrowing heavily to pay its expenses and, at the same time, lending money to South Sea Enterprises. The company was in hock to the tune of $2.25 million—almost $13 million in 2009 dollars.

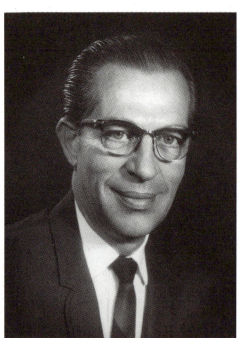

Stefan Tenkoff, Ph.D., 1960. NPI's president from 1962 to 1972.

It seemed simple to Dr. Tenkoff: the company had to live within its means. It was essential to get back to basics—even if that meant operating the same way as it had over 10 years earlier, when sales were at about the same level. Whether he wanted to or not, Dr. Tenkoff set out to undo the work of Luther Hester and Fletcher Kettle—and the bank was doing everything it could to make him want to. The vice president and branch manager along with two representatives from the bank's headquarters came over to NPI to review Dr. Tenkoff's actions. If things didn't shape up quickly, my father could lose his company. Dr. Tenkoff gave the bankers a schedule promising that the debts would be paid off within 24 months.

Dr. Tenkoff had to lay off 200 employees—the first layoffs in the company's history. He shut down production for three out of four weeks in order to allow the stocked inventory to sell. He shut down the acerola operation in Hawaii. He helped wrap up business in the South Pacific. The hotel Les Tropiques stayed in business for a while, but unfortunately the expanded project my father visualized never materialized due to the lack of agreement between American investors and the French governmental agencies involved. My father eventually instructed Dr. Tenkoff to sell off all the South Pacific assets, except Moorea. Dr. Tenkoff also put the research programs on hold, except for the development of a microbiological control of insect pests. Dr. Tenkoff also established a contract manufacturing arm of the business that could manufacture materials for other companies. Humbling in a way, but it helped turn the corner.

CHAPTER TWENTY TWO: WEATHERING THE STORM

The End of an Era

Dr. Tenkoff's close-to-the-wire measures returned a stability of sorts. With careful management, he was actually able to pay off the loans as promised. But it didn't turn sales around. Sales continued to plummet and Amway continued to grow. At a 1962 "Pow Wow," Basil Fuller noticed some of his distributors wearing their Amway pins instead of their Nutrilite key pins. It was a vivid symbol.

The problem, clearly, was in the marketing end. If NPI had been left in disarray, it had been worse for Mytinger Corporation, which had arisen out of M&C's ashes and had become incorporated on February 2, 1960. Out of the four men who had run M&C, only one, Dug Duggan, was really a businessman. He was now gone, along with Bill Casselberry who cashed out his profit-sharing and retired to Santa Barbara. Now without the savvy input from these men, the corporation was increasingly adrift in the changing marketing climate of the '60s and seemed to have ground completely to a halt. The morale problem at Mytinger Corporation was affecting the field. One of Mytinger's employees told Basil Fuller that she went into the conference room and saw Bob Mytinger's secretary cutting out a dress pattern on the conference room table. "Does that tell you something?" asked Basil.

He drove up to Nutrilite to meet with Dr. Tenkoff. "It's pretty sad over there at Mytinger Corporation," he said.

Dr. Tenkoff decided the time had come to buy out Mytinger Corporation. Lee Mytinger put up stiff resistance, but the longer he fought, the weaker his position became as sales continued to fall. In the troubled year of 1959, retail sales of NUTRILITE Food Supplement was almost $12 million; Edith Rehnborg Cosmetics added $6.6 million. The next year, sales dropped to less than $10 million for NUTRILITE Food Supplement and less than $5 million for Edith Rehnborg Cosmetics. Sales fell another 20 percent in 1962 and were on track to bottom out in 1963 at around $8 million—total. After four years under Lee and Bob Mytinger, total sales had dropped by 60 percent. My father couldn't stand the idea that the exclusive contract with Mytinger Corporation was actively preventing NPI from recovering.

Dr. Tenkoff said to my father, "Look, Mr. Rehnborg. I'll handle it. I'll get the deal." And he did: for the remarkably cheap price of $800,000. My father was at first upset that the deal was only for the distributor organization and inventory and it didn't include the building or equipment. He nearly refused to sign. But Dr. Tenkoff was convinced that only the distributor organization was needed and patiently talked my father into signing the contract.

On May 1, 1963, after nearly 20 years in association with first M&C and then the Mytinger Corporation, things were again, finally, under one roof at NPI. The buyout of Mytinger Corporation would turn out to be the key to putting sales growth back on track. With the buyout, some highly capable people, people like Barney Bailey, Ruth Dye, Dick Kline, and Cliff Claus, who had worked for Mytinger Corporation, would come over and run the sales and legal side at NPI. The storm had been weathered. Nutrilite survived, battered, but intact.

Total Retail Sales of NPI's Products

Year	NFS	ERC
1960	$9,657,000	$4,831,000
1961	$7,611,000	$3,894,000
1962	$6,580,000	$3,575,000
1963	$5,436,000	$2,901,000

NPI denotes Nutrilite Products, Inc.; NFS, NUTRILITE Food Supplement; and ERC, Edith Rehnborg Cosmetics.

"*After a storm, a rainbow.*"

—Anonymous

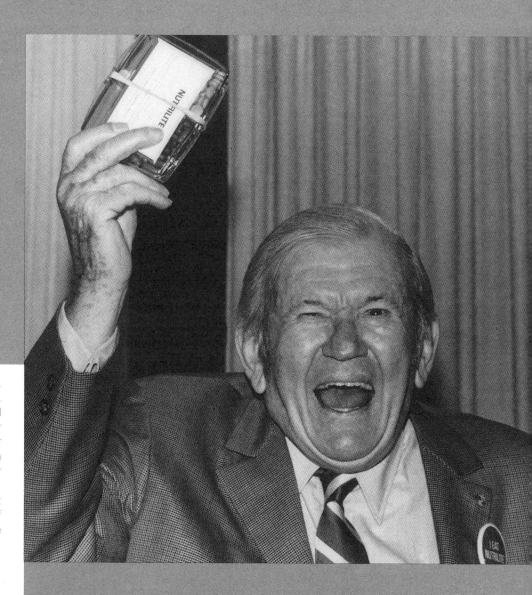

My father at a Nutrilite convention, circa 1965. At these conventions, distributors and staff members could challenge one another to show their pocket carriers of food supplement or take a mock 'penalty.' At this Fiesta in Los Angeles, I challenged my father in front of the ballroom audience, whereupon he whipped out his 'pocket carrier'—a whole container of NUTRILITE Food Supplement—to the delighted cheers of all present.

Chapter 23 | Passing the Torch

There were many changes taking place at Nutrilite in 1964 as the company once again took sales and distribution under its wing. Besides food supplements and cosmetics, the company had also diversified into other product lines, such as household products that helped lend greater stability to the company.

My father spoke with distributors about the changes taking place as a result of the purchase of Mytinger Corporation. At the Fiesta de Oro Convention in Los Angeles, California, on June 20, 1964, he explained to the gathered crowd of distributors:

> *Business like all living things, grows by surges. Our business has just reached the point for a vast movement forward. It is now a big little company. In a few months it will become a little big company, and in the course of a very few years will become a big, big company…*
>
> *For me, who has seen our company grow, this is a grand sight. I know absolutely that even greater growth is in the immediate future, and I know equally surely that the advance will come by means of the same, simple procedures that meant your greatest advances in the past—to sell by pursuing the 'soft sell,' with truth and sincerity the guiding principles. I wish you well, and I am cheering you on.*

My father had worked hard his entire professional life and enjoyed every minute of it—the thrill of knowledge, discovery, and invention, and working toward his goal of making a difference in people's lives all over the world. However, while in his 70s he realized that the time would soon come for him to retire from public life.

While my father was in Tahiti and I was in graduate school, I had written him a letter expressing my desire to play an active role in NPI's future to help him carry out his plans as he intended. My father dashed back a response:

Your letter made me feel a surge of tenderness and affection and of pride that destiny has treated me so well. Your paragraph about business and the future, and our own sort of relay race in which one generation passes the torch to the next, meant more to me than you could have imagined, aside from meeting a man I have so far known as a youth, who was my very satisfactory son.

By 1964, I had the academic credentials to help lead the company, thanks to my father's continual guidance and some fortuitous advice from Dr. Thomas Jukes, NPI's former vice president of R&D. After graduating with my bachelor's degree in chemical engineering from Stanford University in 1958, I had gone on to their graduate program in biochemistry and had the opportunity to study on the molecular structure and activity of tobacco mosaic virus (TMV). However, after one year of graduate work, I found the results of my research were at odds with what my advisor had theorized. I just couldn't commit to publishing what he wanted me to publish. I explained my dilemma to Dr. Jukes and it was through one of his contacts that I found out about the biophysics graduate program at the University of California, Berkeley. I applied to the program and was accepted.

It turned out to be the best time of my academic life. I found myself on the frontier of a new field of research—lipoprotein metabolism. John Gofman, a respected medical physics professor at UC Berkeley, was the first investigator to identify the blood levels of HDL- and LDL-lipoproteins—the so-called "good" and "bad" cholesterol, respectively—as risk factors for heart disease. Alex Nichols was his top investigator, and I worked closely with Alex. We focused on trying to understand the physics, physiology, and biophysics of heart disease. We worked exceedingly hard, but it wasn't the grind I had heard from others who had gone to graduate school. Alex and I worked 10 to 12 hours a day, but every day we would take a break, go down to the gym and work out for an hour, swim, or play volleyball, and then go to the cafeteria and eat, talk about the research projects, and come back and work. At dawn on Thursdays, we would go over to Tilden Park to play 18 holes of golf with another couple of scientists. We would work on Saturday, Sunday, whatever it took to bring a project to completion. I loved every second of it.

It was while I was working toward my graduate degree that I reconnected with Joan Balling, a former Stanford student (and song girl) I had met earlier while attending Stanford. She was teaching third grade in the East Bay community of Orinda. We were married

Chapter Twenty Three: Passing the Torch

in July 1961 and moved into a weathered apartment with sagging floors, in Berkeley. Although we didn't have lots of money, we had enough to get by thanks to Joni's teaching salary and my earnings as a teaching assistant during the academic year and a research fellowship during the summer. We could even afford to take some ski trips now and then. It was a happy time for us. She was a great supporter of my efforts and a major stabilizing voice in my life.

In January 1964, I received my doctorate in biophysics. However, before I started work at NPI, Joni and I wanted to fulfill one of our dreams. We wanted to see more of the world. During that time, there was an unofficial tradition among American college graduates that reached its peak during the interval between the end of the Korean War and American involvement in Vietnam. Taking advantage of a combination of factors—such as a strong dollar and a favorable exchange rate—young men who had completed their graduate work or military service took off with their wives and knocked around Europe for months, sometimes as long as a year, before returning to accept family and career responsibilities. Those journeys, often made by beat-up truck, motorcycle, or hitch-hiking between youth hostels, campgrounds, and bottom-rate pensiones, were an American counterpart to the German student tradition of wanderjahr, the year of travel, a hiatus of relief and fresh experience.

I had attended rigorous schools for more than 20 years, had published eight academic papers, and completed my Ph.D. dissertation. The prospect of an American wanderjahr had been a sustaining ambition, a longstanding dream of coming-up-for-air before plunging into the prospects at NPI. A pair of my college fraternity brothers, Tom Kemp and Tony Serra, fresh out of law school, had journeyed with their wives in a beat-up Land Rover jeep from Portugal to India, a trip whose most enduring memory had been 102 flat tires. Another fraternity brother, Lloyd Kahn, a former Air Force officer, had puttered through Western Europe with his wife, on a Vespa motor scooter. Every postcard was like a reminder that Joni and I could be doing this, too. Even my father had taken his trip around the world, not to mention all that time in China and the South Pacific, and had brought back a wealth of experience and new-found wisdom. Despite the struggles at NPI, we were having a hard time staying put.

An accident decided it. Joni and I were at the Bing Crosby Golf Tournament at Pebble Beach in 1963, when our car was hit head-on by a drunk Army sergeant stationed at Fort Ord. The impact sent Joni flying head-first into the windshield. She was almost killed. Her injuries were serious enough that she won a $5,000 settlement against the drunk driver, although she completely recovered. It was a substantial windfall for two people who had been supporting themselves by teaching—enough to cover a year of travel. At a deeper level it was a *memento mori*, a reminder that we all must die.

We left in January of 1964 on our round-the-world tour. We bought a Volkswagen microbus and drove all over Europe, with two months of skiing at the outset with another fraternity brother, Charlie Savio. We bought round-the-world air tickets, $1,100 each with stops at 42 cities. We made it all the way to Tahiti. By that time, Les Tropiques, my father's fabulous hotel resort, had become not much more than a bar overlooking the runway at the new airport. It was still popular, but decaying, the way buildings do in the tropics when they aren't cared for particularly well.

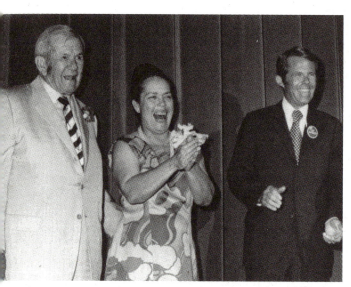

My parents and me at a Nutrilite function, circa 1965.

It was an idyllic time for Joni and me, and we thrived in the laid-back tropical atmosphere of Tahiti. We were going to stay on until the end of 1964, but it got touchy back home. Dr. Stefan Tenkoff was having a difficult time integrating sales and distribution within NPI. Sales were steady, but at such a low level that the company needed some kind of energy injection. My parents called and said, "Please come home, we need you now." I did.

My first "official" job at NPI was as the assistant to Dr. Stefan Tenkoff—NPI's president. In retrospect, it could have been an awkward relationship: the new in-house Ph.D. was the son of the company's founder and chairman of the board and the step-son of its vice president. In practice, the working partnership between the two of us, known as Dr. T. and Dr. Sam inside NPI, proved to be quite effective. While Dr. Tenkoff concentrated on day-to-day operations and manufacturing, I was charged with developing and bringing to market some new NUTRILITE™ products. Together, we focused on rebuilding the business.

Chapter Twenty Three: Passing the Torch

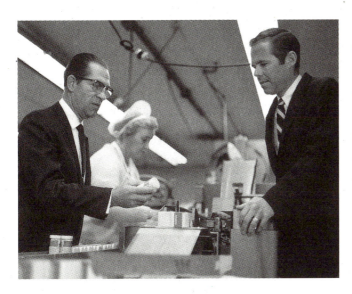

Stefan Tenkoff, Ph.D. and me in the packaging department, circa 1965.

Initially, some of my work focused on the biological control of insect pests and plant diseases, since my experience at Stanford University studying the tobacco mosaic virus fit well with NPI's objectives. To my father, you could control insects by natural predators, poisons, sterilization, and inducing insect diseases. Of these, "the use of poisons … is the least desirable on all accounts." Poisons could kill the pests, but "poisons which can kill insects can also kill birds and animals, and even man himself. There is no question that poisons have been used excessively. Their seeming advantage is that the farmer can see the insects die at once, and this is the result he wanted to have. The much safer procedures take a longer time … as a company NPI is giving very close attention to insect diseases."

I was also deeply involved with food supplement development. At the time, about 15 percent of the nutrition products sold in the country were based on a vitamin B complex. I believed it would be beneficial if NPI had such a vitamin B product with the B vitamins coming from yeast. I thought it was a natural fit considering how successful my father's previous vitamin-B product, OLD SETTLER, had been. I also was able to develop a new vitamin C product that contained bioflavonoids and vitamin C from the acerola my father had been cultivating for several years, first in Hawaii and then later in Puerto Rico; a calcium- and magnesium-containing product; and a natural vitamin E product, among other nutritional products.

The operation was still small enough that products could be shepherded from product concept to laboratory development to manufacturing and into marketing. It was an opportunity that enabled me not only to meet everybody in the company, but to become intimately acquainted with the whole business, all the way from the farms and raw materials to the finished product.

During those early days, I was on the road a lot speaking to various distributor

The Nutrilite Story

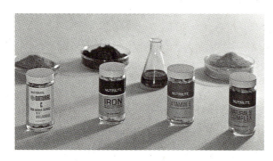

These are some of the earlier products I worked on, 1965. Each packaged product appears with a corresponding raw material in the background: NUTRILITE Natural C with lemon bioflavanoid powder; NUTRILITE Iron with ferrous fumarate; NUTRILITE Vitamin E tocopherol oil from vegetable sources; and NUTRILITE Natural B Complex with golden "wild" yeast.

groups. I guess I was considered the "new Carl"—the young Rehnborg who could energize the sales field. My first speech was in December 1964. I spoke about "The Four Pillars." It was a speech about getting back to basics—and emphasized the importance of exercise, rest, positive mental attitude, and nutrition and food supplements for optimal health. The distributors I met were very encouraging and supportive. They wanted to see me succeed since it was clear that my father would soon be retiring from public life.

For Dr. Tenkoff, the integration of sales and distribution within NPI continued to be a battle. He didn't have much faith in the people who came over from Mytinger Corporation to handle the job, nor did they have much faith in him. He thought he could solve the dilemma by hiring recruiting and marketing people from other companies. However, those new people struggled as well, and the situation grew increasingly frustrating for him. A new sales manager seemed to be hired every six months or so. None of them were particularly successful or had even gone into the field to speak with distributors.

The first sales manager that Dr. Tenkoff hired who actually went into the field proved to be a disaster. He flew into Baltimore to speak with about 300 distributors in Rick Rickenbrode's organization. In his presentation to the group, he wanted to prove that he knew about door-to-door sales. "Just feel my finger," he said pointing to his index finger. "Feel the callus on there from punching doorbells. I know what you folks are up against." Rick didn't think much of his presentation.

At a subsequent board meeting, I told the group that I knew the perfect person for the sales manager job. It was someone that distributors really liked and respected. The person I was referring to was Barney Bailey. When NPI bought out Mytinger Corporation, Barney was one of the individuals who had joined NPI's team. People loved him—he was a big, lovable St. Bernard kind of guy. Barney had run the distributor tours and was responsible for creating the tapes and films that distributors used to recruit new people; however, he had never been in the actual Sales Department. At Mytinger & Casselberry, Inc. and Mytinger Corporation, he had worked in the Audiovisual Department. Management at M&C, such as Dug Duggan, respected Barney's work, but just didn't think of him as a salesperson.

Chapter Twenty Three: Passing the Torch

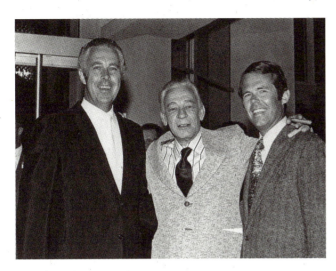

From left to right: Barney Bailey, Rick Rickenbrode, and me, 1965. Call us the Road Warriors. The three of us were on the road a lot, sharing the story of Nutrilite.

Below: John Brockman/ Danny Rogers, 1969.

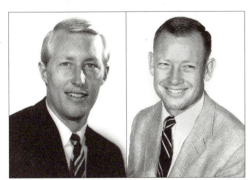

However, I saw the marvelous way Barney had with people and how they trusted him. So we moved him into the top slot in Sales. It turned out to be the right move.

I soon started spending about half my time on the road—talking to distributors about the importance of getting back to basics. I tried to make it fun for people again. I often teamed up with Rick Rickenbrode, while Barney formed a team with Basil Fuller. We would hit the road for two-week stints each month and speak about NUTRILITE products and the business opportunity.

Besides seeing the brilliance of Barney Bailey in Sales, I also was able to recruit other promising young talent like Danny Rogers, a former University of Southern California basketball star, and his brother John Brockman to help us on the road. Danny often tag-teamed with Rick and me—and to make life easier on the road, we began playing practical jokes.

To me, having fun was key. When you are having fun, work becomes play. I love hearing employees laugh in the hallways or distributors sharing a good chuckle ... when I hear that I know they are doing their job. When work is fun, incredible feats can be accomplished. We had some wonderful times sharing the story of Nutrilite. However, I also had some serious points to make during those meetings. One of the most common complaints I had heard was that NUTRILITE Food Supplement was too expensive. During those meetings, I explained why—emphasizing the high quality that goes behind each product that bears the NUTRILITE brand name. Explaining, for example, that the production of a single product like the new NUTRILITE BIO-C Plus, required 326 sheets of paper to be filled out, not counting all the research and development documents and sales and marketing materials. The goal was not to create paperwork, but to ensure quality—something that was of the utmost concern to my father. After reciting 10 note cards of facts, I tried to convey the fact that the production of a high quality, stable, uniform, and saleable product doesn't just happen.

Marty Loos had his own ideas of how sales presentations should be made. He believed many distributors were trying to sell NUTRILITE Food Supplement as if they were doctors, although they had never studied medicine or nutrition. He would read college textbooks about nutrition and body chemistry and was determined to tell the group how the vitamins and minerals worked—without putting them to sleep.

He would stand up on stage with a blackboard like a college professor, writing out how enzymes were formed and showing what happened when vitamins interacted. "The vitamins without the minerals are no good," he would tell a group. "Vitamins are catalysts. They need something to react against. There can be all kinds of combinations …." He combined this information with the story of the Lakeview farm and, in the process, sold lots of product.

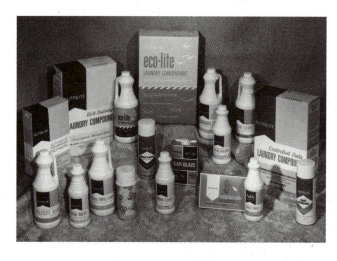

An assortment of NPI's home care products. We had a good environmental image and sold a home care line of products called ECO-LITE which were distributed from 1964 to approximately 1972.

Thanks to the solid foundation of our loyal distributors, our hard work on the road, and Dr. Tenkoff back home stabilizing operations, sales began to pick up, growing over 10 percent for the food supplements in 1968 and even faster for the cosmetics. A new line of ECO-LITE home care products was also doing well.

As the company grew, my family and responsibilities also blossomed. On May 23, 1967, Joni gave birth to our son, Roderick Carl Rehnborg. That same year, I was promoted to vice president and the subsequent year I had added the title and responsibilities of director of R&D. Lots of exciting things were happening.

The company also got a well-deserved boost. In December 1969, the Nixon Administration conducted the first White House Conference on Food, Nutrition, and Health. In Richard Nixon's opening message to Congress regarding the conference, the President stated that "we have awakened to the distressing fact that despite our material abundance, many Americans suffer from malnutrition." A situation Nixon termed, "embarrassing and intolerable …. All of us, poor and nonpoor alike, must be reminded that a proper diet is a basic determinant of good health … We must therefore work to make

CHAPTER TWENTY THREE: PASSING THE TORCH

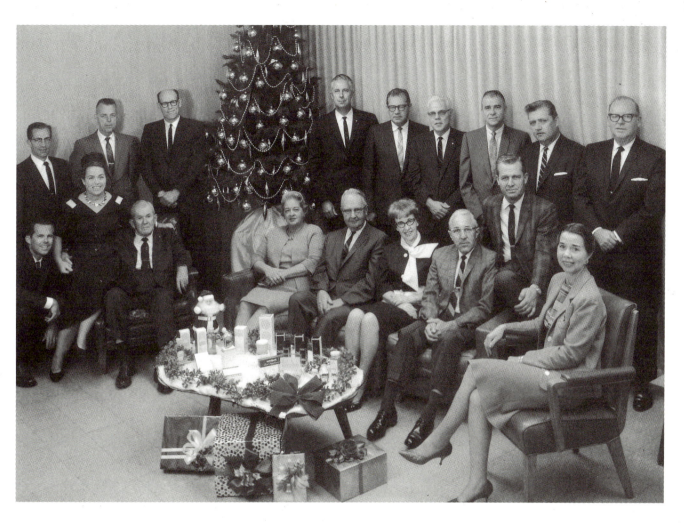

NPI Management at a Christmas party, circa 1966. Top row (left to right): Dr. Stefan Tenkoff; President; Joe Somodi, VP Sales; Barney Bailey, General Sales Manager; Cliff Claus, Sales Manager; Bernie Guthrie, Manager Operations; Roy Carter, Manager Quality Control; Adam Shawula, Package Designer; and Ed Westall, Manager Processing. Bottom row (left to right): Sam Rehnborg, VP; Edith Rehnborg, VP and Treasurer; Carl Rehnborg, Chairman of the Board of Directors; Ruth Dye, Legal Coordinator and Sales Administration Manager; Walt Nelson, Manager Warehouse Services; Penny Sterling, Marketing and Sales Promotion Manager; Maurice Lernoux, Manager Cosmetic Product Development; Merle Umpleby, Manager Marketing Plan Administration and Promotion; and Lee Johnson, Editor *News and Views*.

the private food market serve (all) citizens, by making nutritious foods widely available in popular forms."

This was essentially what my father had been saying, writing, and living for more than 30 years!

The conference, which extended over most of the following year, appointed experts to study the interrelated aspects of food, nutrition, and health. For the first time, Americans were being told that the average American diet wasn't as good as it was supposed to be. The investigations and reports that panels of scientists and educators issued were commented upon and editorialized about throughout the year and beyond. This focus dramatically elevated food, health, and nutrition in the American consciousness.

For NPI, with the bulk of its publicity related to its share of run-ins with federal regulatory agencies, mostly in regard to the content of sales materials, the conference and the impact of its conclusions were like compensation with interest. The timing couldn't have been better. Here was a product, already in place as part of a regular nutritional regimen, that one could adopt right away, with a large body of satisfied customers already practicing what the government had now decided to preach.

For every Nutrilite salesperson and distributor, the initial sales call got easier. The person whose doorbell had been rung became receptive. The explanatory part of the initial call became shorter; educating the customer about the value of good nutrition no longer required reinventing the wheel. Renewals of expiring contracts became simpler: the customer now had third party confirmation of the benefits of what we had been doing all along. As a result of this conference, the health and fitness industry was ignited and the industry was growing and we were growing with it!

Total Retail Sales of NPI's Products

Year	NFS	ERC	HCP
1964	$5,489,000	$3,339,000	$587,000
1965	$5,462,000	$3,722,000	$673,000
1966	$5,807,000	$4,745,000	$682,000
1967	$6,006,000	$4,932,000	$1,156,000
1968	$6,768,000	$5,570,000	$1,236,000
1969	$7,470,000	$5,533,000	$1,151,000
1970	$8,798,000	$5,492,000	$1,465,000
1971	$11,378,000	$5,691,000	$1,905,000

NPI denotes Nutrilite Products, Inc.; NFS, NUTRILITE Food Supplement; ERC, Edith Rehnborg Cosmetics; and HCP, Home Care Products.

Between 1964 to 1965 total sales of NUTRILITE Food Supplement were basically flat. NPI did several positive things in 1965 that would pay off in increased sales during the next couple of years: an Action Award to add an additional percent refund for sales increases, a Vested Interest Plan (VIP) to compensate top field leaders up to half a percent refund based on total group sales increases, more field contact by company representatives, "specials" on a few selected products each month, and by dropping the proposal for NPI to do direct recruiting.

By 1968 several practices were put into place at NPI that positively affected sales. This included being closer to the action by having distribution centers in Illinois and New Jersey that were manned by distributor-orientated staff, greater stability at the corporate level, uniqueness of the product, and the removal of the stigma of "closed territories," which had bothered distributors since its inception in the late 1940s.

In 1969 the First White House Conference on Food, Nutrition, and Health was conducted—igniting the health and fitness industry.

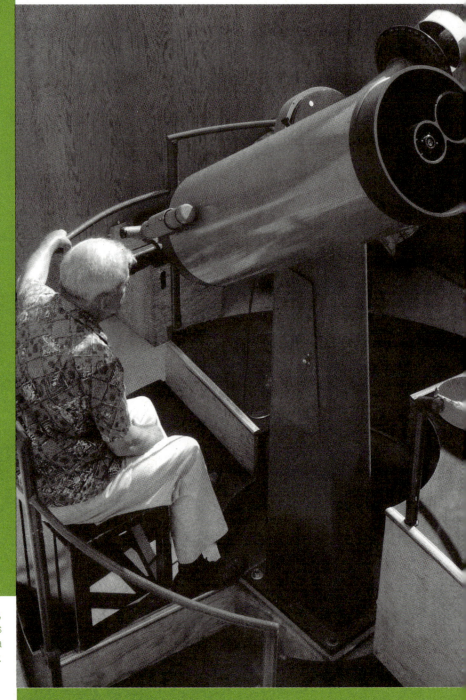

"The spiritual eyesight improves as the physical eyesight declines."

—Plato

My father with his beloved telescope, August 1960. He spent many happy hours in his small "telescope house" in Idyllwild, California where the air was sharp and clear.

Chapter 24 | The Golden Years

As my father approached his 80th birthday, in 1967, there was no question he was slowing down. His first stroke had been followed by three others—"precisely two years and three months apart," he had carefully noted in his journals. Each had taken more and more out of him—not to mention a bout with prostate cancer which, though detected early, involved long and painful treatments.

He would come into the office at most two or three times each week. He was there so rarely that one time he was washing his hands in a restroom, dressed in his Balboa blues, the work clothes he often wore, when a new maintenance man came in. "My name's John," he said. "Do you work here?"

"My name's Carl, and yes, I work here sometimes. I don't come in all the time, but I come in sometimes."

In 1967, he had spent six weeks traveling to hospitals in Orange County to get poked and prodded and irradiated, as he put it, in an effort to cure his prostate cancer. "This adds up to my presently having a poor attendance record," he wrote Dr. Tenkoff. He suggested that, although he wasn't always in the office, he had satellite offices in Newport Beach, Lakeview, and up in his "telescope house" in Idyllwild, and a lot of time on his hands. Could Dr. Tenkoff "bat balls in my direction?" He was quite happy to draw on his own experience to provide advice, "whether or not the advice … was used," he wrote. "This is worth a good try and I would enjoy it."

My father was spending an increasing amount of his time in Idyllwild, a small community located in the San Jacinto Mountains close to the Lakeview farm. Here, the air was sharp and crisp, and it was an ideal place, away from the hustle and bustle of crowds, to study the night sky.

Since Edith was still spending a significant amount of time at Nutrilite, a particularly considerate employee named Katie Berry was hired to help my father out. Katie would help Dad get around, holding his arm gently as he went up and down the steep trail from his observatory to the trailer home in Idyllwild where Katie slept and prepared food for them.

They would spend hours chatting and Katie grew to love my father like a daughter. Dad, too, was very fond of Katie—who was very protective and devoted to him. She loved his tender nature and would tell the story of how he wouldn't allow her to kill the ants that had found their way into the kitchenette. "No, no, no—not that little guy," she said he would say. "He's just hunting for food." So, according to Katie, he would rake them up and "wouldn't have stepped on them for the world."

Out in Idyllwild, my father found peace and comfort studying the heavens above. He didn't consider himself a professional astronomer; however, he was a gifted amateur. He kept copious notes of his observations, such as the one he wrote in 1963:

> *In Aquila, NGC 6709, 18 hours 49, and 10 degrees 17, there is a very pretty cluster of forty stars at a distance of 2,600 light years. It is not noted as remarkable in the catalog, but it is extremely attractive in the glass. Its stars are arranged in streams, and are nearly uniform in brightness. I should record this as one of my favorites.*
>
> *Twenty-six hundred years ago, when the light from this cluster started traveling toward us, was just about the time that the first five books of the Old Testament got their final brush-up into their present form in the Temple at Jerusalem. Some 650 years later Jesus was born. I find myself unable to visualize this distance in space, let alone the much greater distances that are involved in astronomy.*
>
> *I am now looking at the cluster NGC 7062 at 21 hours 21.5, 46 degrees 10, at a distance of 7,800 light years... probably as long a time as the whole of human civilized history. It is far more interesting to regard this grouping and its distance with the awe it calls for and which we rarely give it, than to regard figures without considering their significance. It is a sort of introduction to the staggering distances of the optics in our one galaxy, and the yet more impressive figures for the other galaxies visible on photographic plates.*

Chapter Twenty Four: The Golden Years

Over time, my father had come to believe that by looking at the universe he was looking into the origin of life; finding the mini world by studying its macro version. And while looking thousands of years into the past, he continued to glean insights he could use to shape the future.

As he had done all his life, he continued to write ardently. During his later years, his interests seemed to fall into one of three categories: reflections on life and living, on death and the need to make arrangements for his legacy, and as always on ways to benefit humanity.

While in his 70s, he had penned a 33-page white paper that made its way by route of his good friend Charlie Rhyne to then Vice President Richard Nixon. The paper outlined his concerns regarding the growing population and the coinciding need to feed the masses. "The problem of securing food supplies for an exploding population," he wrote "may be solved by the development of the inexhaustible sea as a food resource, but nothing whatever except just possibly distillation by atomic power will ever take the place of rainfall …."

My father described a world on the verge of apocalypse, either through mass starvation or nuclear annihilation. "The whole thing has become utterly ridiculous," he wrote; "the only way now to stop is just to stop. Any other course is mutual destruction, which at times seems the outcome in any case." Perhaps it had been a mistake not to enforce disarmament unilaterally at the end of World War II, when the United States was the only country with nuclear weapons. "It was undemocratic; it was chauvinistic; it was even warlike;" but not doing so led to the arms race, which had spread to China, France, and Britain.

"We must—we absolutely must—do in One World the things that can turn humanity from a more and more desperate mob into a permanently organized society on our Earth managed scientifically," he wrote. "This requires political unity which only the USA and Russia can create and maintain." If the two superpowers could agree to disagree on politics, but agree on world disarmament and preventing overpopulation, the two greatest contributors to disharmony would be eliminated. Nixon had thanked him for the paper.

My father also continued to reflect on life and living. He marveled at the gift of life. Also while in his 70s, he wrote another essay:

> *The first and greatest of the wonders is the wonder of existence … The odds … which produced you for your individual destiny are as one to a number outside of actual comprehension by a human mind …*
>
> *Have you ever looked out at your world and inside at yourself, and given thanks that you were granted the right … of becoming and living and thinking for your term of years in this amazing universe?*

While my father was appreciative of the gift of life, he wasn't fearful of death. He wasn't a religious man in the traditional sense. But his faith in science and his ability to see both the big picture and the small offered him solace of another and perhaps equally rich order.

Like the stars in the galaxies he studied through his telescope, the individual on earth represented an arrangement and rearrangement of atoms. The available and required materials were used over and over again by a succession of living forms:

> *Because of the numbers of atoms involved in any one organization of a human being, for example, it is exceedingly probable that in the body of any given human individual, at any given time, there are atoms of elements which at some time have been part of the body of every human being who has lived long enough ago for his materials to have been disseminated completely over the earth's surface.*
>
> *Life, seen this way, is both finite, and infinite.*
>
> *Man is an integrated part of the universe, in and of it, made of the same materials and obeying the same natural laws as all the rest of the universe, and a result of the same total evolutionary development as the galaxies themselves.*

Far from being a cause of despair, such facts can be, as they were for my father, a source of "wonder and adventure in the highest degree."

In a way, while he was writing essay after essay, he was wrapping up loose ends. He felt too often people spent more time preparing for short-term departures, but "departures are more carelessly arranged when one goes away forever, if only because one does not usually plan for the event called death." He felt "this is altogether wrong from an emotional standpoint, as well as very wasteful from the standpoint of human interests

Chapter Twenty Four: The Golden Years

involved." Everyone, he felt, had something to contribute that should be given expression. "Then, since one does not know quite exactly the date of his final departure, at least one can make a sort of guess on common human experience, and then, if the record has been compiled earlier than necessary, there is a gain in being able to revise the record now and then to include new insights."

While in his mid-70s, he wrote an essay called "Reflections on Living and Dying." He wrote that he had lived "a full and eventful life and I have enjoyed it completely, and except for a very few, have loved my fellow travelers."

He hoped that he had used the "privilege of living" to give important "donations to knowledge or to controversy."

As he had approached his 79th birthday, he sat down at his typewriter and continued his thoughts about death in a memo about euthanasia. Besides the strokes and prostate cancer, he had his prostate reamed (making a wider passage way through it) for the second time. He felt like he was a "marginal cause," no longer contributing "to the welfare of the human group." His body that had been so sleek and efficient when he walked for miles through China in his pongee suits and dapper pith helmet was now too weak and "too slack and too soft and fat."

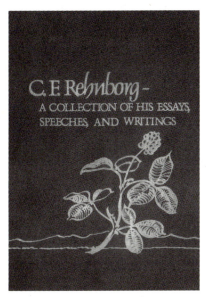

Some of my father's writings, such as the essay "Reflections on Living and Dying," were gathered and published in 1985 in the book, *C.F. Rehnborg: A Collection of his Essays, Speeches, and Writings*.

"In a primitive society," he wrote, "the too-aged one is left beside the trail to fend for himself or die. This even the one left sees not as cruelty, but realism. In a culture such as our present society, on the other hand, he is guarded and tended to a point even damning to the society … Progressively I am more and more disabled. My associates all tell me how well I look, earnestly enough to make it clear that they are affectionate liars. I go to the office two or three times a week, but I am late in arriving and early to leave. I draw a substantial salary, more for what I have done than for what I can do now. I take extended 'vacations,' but I am an effective brake on the activity of my lovely and unselfish wife. I cannot drive a car, I permanently have vertigo and a very shaky balance, and my eyes do not track, so that much of what I see is doubled and unclear." Nevertheless, he wrote, "I am having a wonderful time."

His mind was still on the plankton project. Just a few months later, in April and

May of 1966, he wrote a series of memos to me on growing plankton in lagoons and describing a way to feed the world using a process that relied on the natural temperature and pressure differences of the ocean.

No artificial whale needed, just a nuclear reactor at the bottom of the ocean to pump ice-cold, phosphorous-rich seawater to the surface where it would fertilize the growth of phytoplankton and zooplankton. The difference in temperature between the cold water from the depths and the warm water from the surface could produce low-pressure steam to drive a generator that would power the processing plant. The process would allow plankton to rise to the surface and would in turn make it easier to gather. In fact, he felt you wouldn't even need the nuclear reactor to power the process. You could use the natural temperature and pressure difference to create a current rising to the surface by building a giant tube all the way to the ocean floor—a natural pump that would also generate electricity.

At the time, I read the memos and kind of chuckled. It was a Jules Verne-ish kind of idea. It sounded like a perpetual motion machine, but my father wasn't the only one considering it. Only a few years later, thousands of high-school debaters would propose it as one of their solutions to the energy crisis.

The idea came back to him as he looked out on the placid blue waters off Punaauia the next spring on a trip to Tahiti with Mom, in 1967. He could see the dolphins leaping and the seabirds diving for fish. They were at the top of the food chain. It took as much as 10,000 pounds of phytoplankton, at the bottom of the food chain, to make one pound of fish. With his idea, the plankton would be brought up to you. The system would work just like any turbine-powered plant using fossil fuels, only the sun would create the heat to make the steam. The sea farm would use fertilizer to make plants and animals grow, just like any farm on land, only the fertilizer would flow naturally from 1,000 feet below the surface, the result of natural compost from the dead bodies of plants and animals that had sunk to the bottom. You could build all the facilities out of thick, reinforced concrete to withstand even the worst tropical storms, so that each farm could operate indefinitely. You could drill the channels for the seawater using the same technology oil companies used for undersea wells or that dam builders used for their diversion tunnels. It wasn't far

Chapter Twenty Four: The Golden Years

out. He could even see the independent colonies, kind of like the fishermen of the Aran Islands, making their own fresh water from the steam, generating their own electricity, and even using the organic waste to fertilize their own land farms for conventional fruits and vegetables. It was too big a project for NPI to fund, but my father felt it worth pursuing to have a cheap protein source to feed the world.

He continued to reflect about the changes in technology that had taken place over the past three decades since NUTRILITE™ Food Supplement was first introduced. In a memo written in October 1967, when my father was 80, he described these changes:

> *When NUTRILITE Food Supplement was first being developed, there was no vitamin industry as such, and no vitamin products. Our product became a 'vitamin product' through being swept along by our sales agents and the public news media.*
>
> *When we started, we were not selling a 'vitamin product' but rather a 'food supplement,' and except for the 'vitamin' label under which it is now sold, it is still a 'food supplement.' We should begin once more to talk and think in our own idiom and get back into our own business of food supplements…*
>
> *We are properly committed to extracts and concentrates of plant and fruit materials. The many new items of discovery in the science of nutrition act as the dots in electrotype which reproduce a picture in printing. The picture is the whole relationship of life to its environment. Instead of these details, we need only to look at the whole concept…*

In 1969, at the age of 82, my father officially retired and was made honorary chairman. Even though NPI had its ups and downs, sales had been steady recently and were starting to turn slowly up again. Once again, distributors were growing confident in the company's management. The staff was closer to the distributors than they had ever been, with several sales managers, including myself, spending at least half of our time in the field. Although competition in the dietary supplement field continued to increase, NUTRILITE food supplements were still considered unique and drawing new customers and distributors.

In order to provide a smooth transition and to ensure the company remained on course, he encouraged Edith, who was in her late 60s, to retire as well; however, she wasn't quite ready. Eventually, a stock transfer arrangement was worked out.

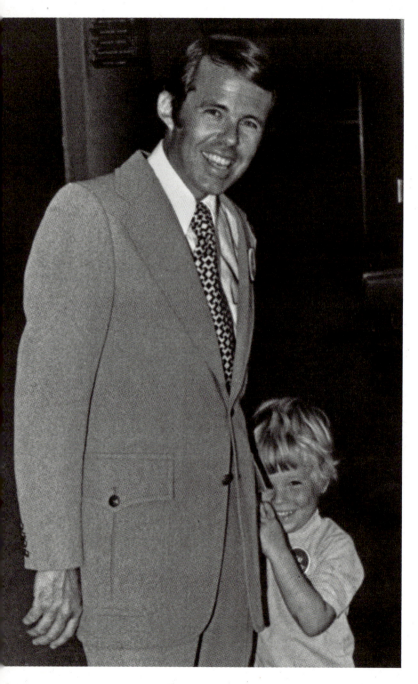

My father spoke with Dr. Stefan Tenkoff, Edith, and me several times about how he wished to settle things. He wanted to give Dr. T certain shares of A and B stock, and also 25 percent of the voting shares. He wanted me to have another 25 percent, and Edith, now chairman of the board, the remaining 50 percent of voting shares. Dr. Tenkoff insisted he wouldn't accept the arrangement "unless it was with the absolute and express approval and acceptance on the part of both Mr. and Mrs. Rehnborg and Sam." Dr. Tenkoff discussed the situation with Mom, pointing out that 50 percent ownership didn't mean control and could result in a deadlock, which would have to be worked out. She assured him that she wasn't worried about it, and the agreement was formalized with the gifts vesting over three years.

With the company business settled, Dad visited Savannah, where his father had once set up a thriving jewelry business. He stayed with his brother Frank's widow. It was both a chance to witness his first total eclipse of the sun and a nostalgic return to his early life among relatives. Following this, he joined a tour of Micronesia with the assistance of Katie Berry. It would be his last long distance trip. As always, he had his dictaphone nearby as he recorded his impressions.

After his trip to Micronesia, the idea of

My son Rod and I at a Nutrilite function, circa 1971. While my father had officially retired from the business, I was spending more time in the field. Accompanying me at one such function is my son. Rod is wearing a pin that was a favorite among distributors proclaiming: I EAT NUTRILITE.

Chapter Twenty Four: The Golden Years

something he was calling Nutrimana kept coming back to him with greater and greater frequency. It was a concept that went beyond nutritional supplementation to that of an all-inclusive foodstuff, a real manna that included protein as well as vitamins and minerals—made entirely from natural plant sources. It would be "a source and kind of food which will sustain the human race in spite of its abuse of the earth's surface until it can make a recovery." He loved the concept and felt that it was really part of the future.

According to his journal, he met with NPI's legal counsel, Ruth Dye, to discuss incorporating Nutrimana and registering the trade name. All the while he continued to refine the religious work that he had published earlier in 1955 and to come up with new ideas that he might be able to fund once NPI was thriving again.

Although NPI was once again growing due, in part, to the loyal and passionate support of our distributors, our efforts on the road, and the increased acceptance within the medical profession of the value of food supplements, the company still had some struggles.

Amway, by contrast, was now the leader in multilevel marketing. One of the secrets of Amway's profitability was that it had a service charge on every order that went out in order to pay for freight and handling. We tried to put some of those increased percentages into place and to upgrade productivity, but were having a tough time doing it. Some of our distributors, or at least some of the leading ones, threatened to revolt.

There were also other multilevel marketing companies springing up—not all of which were doing business in an ethical manner. Just as the development of vitamin and nutrition products aroused the concern of the FDA—a concern based on grounds of quality and safety—the explosion of multilevel marketing with distributors signing up by the thousands every month attracted the interest of the Federal Trade Commission (FTC), the FDA's selling and marketing counterpart. The FTC was looking into multilevel marketing for the same reason the FDA had investigated multivitamin nutrition: an innovative way of doing things had been discovered and was being exploited by the unscrupulous.

The distortion of multilevel marketing by certain individuals in which high-pressure tactics and promises of overnight wealth were used brought increased government scrutiny and consumer skepticism to legitimately run organizations such as NPI, Amway, and others—and burdening them with the task of restoring shaken consumer confidence. It also added resistance to the efforts of my father, for whom the Sales Plan had originally been developed as a lifeline, simply a way to get his product to customers when conventional distribution methods just couldn't reach them.

While grappling with these issues, I continued to spend a significant amount of my time traveling: rallying the troops, talking to people about NUTRILITE products, and building the business. Joni, meanwhile, was essentially raising Rod all by herself. Although she was a trouper, it was putting a strain on our marriage.

One year after Rod was born, we were expecting our second child. I made a special effort to plan an important six-week trip so that I could be home when the baby was due.

Our son came six weeks early. Tucker Upton Rehnborg was big enough at four and half pounds to survive on his own, except for a serious heart defect. Joni's obstetrician told her that she must have been exposed to a virus at the time Tucker's heart was being formed and urged her to move him from Hoag Hospital in Newport Beach to Children's Hospital in Orange, where a team of pediatric cardiologists were among the best specialists available.

Unfortunately, nothing could help our baby. Tucker lived only one more week. Joni and I were devastated. It was hard for Joni to bear, and I felt guilty for being away. The stress eventually took its toll on our marriage.

Meanwhile, Edith was exhibiting rather erratic behavior at NPI that, in retrospect, I believe was due to the combination of medications she was taking. In those days, the side effects of certain drugs were poorly understood. For Edith, the outcome resulted in extremely unpredictable behavior—capricious firings and suspicious thoughts. It attached itself for a while to Dad's caregiver, Katie Berry, whom she summarily fired until cooler heads prevailed, and to Dr. Stefan Tenkoff and me, whom she became convinced were scheming to take over the company.

The outside world had no idea all this turmoil was going on. Back in Grand Rapids, NPI was looking like a prize—thanks to the health and fitness boom. The folks over at Amway were looking with a certain admiration toward NPI. Amway distributors were beginning to clamor for NUTRILITE food supplements, because it was starting to sell widely again.

Chapter Twenty Four: The Golden Years

Part 3
Making a Difference

"The world is round and the place which may seem like the end may also be the beginning."

—Ivy Baker Priest

Advertisement for NUTRILITE Food Supplements, 1971.

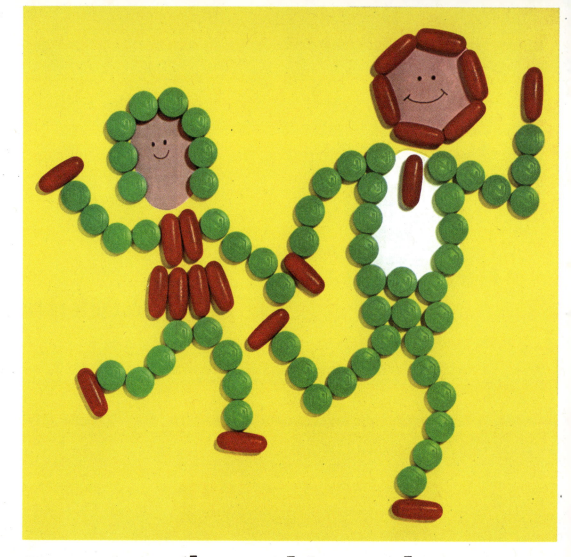

Are you on the road to good nutrition?

Good nutrition doesn't just happen. It takes some mighty careful planning, and that's something a lot of us rarely find the time for. In fact, a government survey disclosed that many Americans (from **all** walks of life) had diets providing less than the recommended amounts of various indispensable vitamins and minerals.

NUTRILITE® Food Supplements can help put you on the road to better nutrition if you're not getting the correct amount of these essential vitamins and minerals.

Get the facts about NUTRILITE in your own home. Check your telephone book for your nearest NUTRILITE Distributor. Or write NUTRILITE, Buena Park, Calif. 90620.

©1971 NPI

NUTRILITE
PRODUCTS, INC.

Chapter 25 | Reunion

Throughout the years, Jay Van Andel and Rich DeVos had been buying NUTRILITE™ Food Supplement and selling it to their group. Although Amway was four times larger than Nutrilite, we would have to send them a bonus check based on the volume of NUTRILITE products they sold. This used to drive Dr. T crazy.

Now, as the health and fitness movement began to burgeon, Amway found itself with a massive distributor organization, but no health products of its own to sell. It had become increasingly apparent that there was a huge market for nutrition-based products not only in the United States, but also overseas.

In the early 1970s, Jay assigned Bob Hunter, Amway's new Director of Research & Development, the task of finding a product equivalent to NUTRILITE Food Supplement. Jay told Bob, "We want it to be just like NUTRILITE. You know, Rich and I spent 10 years in Nutrilite, and we think it's got tremendous potential for Amway, but we've gotta have a product line that's like that."

If anyone could find or develop a competitive product to NUTRILITE Food Supplement, Bob Hunter could. Bob's reputation preceded his arrival at Amway. He had been a research chemist and section head at Colgate in the soap division and had helped develop an amazing fabric that never stained. Unfortunately, the clothes had a big drawback—they were like wearing plastic. They didn't stain, but the fabric didn't breathe, either. But the research led to the development of Handi Wipes[††] and other products. At the time, Bob knew little about nutritional food supplements. "I'm a laundry guy," he said. Jay knew he was a *really* fast learner and told him to look into it.

[††] Handi Wipes is a registered trademark of Colgate-Palmolive Company.

Amway's R&D team went to work on the task, but ran across a major hurdle. They just couldn't find the natural concentrates that set the NUTRILITE brand apart from other dietary supplements on the market. The team could go out in the marketplace, find crystalline (or man-made) vitamins, and bring them together into a tablet or capsule, or even buy an already completed formula, but they couldn't obtain the natural plant concentrates that my father had developed during years of harvesting, dehydrating, extracting, and concentrating nutrient-rich plants. Months of attempts to find alternative sources or duplicate the concentrates proved futile.

After detailed study, Bob felt it couldn't be done cost-effectively. Before he went on vacation in the summer of 1972, Bob stopped by Jay's office and said, "Jay, you know, we're just busting our pick on this thing. We can't find these concentrates anywhere."

Jay said, "Keep at it, there's got to be a way of getting those concentrates. That's what makes NUTRILITE different."

When Bob returned from his vacation, he found that Jay and Rich had talked and they had found a way to get the concentrates—they bought controlling interest in Nutrilite! Bob went back to Jay's office and thanked him for making his job so much easier.

The suddenness with which it happened caught nearly everybody by surprise. If, in real estate, the proverbial three selling points are "location, location, and location," then the equivalent in business is surely, "timing, timing, and timing." And Amway's timing was impeccable.

Amway also made a very generous offer—four times the book value of the company. Being aware of customer and distributor demand for a NUTRILITE-type product, they had accurately gauged what the company was worth to them. Amway would have control, but NPI would still have significant ownership and would continue to operate as a separate company. The plan was that each of the principal owners would sell 51 percent of their holdings.

From my standpoint, the timing felt right. I could see that the company wasn't profitable enough to go international, and the banks wouldn't loan us enough money to expand. I thought Amway might be the key to taking my dad's product around the world. I agreed to the negotiations. My father was involved in a small way, although his health was now rapidly declining.

CHAPTER TWENTY FIVE: REUNION

The deal was wrapped up on August 31, 1972. After nearly 15 years of head-to-head competition, NPI and Amway would unite and work together as a team.

The Nutrilite distributors knew nothing about it. They were caught completely off guard. As Marty Loos remembers it, he and some of the most prominent senior keys were called to a mysterious meeting at a hotel close to the Los Angeles airport. After a night of confusion, rumors, and joking about the purpose of the meeting, the distributors were ushered into a closed-door session in the hotel's conference room.

"We were supposed to hear good news—good news!" said Marty. "Everybody's milling around, all speculating on what this good news was gonna be." Somebody said, "Well, we're going to hear that Barney Bailey is pregnant." They got a good laugh out of that because they all liked Barney.

However, once the meeting began, with all the leaders from the distributor organization shuffling in, the tone of the group changed. At the meeting, Marty remembered hearing the master of ceremony state that, "Dr. Sam, Sam Rehnborg will be getting up and talking to you about something, and please don't judge, please don't make a decision until he's all through." As Marty recounted the situation:

> *All the kidding, joking, and everything stopped like that. I was sitting up front with Dottie, she was on my right, and I was sitting right in front and Dr. Sam was right there, and he comes up, 35 years old or whatever he was, and I took one look at his face. It was as white as a sheet…*
>
> *He got up there and he started off, 'Now I don't want you to make any decision. I don't want you to …' Dead silence. Everybody's petrified. Then he gets into it, that they sold the interest to Rich and Jay. And the women started to cry. Now we're talking about people who have been in the business 30 years—whole lifetimes. Women started to cry. I could hear Rickenbrode down there—he started to curse out loud at the top of his voice. And the others. And that room got icy cold. Now, I've read about that in books. I've never experienced that before. I've never experienced that again. But that room got icy cold. And they open the door and in walks Rich. Rich DeVos. Dead silence.*
>
> *Rich DeVos began talking. He went through it and everybody's dead silent. Then Jay was introduced. The effect was the same.*

Some of the distributors were threatening to quit. Others were urging a rump meeting of dissenting voices that afternoon. Marty, Ned Ross, and other key distributors discouraged this. "Don't you understand? This is a *fait accompli*," said Marty. "It's done. It's finished. It's signed, sealed, delivered. It's over with. Go sell your NUTRILITE products. That's what I'm going to do."

To a number of inconsolable Nutrilite veterans, the people who cared about the product had been sold out to the people who didn't. Marty disagreed. "I know they [Rich and Jay] respect and love Nutrilite as much as I do. They're not going to do anything to hurt it. And as long as I can have NUTRILITE products, I don't care about the rest of it."

Marty Loos hadn't spoken to Rich DeVos in 13 years. Not since that fateful meeting in Lake Louise. But Marty went over to Rich and said, "Rich, I don't like what happened, but I can see the reasons for it, and I want you to know that I'll back you up."

A flurry of announcements were sent out in September 1972, beginning with a telegram to the key distributors, promising that nothing would change until the following year when distributor organizations and product lines would be integrated. The announcement included a brief statement from Mom:

> *It has always been Mr. Rehnborg's dream, and mine, to see NUTRILITE Food Supplements made available to all the people of the world. We are excited by the tremendous potential of this great new move toward that end.*

Barney Bailey, probably the best known man in the field outside of the family, sent a message as well:

> *My goal—as with most of you—has been, and is now, to help others tell as many people as possible about the benefits of NUTRILITE products and the advantage of this method of distribution…*
>
> *But there is a great deal of work left to be done and with Amway we can make still more fine progress. Amway has the facilities, the staff, and the field organization to do the job of helping us more rapidly towards our goal of making NUTRILITE a household word in every home in America.*
>
> *All of us can have an even more successful future with this greatly expanded activity. I'm very much looking forward to it.*

NUTRILITE PRODUCTS, INC.
5600 BEACH BLVD. • BUENA PARK, CALIFORNIA 90620 • TELEPHONE 714-521-3900

September 11, 1972

A SPECIAL MESSAGE TO NUTRILITE DISTRIBUTORS

An event of great importance to all Distributors of NUTRILITE Products has taken place. As of August 31, 1972, Nutrilite Products, Inc., and the Amway Corporation of Ada, Michigan, have joined forces, with Amway acquiring a controlling stock interest in NPI on that date.

This means that the second-largest direct selling organization in the United States will combine with the country's oldest and best known manufacturer of food supplement products, joining the Distributor organizations of both companies into a single powerful selling force whose aim and objective is to become the biggest direct selling company in the world. Fortunately the Amway and Nutrilite Marketing Plans are so similar that only minimal changes will be necessary to weld them into one.

This move was made only after much study and consideration of all the aspects involved. The managements of both companies were convinced, finally, that such a move would be beneficial to all concerned--to the companies, to the employees, and to the Distributors of both organizations. The single powerful sales force that will result will be able to accomplish far more for all Distributors than either would be able to do alone. It has always been Carl Rehnborg's dream that NUTRILITE XX Food Supplement would be on every table in the land, and this move will insure the broadest possible distribution for this great product.

The change will bring about the broad basis of sales volume that will enable NPI to more fully develop and expand its manufacturing capacity, and to exploit its research and development facilities, which in turn will make your opportunity bigger and potentially more profitable. It will insure the future rapid growth and expansion which, in these years of spiraling inflation and constantly increasing costs, can much better be accomplished by a larger company such as Amway.

It is important for you to know that Nutrilite Products, Inc., will continue to be a separate corporate entity with its own management, and that the company will continue to manufacture NUTRILITE Food Supplements and cosmetics, as

- over -

NUTRILITE® FOOD SUPPLEMENTS • Edith Rehnborg Cosmetics • NUTRILITE HOUSEHOLD PRODUCTS

---

well as being responsible for the development of new food supplement and cosmetic products. The only difference is that NUTRILITE products will be distributed by Amway Corporation after December 31, 1972, instead of by NPI. Distributors will continue to order and receive products from their Keys or Sponsors in the same way as before. The Distributor organizations and product lines of the two companies will be integrated early in 1973, and you will receive all necessary details and information prior to that time.

We believe that NUTRILITE Distributors will benefit in numerous ways as a result of this new combining of forces. You will have a far wider range of excellent products to sell, with tremendously expanded potential. There will be much faster delivery of merchandise from more than 33 warehouses, a commercial sales program, greatly accelerated advertising, a wider range of sales training and audio visual materials as well as customer literature, and an expanded sales rally and meeting schedule. Other benefits will include stepped-up publicity and more influence in both legal and political matters. Amway has just concluded, as of August 31, the most successful fiscal year in its history, with retail sales volume in excess of $180,000,000.

We are tremendously excited about the prospects for the future, and we would like to quote from Amway's announcement: "...Nutrilite...will dedicate itself to the role in which it excels--the manufacture of top quality food supplements and other quality products. Amway will continue in the roles that have brought it to its great success--the operation of the Amway Sales and Marketing Plan through the Amway distributor organization, and the manufacture of top quality home and personal care products for distribution through that organization. Amway's superb technology in the manufacture of detergents, along with Nutrilite's unmatched expertise in the manufacture of food supplements, and the combined technology of both companies in the manufacture of cosmetics and personal care products will give the combined distribution organization the greatest line of fine products of any marketing organization in the world."

As you can see, you will be a part of one of the largest and most successful selling organizations in the world! In the meantime, what about the months prior to December 31, 1972? You have a tremendous 1972 Christmas Gift Line to sell, and an exciting 38th Anniversary Recruiting Campaign to kick off the fall season! We urge you to go right on doing the great job you have been doing, selling NUTRILITE Food Supplements, EDITH REHNBORG Cosmetics, and NUTRILITE Household Products! Nothing would be greater than for you to come through with the biggest and best Christmas gift selling season we've ever experienced! Keep right on selling, recruiting, and training...and during the next 3 months we'll be getting the information to you that will open a whole new world of selling to you as of January 1, 1973!

Sincerely yours,

NUTRILITE PRODUCTS, INC.

Sam Rehnborg

Sam Rehnborg, Ph.D.
Executive Vice President

A special message to Nutrilite distributors, September 11, 1972.

Dr. Tenkoff wrote a more detailed explanation of the issues for the key distributors. NPI's prime consideration was the good of all the distributors, because they were the ones who made the company and the products successful. Their opportunities were limited as long as they were tied to a small company, making it hard to fulfill the dream that my father had of the broadest distribution possible of our products. "We anticipate, with excitement and certainty, to double, triple, and even quadruple volume rapidly, which will put Nutrilite at the zenith and this is what you and we all want and are working towards. Let us all band together in our new association for our mutual growth and glory."

I also sent out an announcement assuring all distributors that, since the Amway and NPI Sales Plans were so similar, only minimal changes would be made to weld them into one. NPI would still manufacture the food supplements and cosmetics. "The only difference is that NUTRILITE products will be distributed by Amway Corporation after December 31, 1972, instead of by NPI," while Nutrilite distributors would have a wider range of products to sell, faster delivery of merchandise from more than 33 warehouses, and improved advertising and merchandising support.

In the late fall of 1972, Amway paid for all key distributors to fly into Ada, Michigan for a two-day meeting. It was a powerful and very effective meeting and helped pave the way for NPI and Amway to work together.

The huge issue had been settled. I knew in my heart that what I told distributors was true: having far more distributors, including those in the United Kingdom and Canada, would ultimately mean far more people benefiting from NUTRILITE products. I also knew my father, who was in very poor health, would be pleased with the outcome. Besides, Amway had already proven to be much more successful than NPI at utilizing the Sales Plan.

After the New Year, preparations were in full swing to begin merging the distributor organizations. Barney Bailey went up to Seattle in January 1973 for the first combined meeting with Amway and Nutrilite distributors. It's a day etched in my memory—Friday, January 26, 1973—although I was more than 1,000 miles away from the meeting.

I was actually back home and, more precisely, by my father's bedside. As the company he fathered and the one he step-fathered were in the process of beginning combined operations, he had been admitted to Hoag Hospital in Newport Beach.

He was 85 years old. He had lived a full life and had the courage and conviction to

Chapter Twenty Five: Reunion

blaze his unique path in the world. Now he was dying in a world that, in his lifetime, had been transformed around him and, to a significant degree, by him. Balboa Island, a few miles south, a seasonal community where he had spent countless hours in the back of the sail loft crafting his food supplements was now a posh, year-round yachtsmen's paradise, where people from all over the world came to sail, party, and fish. His first tiny alfalfa farm in the San Fernando Valley had been replaced by rolling acres in the San Jacinto Valley. Its produce, grown and harvested according to methods he pioneered, was transformed at a nine-building manufacturing complex he had built in Buena Park into nutrition products used throughout the United States and soon, with Amway's help, around the world. He had made his mark on the present and pointed the way to the future, not only in his discoveries and application of the value of plant life in nutrition, but in his exploration of the practicality of plankton as a source of protein, hydroponics as a means of cultivation, the importance of forest preservation and reforestation, and his love of humanity that was exemplified in his approach to living and life's work. The world may have caught up with my father in the recognition and popular acceptance of some of his ideas, yet he remained on the cutting edge in others.

As he lay in his hospital bed, my mother kept vigil either at his bedside or in the hallway outside his room. Protective of my father, she was his gatekeeper, monitoring who got to visit and for how long. The doctor recommended that his life support be removed and we consented. Katie Berry said her goodbyes earlier and felt my father squeeze her hand. It was the only way he had left to communicate; the tubes in his nose made it impossible to speak. Dr. Tenkoff also visited, but wasn't sure if my father, who was heavily medicated, recognized him. Joni visited as well.

In many ways, he had already said his goodbyes and was at peace knowing the end was near. Nearly a decade earlier, he had written: "Personally I do not consider death, which is the absolutely inevitable final episode in the life of a human being … is in any way gruesome. Further, I would like to say goodbye to my family and friends, if only to tell them how much more I love them than it was conventional to show, and how honored and enriched I was to have them for my associates. Certainly if death is the end of one's existence, and the beginning of nonexistence, it is a completely dreamless sleep and therefore an untroubled sleep."

The Nutrilite Story

While I sat there by my father's bedside, holding his hand, the untroubled sleep descended on him. I'll never forget when he stopped breathing for the last time and the pained expression on his face disappeared and the peaceful mask of death enveloped him. It was a sad but moving moment for me, and I was happy to see him on to better places.

My father's passing went unremarked in the media that January, as it had been a particularly busy news month. Richard Nixon was inaugurated for his second term. The Watergate burglars, who would bring Nixon down, were arraigned in court. The Government of North Vietnam agreed to an armistice ending the war with the United States. And, Lyndon Johnson, who had dramatically escalated American involvement in the war and whose presidency was destroyed by it, died.

There was no funeral or memorial service, as my father had specifically requested. Instead, he was cremated, and his ashes were scattered from an airplane over the Pacific, where he had sailed, first in rented boats and later as an experienced sailor in ketches and yawls of his own. The redwoods could have been an alternative, but that would have involved a lot of red tape and the ocean was faster. He definitely wanted to get back in the action in the universe as quickly as possible. In this, we kept faith with my father's own belief in ultimate reunion: that man "is an integrated part of the universe … made of the same materials … and a result of the same total evolutionary development as the galaxies themselves."

My father, barefooted and wind-tousled, enjoying one of his favorite pastimes—sailing aboard his 30-foot sailboat, the *Scandal*, 1952. Much of his inspiration was drawn from the sea.

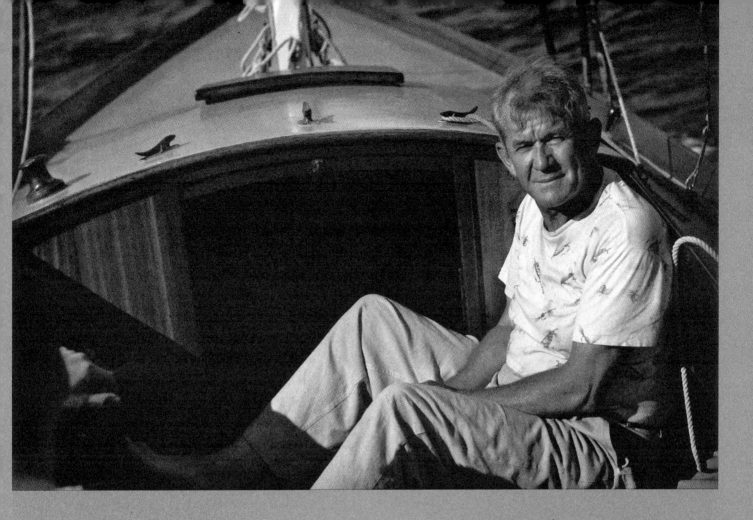

"… having met many of the great men of our time, I can say that Carl Rehnborg was truly one of the greatest. Our earth is a better place in which to live because of his quiet but lasting contributions to all humanity. Few indeed have contributed more. He possessed the attributes of greatness which characterize the leaders of our nation and the world, even though he led the life of the quiet scholar, a multifaceted and compassionate individual working alone on the critical problems of humankind. He did not reach for headlines but did the hard, difficult research work … which is his trademark of greatness in the history of mankind.…"

—Charles S. Rhyne

"Twenty years from now you will be more disappointed by the things that you didn't do than by the ones you did do. So throw off the bowlines. Sail away from the safe harbor. Catch the trade wivnds in your sails. Explore. Dream. Discover."

—Mark Twain

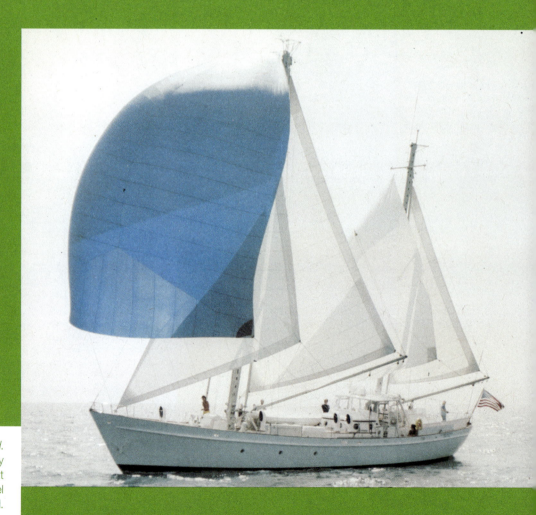

The *Firebird*. Built in 1967 and completely overhauled in April 1979, I spent three years aboard this vessel circumnavigating the world.

Chapter 26 | My Sabbatical

I had agreed to stay on as part of the NPI management team, but found myself at a crossroad. My father was gone; the company he founded had been sold; my own marriage was broken; and the sale to Amway Corporation would bring a new set of responsibilities.

Before assuming my new position, I was determined that I would use the breathing space to keep a promise I had made to myself when I was a young boy. I wanted to see more of the world. It was a dream that had been cut short years earlier. My father had taught me sailing; now, as an experienced sailor, I decided that I would sail around the world.

I broached the idea to Jay and Rich in 1974, and they were very supportive and encouraged me to go for it. "If you don't do it now, you'll never do it."

It took me about one year to get ready for the voyage, finding and preparing the boat and recruiting my companions. I also took special photography courses and purchased cameras for above and below water so I could document my journey. All the while, I continued to speak at meetings helping to ease the transition to Amway by reaffirming continuity with NPI and my father.

The level of activity and excitement surrounding Nutrilite stepped up immediately following the acquisition. Beneath the cheers, however, were the inevitable jitters. The deal had been done, but would it really work as promised? Would the two partners be able to work together? Would NPI still retain the independence it had been promised? Could the very different marketing styles of the Amway and Nutrilite distributors be smoothly merged?

The transition path to join the two companies was a little rocky at first. For one thing, the distributor organizations were very different. Nutrilite distributors were product-orientated, selling a unique item that customers associated with personal health and well-being. They were passionate about the product, optimal health, and nutrition. Amway distributors were just as passionate, but the passion focused more on the business end—on selling product, free enterprise, being their own boss, and the business opportunity.

Secondly, there were also questions at the management level, a collision of corporate cultures. Each thought that its approach was superior. Dr. Tenkoff, who had assumed overall operational responsibilities from the time of my father's first stroke, found that ultimate decision-making authority had shifted to Ada, Michigan. He was no longer able to give the final managerial answers that he had been accustomed to making. This situation grew increasingly frustrating for him.

A fire at the Lakeview facility disrupted production, but the plant was put back in shape after a short repair period. There were also some product challenges. For example, both companies had a cosmetic line. NPI had Edith Rehnborg Cosmetics; Amway had Artistry. It didn't really make sense to have both lines, but which one to keep? After rounds of discussions, Edith Rehnborg Cosmetics was eventually discontinued and phased into the ARTISTRY™ line.

Another concern had to do with the food supplement offerings. The marketing staff at Amway wanted to sell the low-potency, low-concentrate product, NUTRILITE™ 100, a one-a-day type vitamin, thinking that it would be easier to sell since distributors wouldn't need any special nutrition knowledge. Bob Hunter was skeptical. The product was sugar-coated and packaged in an apothecary jar. Bob insisted that the natural concentrates were very meaningful and that Amway marketers needed to listen to their counterparts in Buena Park.

As it turned out, it was NUTRILITE DOUBLE X™ supplement, the traditional product based on natural concentrates that spearheaded market expansion. The first year alone, after the acquisition, the rollout volume for NUTRILITE DOUBLE X had quadrupled. "The margins were better," according to Bob "and people got better responses, and it just grew."

As anticipated, NUTRILITE sales accelerated when the product was wedded to the Amway distributor system. Any questions as to whether people who sold household products could effectively present and sell a nutritional regimen were quickly resolved,

Chapter Twenty Six: My Sabbatical

thanks in part to the NPI sales force, steadfastly led by the ever-ready Barney Bailey and the veteran distributors, as well as to the increasing awareness of the importance of nutrition to good health.

It was in the summer of 1975 that I sailed out of Newport Harbor, in the company of a friend and his family, in what would turn out to be an odyssey that would help to establish the groundwork for both my future life and that of Nutrilite. The journey was a combination of world and self-discovery that included elements of adventure, study, father-daughter and father-son bonding, and an extended guys' night out. I brought all my old science books and revisited all my early science and nutrition studies. Part of the thing that I really wanted to do was to get back to basics on science. I was also immensely interested in the cultures of the world, so I had a huge library of books about all the places we were going to visit. I had this underlying desire to study the cultures, eating habits, and nutritional patterns of people around the world because one of my dreams was to take the NUTRILITE brand around the world.

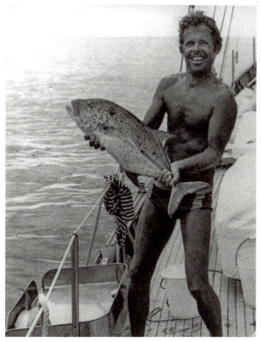

Sailing aboard the *Firebird*, late 1970s. It was great fun and a wonderful learning experience.

Using the navigation and astronomical skills first taught to me by my father, I was in many ways re-experiencing his firsthand education by means of travel. I took copious notes and photos.

For part of the trip, I was accompanied by my daughter, Lisa, and son, Rod. By this time, Lisa was an adult and working in San Francisco, while Rod was eight years old and would join me during his summer and school breaks.

It wasn't until after we reached Tahiti that the crew assumed its final working form: four reasonably compatible men on what became a remarkable sailing adventure around the world.

There were a few hitches along the way. One was that I improperly calculated the downtime of maintaining a vessel the size of the 84-foot *Firebird*. In the United States, you could get a sailboat hauled and painted in a couple of weeks. However, in other parts of the world, it takes considerably longer. When we hauled the *Firebird* out of the water in Tahiti,

Sydney, and Malta, it took a lot longer—months, in fact—and we had to do a lot of the work ourselves. Since there are certain regions you want to be in at a certain time of the year for weather, it really fouled up our sailing plans. The result was our planned two-year voyage ended up being three.

As the *Firebird* made its ports of call, 39 in total, I remained in contact with NPI. Six months after I left on my voyage, Amway and Dr. Tenkoff had reached a mutual decision that he would resign. After two decades of faithfully serving the company and bringing it successfully through its darkest hours, Dr. T could retire with a sense of a job well done. In March 1976, Bob Hunter was sent to California. He was put in charge of NPI as its Executive Vice President and Chief Executive Officer.

I had met Bob earlier—during the merger. I thought he was difficult to deal with at first, but he was a very smart scientist. As soon as he came out to California, he went to Lakeview. From his recollections of what he had seen four years earlier—during the negotiations for acquisition—he felt that very little had been done to improve the Lakeview plant. He had a deep appreciation of the significance of the natural concentrates developed by my father because all his efforts to duplicate them had failed. According to Bob:

> *I looked at Lakeview and said, 'This can't be. This is where the business starts, and this is where the heart and soul of Nutrilite is. We can't let it run down.' The equipment was getting old, leaky, and rusty and needed to be renovated.*

Bob had Lakeview spiffed up for tours. Bob was advised by his colleagues in Ada to review senior management staffing. According to Bob, "These people had a tremendous amount of knowledge and experience. I felt that they could help me. I probably needed them more than they needed me. We began to have regular staff meetings and built a good team spirit. A retirement plan was put into effect with several of the veteran NPI staff staying active in the company into the 1980s."

Also, for financial reasons Amway wanted to increase their ownership share of NPI to 80 percent or more and Bob began negotiating with the existing minority stockholders. My mother was agreeable to a buyout. Dr. Tenkoff, who Amway management had expected would be difficult, agreed to accept whatever offer my mother and her lawyers decided was fair market value. I was the only one who declined. I felt it was still a family business, and I wanted to hang in there for the long haul. I wasn't pressed further.

Chapter Twenty Six: My Sabbatical

Throughout all this—the management transition from Dr. Tenkoff to Bob Hunter, the negotiations for an Amway stock buyout, and the renovation of the Lakeview plant—I was in contact with what was happening. At every port, I would get a packet about NPI—about the research and the people—so I was able to keep up to speed with what was happening back home and send in input on products and concentrate philosophy. Bob Hunter and I exchanged taped messages frequently. I also kept in touch by radiotelephone with my family, particularly my daughter Lisa. When she wasn't in to receive my calls, I would get the news from her lively roommate, Francesca Cresci.

Amway was planning to introduce NUTRILITE food supplements in some of the places that I was visiting: Australia, Japan, Malaysia, and China. Each country represented a different marketing challenge with a different set of regulatory requirements. Taking the long view, Amway management decided not to enter any market until it could be done right, which required jumping through a seemingly endless series of regulatory hoops. In some countries, this meant reformulating the products and changing the product's potencies. This painstaking, determinedly ethical approach was to produce enormous benefits over time, but it required the resources and staying power that NPI, as an independent organization, simply didn't possess on its own. Amway made it possible.

As I was visiting these countries, sampling cultures on an individual basis, I was able to see firsthand the differences between people and places, and learn how their governments worked. You can't learn all that from books, no matter how many you have. Every restaurant meal, visit to someone's home, or simple shoreside trip to pick up supplies was an opportunity to learn something about how people felt about food, health, and nutrition.

I met some wonderful people along the way. But inevitably, the time would come when I had to lift anchor and move on.

I knew I was coming back. Jay and Rich had told me that when I returned, Bob Hunter would stay on as Chief Executive Officer. Meanwhile, I would rejoin the team as senior vice president of marketing development & research and in that capacity help take the NUTRILITE line around the world. It was something that I was really looking forward to.

In July 1978, the *Firebird* at last entered Emerald Bay in Laguna Beach, California where Joni had found a house for me to rent. I called from San Diego to let her know when I would arrive, and my family and a group of my friends were gathered on the beach to greet me.

Once arriving, I tossed out the anchor, jumped into the water, and swam to shore.

On returning, I plunged immediately back into the corporate culture. Within two weeks, I was addressing 25,000 distributors at an Amway convention in Long Beach. I had to get new shoes for the occasion because my regular shoes wouldn't fit. It had been several years since I last wore shoes, so my feet had spread. I spoke to the distributors about my voyage and about my dream for the NUTRILITE brand. Refreshed and recharged, I was ready for the opportunities and challenges ahead. It was a great joy to be back.

Just after my return, something else happened that would help determine the course of the rest of my life. I met my daughter Lisa's roommate, Francesca Cresci, and that was the end of me. She was a former Miss San Francisco, and to this day is still incredibly beautiful with an infectious wide smile and sparkling brown eyes. But, what really moved me was the fact that we liked to do everything together: tennis, surf, volleyball, ski, dance, run, hike, laugh, and she liked to be around people. It was just unbelievable; we got along so well, even though she was 17 years younger. On April 6, 1980, Francesca and I were married. A few years later, we were blessed with two incredible daughters—Kori who was born in 1983 and Jenna in 1986. Sometimes I have to pinch myself. I count myself one heck of a lucky guy.

CHAPTER TWENTY SIX: MY SABBATICAL

"Nothing great was ever achieved without enthusiasm."

—Ralph Waldo Emerson

Nutrilite Products, Inc. celebrates its 50th anniversary, September, 1984.

Chapter 27 | Coming Full Circle

It was great to be back. Every day was full of opportunity and challenges, and I loved coming to work every day.

Bob Hunter and I worked closely together on many aspects of running the company. As I soon found out, we had similar visions and compatible styles. Bob was a brilliant scientist and a smart businessman. In a way, he was *Mr. Inside* as he focused on the operations of the company, while I became *Mr. Outside* as the company's spokesperson. During the process of working together, we really hit it off and became great friends.

After two years of working in sync, Bob returned to Ada, Michigan, where he was promoted to Executive Vice President, Corporate Development. He was also given the additional responsibility of Policy Administration and oversight for Amway's outside operations like the hotels and Nutrilite. It was a big opportunity for him. So, while Bob was gone physically, we still maintained a close working relationship with respect to Nutrilite.

It was during this time, in 1983, that I was named President and Chief Executive Officer of Nutrilite. Due to major management changes in Ada, Bob returned to California in 1984. Together, once again, we formed the Office of the President and were able to lead NPI into one of its strongest growth phases to date.

During this time, we stepped up our marketing and management efforts. Amway's marketing staff members visited us frequently, and the business flourished as we worked closely together. Not only did NUTRILITE™ become a major brand in Amway's product line of offerings with sales of almost 15 percent of Amway's total in 1987, but NUTRILITE products exploded into the international markets—as had been my father's original intention.

Dad would have been very pleased to know the extent to which his food supplement had taken wings. Decades earlier in the 1950s, he had traveled abroad planning to set up distribution systems in Europe and Asia, but his efforts were opposed by Mytinger & Casselberry, Inc. Eventually, he shelved the idea as sales began to drop in the late 1950s and 1960s. However, with the marketing muscle of Amway and a product that had stood the test of time, it had become a reality. NUTRILITE products were spreading around the world. The first international market to open was Canada, which occurred in 1974, soon followed by Australia, Malaysia, and Hong Kong. By 1984, NUTRILITE food supplements were also available in the United Kingdom, Germany, Taiwan, and Japan. I had the great pleasure of introducing the NUTRILITE brand to each new market. It has been a most rewarding and exciting experience.

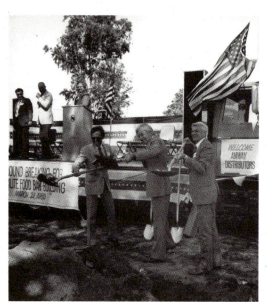

From left to right: myself, Jay Van Andel, and Robert Hunter, 1980. Breaking ground on NPI's 20,000 square foot food bar plant in Buena Park, California.

In order to keep up with the growing demand created by these new markets, NPI's headquarters and manufacturing facilities began to expand in a dramatic fashion in the late 1970s and early 1980s. A new packaging building was completed in 1980, a food bar facility was created in 1981, and a 35,000-square-foot warehouse was erected in 1987. In 1988, we acquired additional property in Buena Park and built a large 134,000-square-foot packaging and warehouse center on the other side of the Southern Pacific railroad tracks. It was an exciting time for the Buena Park area.

Meanwhile, the farm at Lakeview was refurbished, brought up-to-date architecturally, and a new protein manufacturing facility was established on-site.

Formal strategic planning and performance teams were also introduced to help guide the company into this future. This had a very positive impact on business growth, as well as on employee morale.

In the 1980s, I had attended scores of business seminars and read many business and management books in my goal of making Nutrilite one of the best managed companies on the West Coast. One business management philosophy that appealed to me immensely and seemed to make sense for NPI was the Japanese management philosophy often

Chapter Twenty Seven: Coming Full Circle

referred to as *Kaizen*. It's a philosophy based on continuous improvement. The logic being that if you practice continuous improvement at every level of the company, from managers to workers alike, then tiny, little changes add up to very big improvement over time, and you have a mentality that allows you to be ready for the big breakthroughs when they present themselves, as well. One of the best examples of a company practicing this is Toyota, which has been doing it since the 1950s. *Kaizen* gets a lot of credit for making Toyota the largest automobile company in the world.

At Nutrilite, we began our efforts at *kaizen* by bringing participative management to the employees and by giving them a piece of the action through avenues such as a good bonus structure and profit-sharing. It had a great appeal to everyone.

My father always believed in profit sharing and had set it up in 1954 at a time when it was almost unheard of—but he had created it on his terms, and it was much more paternalistic in nature. Dad wanted to share the profits of the company, but it was always done with the thought of looking out after his employees in a positive way. It was a wonderful program, but I wanted to move the company toward a slightly different type of management—one that was more participative in nature and would give employees more responsibility for their individual jobs and employ continuous improvement techniques throughout the company.

In order to accomplish this, Bob and I established a management team called the President's Team, which was headed up by the Office of the President. The team consisted of the top management in the key departments of the business, such as Research & Development, Operations, Marketing, Sales, Human Resources, and Quality Assurance. Working together, we developed a strategic plan for NPI—one that was based on a vision of where we wanted the company to be by the year 2000. During this process, we identified seven key areas that we wanted to continually improve upon. These key areas were featured in every discussion of the future we had with employees. Then, we reached out to all of them—from the employees in the agricultural fields to the employees in the laboratories, to the employees in operations, and beyond. We encouraged them to tap into their experience and insight for ideas on how to make the company better and to move it more speedily into the future.

Did You Know

… NPI's strategic plan in the 1990s focused on seven key result areas? These areas were the focus for continual quality improvement throughout the company and included the areas of:

- Human Resources
- Sales and Profits
- Science and Technology
- Marketing
- Manufacturing
- Facilities
- Information Systems

Performance teams were formed. Every employee participated in at least one performance team that met on a regular basis. These teams collected ideas on how to improve performance through continuous quality improvement in one or more of the identified key areas. The ideas were then communicated throughout the organization. Everyone in the company was involved and had a stake in achieving these continuous improvement goals. And, everyone benefited when goals were met through increased bonuses and profit sharing.

We also implemented a custom designed 15-month course for Nutrilite's managers and up-and-coming supervisors and professionals. The course helped key people improve their perspective on their role in the company and how they could improve its progress. In the process, the role of managers and supervisors changed. Instead of management telling, directing, or controlling employees, the shift was one toward that of management functioning as team leaders and process managers who facilitated such functions as problem-solving, coaching, evaluating, and planning. The end result of all this was that employees assumed more responsibility for what they were doing, learned how to function more effectively as work teams, and got more involved in where the company was going. It was amazing to see the impact that this had on morale throughout the company and on our corporate culture as a whole. It was very positive.

During this time, my children Lisa and Rod also joined the Nutrilite team. Lisa joined in the fall of 1986, and I couldn't have been more pleased. Ever since she was a high school student, I had asked her if she was interested in coming to work for the company. She always seemed a bit hesitant, concerned about her nutrition knowledge (or lack thereof), of working in a large corporation, and of the amount of travel that would be required. She was also

Chapter Twenty Seven: Coming Full Circle

nervous about speaking in front of the large audiences she had seen me address ... as well as the added responsibilities of being the granddaughter of the founder. It was my mom Edith who helped seal the deal. During one of their ongoing Sunday morning coffee conversations, Lisa broached the topic to her grandmother, who thought about it for a moment and promptly said, "Oh yes, you can do it. I want you to do it!" It turned out to be just the nudge my daughter needed at that time in her life.

Lisa started off in a training program and soon became acquainted with every department at NPI. A six-month stint in Ada, Michigan, provided her with an even deeper appreciation of the business. She worked closely during this period with Barney Bailey, whose in-depth knowledge of intricacies of the business made him an ideal guide and mentor. She also worked very closely with Penny Sterling, a dynamic woman who had joined us from Studio Girl Cosmetics. Penny was a one-woman marketing department. She was extraordinarily knowledgeable about the products, nutrition, sales, and marketing. When Barney and Penny retired, Lisa became the manager of Nutrition & Sales Services. The position soon blossomed to encompass guest relations. Today, she is in charge of Nutrilite's corporate culture and works closely with employees to ensure that the corporate culture originated by my father continues on into the future.

My two eldest children, Rod and Lisa, and me, 1993.

My son, Rod, also came aboard. His first job was in 1983 at the age of 16, washing buckets in the tableting department and spreading raw material on dehydration trays in the granulation department. A couple of years later, he started at the University of California at Berkeley, majoring in history and studying Italian. During the summer of his sophomore year, he worked for two months for Amway in Milan. While working in the distribution section, he realized that he should probably study something more useful for business than European liberal arts. When he returned home that summer, he decided that, although he was not willing to go as far as changing his major to one of the hard sciences, he could at least switch his geographical focus to Asia. Asian studies seemed to be more practical for the future, certainly so if he were to join Nutrilite, which was starting to grow sales in Asian markets rapidly. He changed his major to Japanese history, spent a semester at a university in Osaka, Japan, and started learning Japanese.

When Rod graduated from Berkeley, he went to Tokyo and joined the marketing department of Kato Spring, a maker of precision parts for the electronics and automobile industries. He was the only non-Japanese employee of the company and had a unique learning experience for two years. In 1993, he returned to California and joined NPI's marketing department and worked as a product manager for products sold in Japan. After a year or so with us, he decided to get some academic training in business and was accepted to UCLA's Anderson School of Management. During his graduate schooling, he worked one summer as an intern for Amway in Japan and was very impressed with the operations there. The following year he returned to Asia, this time to Vietnam where he led a group of graduate students on a two-week business tour of that country. Accompanying him on the trip was his girlfriend, Gweneth. It was in Vietnam that he proposed to her, and after they returned home, they were married.

Once Rod graduated from UCLA with a master's degree in business administration, he followed Gweneth to Boston for her graduate studies in International Relations at Tufts Fletcher School of Law and Diplomacy. Rod joined the large pension fund TIAA-CREF where he helped run their Japanese stock fund. He commuted back and forth between Boston and his job in New York for two years while Gweneth finished her studies. In 1998, Rod and Gweneth returned to Los Angeles, where he joined another investment fund, but also worked with us consulting about Japan and other Asian markets and participating in a number of distributor events. Meanwhile, Gweneth joined Nutrilite. She worked for two years as the director of the Center for Optimal Health at Nutrilite and helped get that program off the ground.

Chapter Twenty Seven: Coming Full Circle

In 2007, Rod was recruited by a London-based investment fund to manage their Japanese stock fund. After a year in London, Rod was transferred by the company to Hong Kong, where he, Gweneth and their three children now live. He still works closely with Nutrilite in the different Asian markets, and, hopefully, one day he and Gweneth will return to Nutrilite in some major capacity.

During this time, new markets were continuing to open for the NUTRILITE brand around the world, the biggest of which was the launch of the NUTRILITE brand in China in 1998. For some time prior to this, the use of NUTRILITE food supplements had been expanding in the Asia market among non-Chinese, particularly those living in Hong Kong, Taiwan, and Malaysia.

The China market turned out to be an enormous one for Amway, and Amway rapidly became one of the top direct-selling companies in China. However, it was not without some challenges. The opening of China brought a dramatic cultural conflict for the Chinese people: 50 years of strict, anticapitalist state regulation versus 4,000 years of holistic health tradition and an equally long history of Chinese entrepreneurial skill. Nutrilite's expansion in China was both protean and dramatic in ways that Chinese authorities hadn't seen in over a half a century. This was capitalism, but with a difference: instead of a major corporation with a heavy visible presence, NUTRILITE products were expanding through lightly capitalized entrepreneurs in a tremendous release of individual energy that had been stifled since the late 1940s. Unfortunately, this newfound entrepreneurial spirit led to a proliferation of unscrupulous pyramid fraud operators looking to take advantage of those individuals seeking real and legitimate business opportunities. These frauds caused an extreme breakdown in the culturally relevant social order.

Alarmed, in April 1998, the Chinese government rather than taking the time to adopt laws distinguishing legitimate direct selling from fraudulent pyramid operations, chose to simply ban all direct selling, including Amway Asia Pacific Ltd. and other direct marketing organizations from door-to-door sales. Under a new system, Amway was granted a special license together with 10 other foreign invested companies to sell NUTRILITE food supplements, as well as dishwashing soap, window cleaner, and other items through retail stores and salespersons assigned to the stores. In December 2005,

Did You Know

… in 1994 Amway Corporation purchased the remaining shares of NPI and Nutrilite became a division of Amway? This decision ultimately changed the face of business as new technology and systems were put into place. It was the stimulus to take the NUTRILITE brand to the next level.

… Amway China is now the biggest market of any country for the NUTRILITE brand, with sales in excess of $1.3 billion in 2008? In addition, the Chinese version of the NUTRILITE trademark [纽崔莱 (NIU CUI LAI)] has been granted "Famous Mark" status, giving the mark expanded trademark protection.

China, as part of its obligation to join the World Trade Organization, adopted the Direct Sales Management Regulation under which Amway was subsequently issued a direct selling license on December 1, 2006. This has worked very well, and today Amway has more than 200 shops throughout China.

Soon after the NUTRILITE brand entered the market, Lisa and Rod joined me on a memorable trip to China where we had the opportunity to retrace my father's earlier steps in order to do a video about his life. Lisa loved that trip:

> *It was wonderful tracing grandpa's footsteps. It was different than I imagined. Before the visit, everything I had seen—photographs and videos—were in black and white or in grey tones. However, once in Shanghai, everything I could see was in Technicolor. It was the most amazing thing to me. Tree-lined streets and open markets with colorful fruits and vegetables meticulously displayed. Beautiful neighborhoods and parks. So lovely, so green. And the people, so loving and friendly.*

During the filming, we visited the places where my father had lived and worked. We could feel his presence as we visited one particular garden and imagined him foraging for leafy greens. Some of the International Settlement remained intact—similar to what he had experienced. It was a moving occasion for us as we reflected on his time in China and what he had learned there nearly a century ago.

In 2005, NUTRILITE DOUBLE X™ supplement entered the Chinese market and was met with warm recognition at the various rallies that Rod and I attended and addressed. With the introduction of DOUBLE X into the land whose holistic approach to health had inspired it, my father's — and Nutrilite's — story had come full circle.

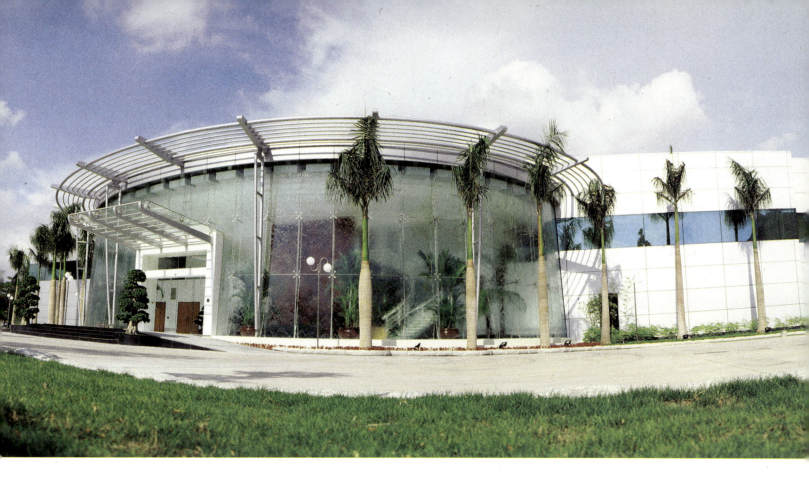

Manufacturing facility in Guangzhou, China, 2004. This beautiful and state-of-the-art manufacturing facility opened its doors in 1995 and is where more than 170 Amway products, including NUTRILITE brand food supplements, are manufactured.

"We are only beginning to comprehend the extent of our dependence on the compounds synthesized in plants … the chemistry of the life process of an animal is determined by the chemistry of a plant."

—Carl F. Rehnborg

In September 2009, the NUTRILITE brand celebrated its 75th anniversary in business. From the beginning, the concept of balance has resonated strongly for the brand.

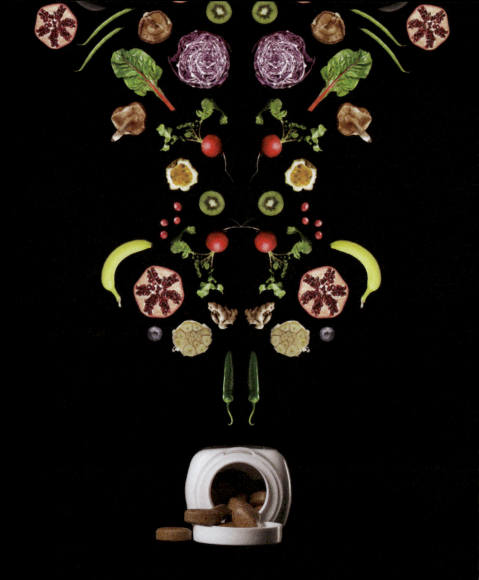

NUTRITIONAL BALANCE IS SECOND NATURE TO US

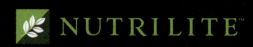

Chapter 28 | The Perfect Balance

Now that NUTRILITE DOUBLE X™ Food Supplement has launched in China, people often ask me, "Does this mean it's the end of the dream?" This generally gets my heart racing and my blood boiling, and I like to say, "Of course not, the dream is far from over." As a matter of fact, we're just at the beginning and still have a very long way to go.

It has been almost 100 years since my father had his seminal insights about a plant-rich diet as a key foundation for health. During that time he recognized that while both a plant-rich diet and supplementing the diet were important, they were also a part of the larger optimal health picture that was really geared at helping people take responsibility for their own health. That meant not only good nutrition and a plant-based diet, but also exercise and positive thinking.

How clear the wisdom of his early insights now seem. Here we are today, years later, and the foundation for optimal health has become more important than ever. Chronic, age-related health conditions such as heart disease, cancer, and diabetes are alarmingly on the rise. This is the case in almost every country. Despite these daunting public health statistics, there is exciting news. Optimal health is within reach of every individual. A vast body of research, including our own, recommends a diet rich in fruits and vegetables, frequent and regular physical activity, healthy ways to cope with stress, and healthy lifestyle choices as effective ways to optimize health and minimize health risks. The benefits of these types of changes are quickly evident and have the potential to manifest and multiply over a lifetime.

Today at Nutrilite, you'll find that we position our products in the context of an overall approach to optimal health—just as my father had proposed. We design and develop our products to supplement a healthy diet from the best nutrient-rich plant materials available. In fact, this attention to plant quality is such a fundamental part of the NUTRILITE™ brand, that we've incorporated it into our tagline: "BEST OF NATURE. BEST OF SCIENCE."

We have a firm commitment to continue to incorporate the best of nature and science into high quality, scientifically sound products to help consumers travel on their path toward optimal health. Over the years, both areas have been in a constant state of evolution as new information becomes available on the importance of nature and science in helping people achieve optimal health. I firmly believe that the tremendous growth in recent years in understanding both nature and science will catapult the brand into an exciting new age where more and more people will be aware of its significance and its impact on health.

Best of Nature

The rapid expansion of the Nutrilite farms in recent years makes the "Best of Nature" platform more robust than ever. It all started with my father's first farm, a 3.6-acre (1 ½ hectare) plot bought back in the early 1940s in the San Fernando Valley. It was there that he experimented and developed the first foundations of what we call Nutrilite Farming Practices. These earlier practices were adopted to protect the plants from pesticides and herbicides so that they wouldn't harm the people who consumed them later. Today we continue in his mission, and have farms not only in Lakeview, California but also in Mexico, Washington state, and Brazil, and each is certified organic. Not only are they certified organic, but in recent years we have raised the bar beyond organic standards by implementing what we call "Sustainable Farming and Permacultural Practices." Sustainable farming and permacultural practices perpetuate and enhance the health and vitality of the entire farm: soil, water, air, plants, and the people who live around and work on the farm. We do this because when this is done, a "perfect balance" is achieved and everyone benefits. The end result, of course, is to produce the most nutritious crops and plant materials for use in our products to better enable people to maintain a plant-based diet as they move toward optimal health.

The focus of the Lakeview farm has evolved over the years. Historically, it was the

Did You Know

… NUTRILITE is the only global brand to grow, harvest, and process plants on its own certified organic farms?

Based on an independent review in 2008 by international research firm Euromonitor Consultancy.

… ideas that my father grasped intuitively long ago have since been verified in the formal scientific community? For example, BIOTROL, the first commercial biological pest control introduced by Nutrilite Products, Inc. at a time when nonchemical methods of fighting insect pests were virtually unheard of, has since been joined by organic and "less toxic" methods of pest control that now account for almost half of the home and garden market, according to the U.S. Environmental Protection Agency.

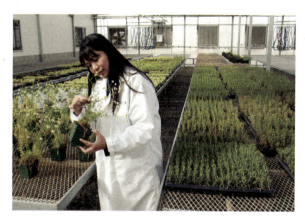

An experimental green house in Lakeview, California, 2003. The majority of our agriculture research takes place at Lakeview's Agriculture Research Farm. Tours are available by appointment.

"workhorse" farm where many of the long-term crops were grown. However, with encroaching development near the property in recent years, the majority of the original 2,000-plus acres (800-plus hectares) has been sold. Today, Lakeview serves as our primary agricultural research station, and it is the center of knowledge and innovation in agricultural research that supports the needs of our farms around the world.

In addition to an ongoing focus on Sustainable Farming Practices, our Lakeview facility also serves as the heart of our concentrate development efforts. Here our researchers are leading the way to improve existing plant concentrates, identify new plant materials from around the world, and experiment with growing and harvesting practices that optimize the phytonutrient content found within the plants we grow. It is an extraordinarily exciting time of discovery for our researchers.

Since my father's time, the number of plant concentrates found in our food supplements has soared—from only a handful in the early 1930s to more than 130 today.

Our ability to control the quality of these concentrates has also evolved significantly, perhaps most dramatically since the turn of the century. Since my father's time and until recently,

THE NUTRILITE STORY

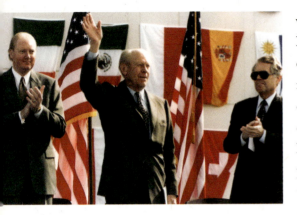

Former United States President Gerald R. Ford (center) helps dedicate the new Powder Drink facility at Lakeview, California, 1998. Accompanying him on the podium are Dave Van Andel and myself.

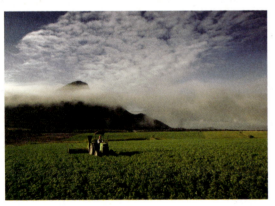

Rancho El Petacal, Jalisco, Mexico, circa 2004. By the year 2000, the El Petacal farm had grown from 900 acres (364 hectares) in 1992 to 1,400 (566 hectares).

we operated on the principle of vertical integration. Simply put, this means having control from seed to finished product. However, with the increased demand for product and with the increased number of breakthroughs regarding phytonutrients around the world, we found that we could no longer effectively operate in this vertical integration fashion alone. In an effort to continually improve what we are doing and to expand our capability to deliver high quality plant materials, we developed the NutriCert™ program. This program uses horizontal integration, which allows us to find farmers with farming values similar to ours and train them to grow crops according to our strict farming practices, including organic specifications. It allows Nutrilite to be more responsive to the needs of the market and ensures maximum control over our plant concentrate supply chain—while providing knowledge in sustainable farming practices to local farming communities. It's a win-win situation that appeals to everyone.

Besides the strong emphasis on research and development, Lakeview is also an education and training facility. Children from nearby schools come to raise organic vegetation for school projects. It's also a favorite destination choice among distributors from around the world. While touring the facility, distributors have a chance to visit our experimental greenhouses, test plots, and earthworm beds to learn more about the innovative sustainable farming practices we employ. They also have the opportunity to see firsthand how we turn the plants we harvest into the concentrates for use in our products. It's a fun hands-on learning experience that they can share with their distributors and customers when they return to their respective markets to help them better understand the unique benefits of our products.

Visitors also have a chance to visit the Carl F. Rehnborg Museum. Housed in the Quonset hut (which was moved from Buena Park to Lakeview in the 1950s), it holds my father's living quarters and conjures up memories from decades ago. The museum also contains an assortment of historic documents, products, and equipment. From past to present, visitors can tour our immaculate agricultural and manufacturing facilities to better understand how our products are made.

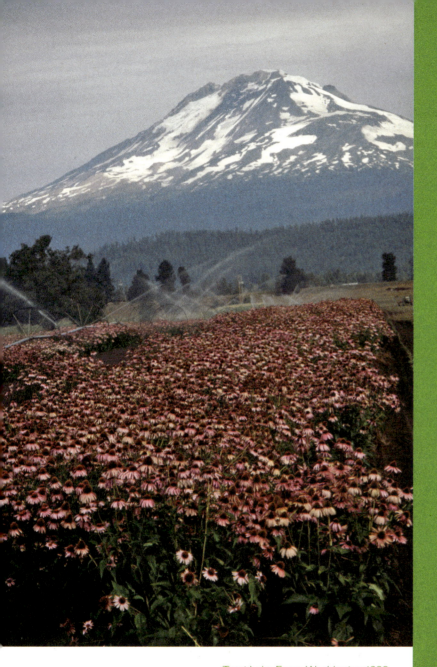

Trout Lake Farm, Washington, 1998. Located in the foothills of the Cascade Mountains, the farm's irrigation is provided by the White Salmon River, fed by glaciers from the mountains.

Did You Know

... in 2004, Nutrilite began the NutriCert™ program? The program establishes sustainable, organic farming guidelines for farmers interested in growing crops for NUTRILITE brand supplements. The five main principles of the program include:

(1) Encourage Diversity – on the farms, cultivate vegetation in layers (such as herbs, bushes, and trees in the same field), and practice green soil cover, crop rotation, intercropping, integration with animal husbandry, the use of beneficial insects and microorganisms, green manure, and forest and native vegetation.

(2) Build Soil – use composted manures and crop residues, rock powders, mineral fertilizers, and beneficial microorganisms; erosion control; mulching; good use of irrigation and water resources; and no soil burning.

(3) Don't Contaminate – use integrated pest management techniques; adhere to organic certification standards; and protect from neighboring and eventual sources of contamination.

(4) Ensure Traceability – every action performed on the farm must be documented and controlled. Input records, seed lots, crop rotations and more provide quality assurance in the final product.

(5) Build a Healthy Social Environment – on the farms and in the surrounding community, provide farm employees and their families the opportunity for personal development, healthcare and education.

The Nutrilite Story

Freshly gathered acerola cherries at Fazenda Nutriorganica, Ceará, Brazil, circa 2005. Acerola is grown year round. Harvested when green at the peak of their vitamin C content, they are dried at the onsite production facility and then shipped to Lakeview, California for processing into NUTRILITE exclusive concentrates. Other crops include passion fruit, pineapples, guava, and tropical herbs.

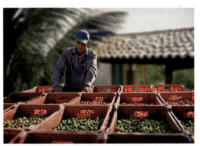

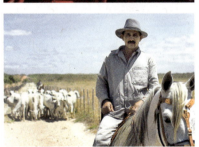

Worker at Fazenda Nutriorganica in Ceará, Brazil, circa 2005. Over 300 head of cattle on the farm provide natural fertilizer for the crops.

Our farm in El Petacal, Mexico, is devoted to the long-term production crops that used to be grown at Lakeview, plants such as alfalfa, parsley, spinach, broccoli, and citrus. Located near the Pacific coast in southwestern Mexico, the farm boasts a wonderful and unique growing climate with plenty of sunshine and water—the perfect conditions for growing the nutrient-rich crops that we use in our products.

This farm has become an integral part of the community. For example, here we run a Cultural and Education Support Center that provides basic education on nutrition and ecology. In addition, we hired Dr. Sandra Romo—El Petacal's only medical practitioner—as a staff physician in 1996 to help transform the quality of life for the roughly 600 people in this tiny mountain village. With her hard work, passion, and commitment, Dr. Romo has been able to bring essential healthcare services previously unheard of to the community, including dietary counseling, childhood immunizations, pap smears, pregnancy checkups and delivery referrals, and trauma care. According to Dr. Romo, "It has been an exciting opportunity to put together a clinic serving a community that had no medical service whatsoever. I could equip it as I wanted, and I was given the time I need to serve Nutrilite workers and their families as well as the larger community."

This is what Sustainable Farming and Permacultural Practices are all about.

Besides the farms in California and Mexico, we also have the largest certified organic herb farm in North America: Trout Lake Farm. It's located in a pristine valley in south central Washington state. This farm comprises an expansive 700 acres (283 hectares) where more than 70 botanicals and three million pounds of herbs can be grown annually. Here, such herbs as echinacea, rosemary, peppermint, and nettle are harvested for use in NUTRILITE food supplements. We are also growing nutrient-rich blueberries and are exploring the possibility of growing other types of berries for use in our products as well. Just like other Nutrilite farms, the Trout Lake farm also supports many local community projects including the Trout Lake Fair, the local baseball league, the area arts council, and the local public school.

In 1998, Nutrilite acquired its largest farm, Fazenda Nutriorganica in Ubajara,

Chapter Twenty Eight: The Perfect Balance

Ceará, Brazil—just three degrees south of the equator. This property spans an expansive 4,100 acres (1,658 hectares). From the start, we partnered with the state of Ceará to obtain farmland and critical support with water. In return, we agreed to help create jobs and learning opportunities for the local community. I'm happy to report that, to date, we have exceeded the government's expectations in this area.

One of our goals in Brazil was to identify the acerola variety with optimal nutrient content and production yield. To do this, we screened over 70 varieties of acerola trees. Once we identified those trees with the highest nutritional value and yield, we planted more than 100,000 trees making our Ubajara farm the single largest organic acerola farm in the world. In addition, we have provided the local farmers—farmers who are part of the NutriCert program—with these healthier acerola seedlings along with nutrient-rich compost to help ensure their success. The Brazilian government loves what we are doing. Land that was once desolate and idle now flourishes with healthy crops.

We've also begun a reforestation program along the banks of the nearby Jaburu River that has helped increase biodiversity and maintain the natural equilibrium of the surrounding area.

In addition, we have focused our efforts on building a healthy social environment around the farm, providing employees and their families with the opportunity for personal development, including education and training. The results have been very positive. Story after story has poured forth describing the powerful impact the company is having on people's lives—from improving self-esteem and better socializing to advancing education.

According to Neal Brophy, who has managed the Nutrilite farms since 2001 and has been with the company for more than two decades, "It has boiled down to getting the right people in place," people with the passion to do the right thing. This is the case for many Nutrilite employees. One such person is Richard Charity, Farm Development Manager, whom Neal refers to as "the Pied Piper" of the Brazilian farm. According to Neal, "He's reaching out to the people and community and making the farm more than just a workplace, but rather a second home and a place full of positive energy."

Besides being full of positive energy, the Ubajara farming operation is full of learning opportunities for the community. For example, we have sponsored a local public school, which sits on the farmland. The school is equipped with computers and allows the

The Nutrilite Story

local children to expand their knowledge and vision. Here, children are inspired to learn more about science, agriculture, and working with nature. One enterprising 14-year-old boy who attends the school wrote a fantastic paper on his memories of his community environment, most of which were the farm itself. The essay was such a success, he had the opportunity to travel and meet the president of Brazil. A year later, a nine-year-old girl that participated in a drawing contest for schools nationwide, also left her insights into the importance of sports and education in the fight against drug abuse; she also accepted the prize from the president's hands. That's exactly what Nutrilite is about: making a difference, one person at a time, by giving people the tools they need to reach their personal best.

"We need to continue to transform our farms and the communities around them," commented Neal. "We are making it better for the local community. We can be really proud of what we're doing."

The whole goal is to make each farm sustainable. "I want these farms to be living organisms long after I'm gone," adds Neal.

That's exactly what my father would have wanted.

Did You Know

... in the 1950s Nutrilite sponsored children's nutrition assessments at Stanford University to understand the impact of nutrition on cognitive function? Later in 1989, the C.F. Rehnborg Professorship in Disease Prevention was established at the Stanford University School of Medicine. The C.F. Rehnborg Professorship was endowed with contributions from the Rehnborg family, Nutrilite Foundation, and Amway Corporation, and perpetuates ideals of my father by helping, encouraging, and advancing the study of disease prevention.

Nutrilite has collaborated with other prestigious institutions over the years including: Kyoto Prefectural University of Medicine in Kyoto, Japan; Sun Yat-sen University in Guangzhou, China; Yonsei University in Seoul, Korea; the Center for Genetics, Nutrition and Health in Washington, D.C.; and the California State Polytechnic University in Pomona, California.††

†† The listed institutions provide independent scientific research services to the Nutrilite Health Institute (NHI). The research is funded by NHI and the inclusion of these institutions is not an endorsement of NUTRILITE branded products.

Chapter Twenty Eight: The Perfect Balance

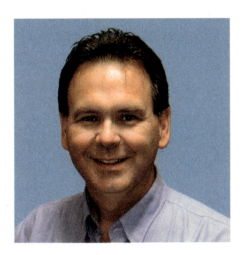

Neal Brophy
Director of Global Agribusiness, 2009.

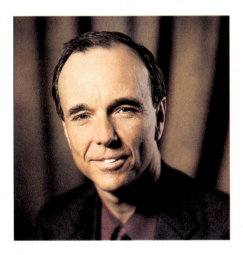

John Lindseth
Vice President of Nutrilite Operations, 2008.

Best of Science

Equally important to our investment in organic, sustainable, and permacultural farming practices, and development of nutritious plant concentrates, are our investments in research—our "Best of Science" platform.

Probably our most significant investment in science was the creation of the Rehnborg Center for Nutrition & Wellness. Established in 1996 and renamed the Nutrilite Health Institute (NHI) in 2002, it's basically a corporate university within the Amway organization.

The spark for the Institute occurred in the 1980s as the business began to grow rapidly around the world. While studying business management philosophies during that time, I found that a number of successful companies, including Disney and 3M, embraced a corporate university concept where they had dedicated groups of people who were focused on the company's future—exploring options on how to do things better, ensuring a strong knowledge base, and educating their employees and people on how to best carry forth those new ideas.

In the early 1990s, a Nutrilite employee broached the topic of a corporate university, and the timing was right. It made sense, and we moved ahead rapidly to get it into place. We established the Rehnborg Center for Nutrition & Wellness. I took on the role of its president, and in order to ensure a smooth transition and to allow me to focus on the development of its strategy and my role as Nutrilite Global Brand Ambassador, John Lindseth came to California in April 1996 as Director of Nutrilite Operations. With a job well-done, about one year later, he was promoted to Vice President of Nutrilite Operations.

In order to fulfill my father's and my plan for a strong scientific focus, Dr. George Calvert was asked to lead the science team for the Rehnborg Center. Under the combined leadership of Dr. Calvert, Robin Dykhouse, and Audra Davies all areas of

The Nutrilite Story

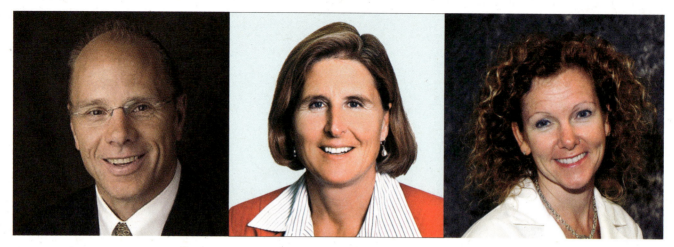

George D. Calvert, Ph.D. Vice President, Research & Development and Supply Chain, 2008.

Robin Dykhouse, Vice President, Consumables Research & Development, 2008.

Audra Davies, Director, Nutrition Product Development, 2008.

scientific credibility from clinical studies, bio-assays, product development, varietal screenings, agricultural methods, concentrate, and phytonutrient identification and analysis with chromatography and nutrigenomics were accelerated to set the highest level of scientific excellence in Nutrilite's history.

Filling the original vision, the Nutrilite Health Institute, as it is called today, is involved in cutting-edge research, maintaining and expanding an extensive knowledge base, and providing continuing education and training for staff and distributors around the world. The focus of the Institute is on phytonutrients, nutrition, and optimal health. It also keeps intact two of my father's deepest wishes. First, it allows visiting distributors to see firsthand what we're all about, the care with which NUTRILITE products are made, and the science behind them. Second, it establishes the formal research center that had been one of my father's greatest unfulfilled dreams back in the 1950s.

In sharp contrast to my father working alone in the Balboa boat shed, there are now more than 100 dedicated scientists, researchers, and educators supporting the Nutrilite Health Institute and the NUTRILITE brand and within the entire Amway family we have 500 scientists working collectively in 65 laboratories to develop products that make a difference.

All told, our scientists within Amway have more than 100 advanced degrees across a wide range of disciplines: biochemistry, chemistry, microbiology, molecular biology, food science, horticultural and plant sciences, and

Did You Know

… NHI scientists have collaborated with scientists from Interleukin Genetics to confirm the link between nutrition and genotype? Together, they studied the effect of an herbal formula on the production of Interleukin-1 (IL-1) in healthy adults. IL-1 is a powerful mediator of the inflammatory response and an emerging predicator for heart health. People who are IL-1 positive produce more IL-1 and another marker of inflammation, C-reactive protein (CRP).

The researchers screened the participants to confirm their IL-1 genotype and randomly assigned them to take either the herbal blend or a placebo daily for 12 weeks. The blend contained four herbs—rosehips extract, blueberry and blackberry powder, and grapevine extract—selected from hundreds of plant extracts based on their ability to reduce the production of IL-1 in laboratory studies.

Results of this groundbreaking research were published in the prestigious scientific journal *Nutrition* in 2007. In almost half of the participants who were IL-1 positive—and predisposed to produce more inflammatory markers—the herbal formula was able to reduce IL-1 gene expression by 60 percent, IL-1 production by 40 percent, and CRP production by 20 percent or more. All of these results were statistically significant compared to the placebo. These findings indicate that the herbal blend helped balance IL-1 gene expression and help maintain healthy CRP levels already in the normal range.

This study is just one example of NHI's commitment to developing nutritional products that work with an individual's genetic makeup to help them better achieve optimal health and perfect balance.

toxicology—to name a few. As of 2008, we have 32 employees with doctorate degrees. All totaled, there are approximately 4,500 years of total R&D and quality assurance experience represented in the organization. Needless to say, if there's a technical challenge confronting us, we have a wealth of expertise to find a solution.

Also helping to guide our efforts is NHI's Scientific Advisory Board. Established in 2004, the board brings together leading experts in the fields of nutrition, health, and genetics around the world. This prestigious 10-member panel provides invaluable experience and insight during the development of NUTRILITE brand products and is instrumental in guiding the brand into the future.

The focus of our research from the very beginning has been on the understanding of the key concepts that contribute to optimal health, in particular, the role of a plant-rich diet in sustaining and balancing the body's myriad functions. Almost 100 years ago, my father had theorized there must be hundreds or thousands of compounds in plants that were important in human nutrition. We have been studying these for a very long time, identifying them in different plants, understanding their structure, and then how they function to support health. It continues to be the primary thrust of our research. Interestingly, phytonutrient research is now recognized around the world as having a very high impact on human health. I am proud to say that we were there when phytonutrient research began, and we are at the leading edge now, and we plan and intend to lead the way into the future. It seems with each passing day there is a new discovery in phytonutrient research that further confirms the potential for plants and a plant-rich diet to optimize health and reduce risks.

One new field of research that supports our work is that of *nutrigenomics*. This realm of study examines the interactions of genes (our DNA) and nutrients and their effects on health. It's an incredible

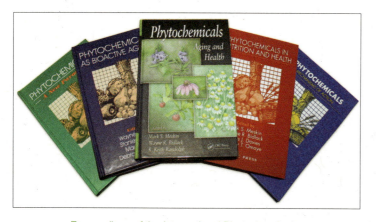

Proceedings of the *International Phytochemical Conference*. Since 1996, Nutrilite Health Institute (formerly the Rehnborg Center for Nutrition & Wellness) has partnered with California State Polytechnic University, Pomona, to host the biennial conference, which provides an excellent opportunity to bring nutrition and phytochemical experts together to explore and exchange ideas in this exciting field of research.

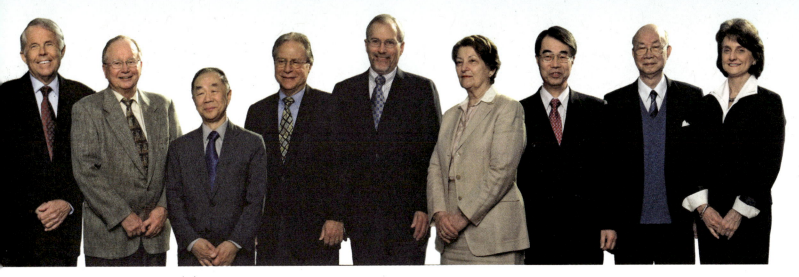

NHI's Scientific Advisory Board, 2006. From left to right: Sam Rehnborg, Ph.D., Thomas Slaga, Ph.D., Junshi Chen, M.D., Kenneth Kornman, Ph.D., D.D.S., Stephen Fortmann, M.D., Artemis Simopoulos, M.D., Hoyoku Nishino, M.D., Z.C. Ho, M.D., Ph.D., and Ruth DeBusk, Ph.D., R.D. (not shown, Young-Joon Surh, Ph.D.)

Did You Know

… a study found that one's lifestyle choices (food choices, response to stress, smoking, exercise, quality of relationships, social support network) may actually change gene expression in hundreds of genes in only a few months?

field and carries enormous potential to make a difference in peoples' health. Certainly, this is where we are finding that phytonutrients have a major role to play. We have been pioneering in nutrigenomics since the mapping of the human genome was completed in 2003. We knew at that time that this accomplishment would set the stage for a rapid increase in the ability to investigate the role of genes and nutrients in health and disease, something that most medical people had known was there, but had difficulty measuring.

To facilitate our entry into this arena, Amway Corporation partnered with Interleukin Genetics, a biotechnology company with strong technical expertise in genomics and a proven ability to develop diagnostic and therapeutic products. Together, we have developed technology to help people use their DNA—their own genetic material—to identify certain unique health risks. Once people know these risks, they can apply targeted nutritional and

THE NUTRILITE STORY

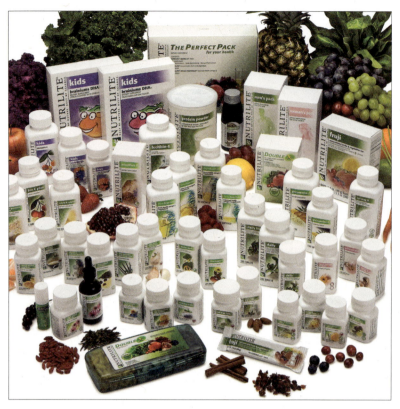

Sampling of NUTRILITE brand products, 2009. We know that consumers demand choices, so we are actively looking at different delivery forms; not just tablets and capsules that one swallows, but gels, liquids, chews, sticks, twist tubes, sprays, powders, bars, and quick melts.

other optimal health solutions to better protect their health.

While my father could only speculate on the many mechanisms contributing to optimal health, we now are using science's most powerful tools to develop tomorrow's plant-based solutions. We've certainly come a long way in our understanding of the function of the phytonutrients in our products. Now, armed with this knowledge, we have been able to create even better products that deliver greater benefits.

We have made significant investments into these new technology tools as well as continue to strengthen our internal and external scientific resources. One key way we leverage this Best of Science power is by identifying and substantiating the functions of ingredients and products. We refer to this process as the *efficacy substantiation continuum*. Whereas we historically relied primarily on third party literature to substantiate ingredient and product function, we now have moved to a bio-directed model. This includes high throughput bioassay screenings to discover new ingredient functions, bio-directed fractionation (an experimental design that aims to determine the components in an ingredient responsible for a specific effect), consumer research to identify key product experience and functional attributes (which includes identifying unmet consumer needs and testing the product to ensure those needs are met), and human clinical trials where the function of an ingredient or product within the human body is evaluated

Did You Know

… as of 2009, we have completed 50 clinical studies on NUTRILITE concentrates, products, and prototypes? We also have more than 170 granted patents and patent applications worldwide supporting more then 250 products. Product innovation remains a hallmark of the NUTRILITE brand and will always be an important part of our "BEST OF NATURE, BEST OF SCIENCE" heritage.

For additional information behind the science of NUTRILITE brand products, see Appendix 4: Best of Science (Publications List).

---

under carefully controlled conditions. This continuum allows us to target a specific functional outcome, establish mechanism-of-action targets, research and screen hundreds of ingredients in bioassays reflecting the mechanistic targets, identify active compounds through biofractionation and move to human clinicals with more confidence in our outcomes.

We didn't have these capabilities in 2000. Since that time, we have successfully applied these research tools on three products developed to support heart, bone, and upper respiratory health. These positive results indicate that this model is predictable—a critical component for our success as well as a unique competitive advantage.

Owing to our investments in all these research areas, we have established ourselves as a leader in nutrition and optimal health. Groundbreaking? Pioneering? Absolutely! Just as my father's discoveries were groundbreaking in his time.

Best of You

We've come a long way since Dad's time and will continue to forge ahead combining the "Best of Nature" and the "Best of Science" to help people all over the world become their "Best of You." We have no intention of resting on our laurels—there are just too many more exciting discoveries to be made.

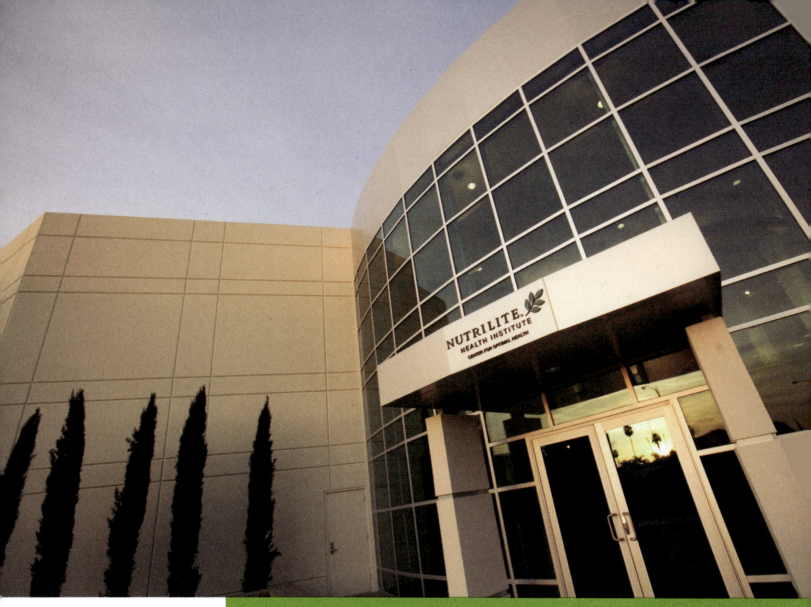

The Nutrilite Health Institute's Center for Optimal Health, 2006. Completed in 2005, this first class 33,000 square foot facility is designed to motivate lasting lifestyle change and houses various interactive product, history, science, and nutrition-related exhibits.

"There is nothing like a dream to create the future."

—Sam Rehnborg

Chapter 29 | A Look at Today and a Glimpse into the Future

As I sit in my office and reflect upon where we are and where we are going, I can't help but smile inwardly. Just one glance out the window and I can see Nutrilite employees gathered together laughing. It's a happy place, a place where people enjoy working. Dad would have liked that.

Across the courtyard, the Nutrilite Health Institute's Center for Optimal Health, completed in 2005, sparkles in the summer sun. As you enter the foyer, an inscription that captures the essence of healthy living welcomes you: "Optimal health compels you to choose every day to be your best by selecting the right foods and supplements, engaging in exercise and rest and incorporating healthy habits and balance in everything you do." To be sure, the Center was created with one goal in mind: helping people lead healthier lives.

It's a goal my father was passionate about. It's a goal I'm passionate about, and it's a goal that Amway has given top priority. I couldn't be any prouder to be part of a company that shares my father's core values and provides products, programs, and opportunities to help people reach their personal best.

As president of the NHI since its inception, I've had the privilege of traveling the globe to share this message of optimal health. During the course of my travels, I've had the good fortune to speak with hundreds of thousands of people every year, encouraging them to take action and embrace the concepts of optimal health. I'm pleased to report that this movement, which is the cornerstone of helping people to lead happier, healthier lives, is gaining momentum.

Today, we are seeing more people beginning to take responsibility for their own health and well-being. It has become a top priority. People are exercising more these days, and they are choosing to eat a healthier diet by selecting more fruits and vegetables and fewer processed foods. Even the word "phytonutrient" seems to be popping up everywhere, from the daily news to mainstream advertising. All of a sudden, we now recognize phytonutrients in our orange juice and even in our ketchup. Type the word "phytonutrient" in an Internet search engine and hundreds of thousands of references will come up. These phytonutrients are what my father referred to decades ago as "associated food factors."

Can you imagine what would happen if enough people embrace the idea that healthy living is important in their lives and consequently make healthful changes to their diet and lifestyle? We would reach a point where more middle-aged adults automatically equate healthy aging with being active and maintaining a healthy body weight. We would see children and adults reach for fruit rather than junk food; city planners would automatically include sidewalks, bicycle lanes, and other features to promote active lifestyles among their citizens; and insurance companies would reward healthy behaviors that help reduce the risk of disease, rather than only paying when people became sick or injured. In the process, we would save millions of lives and billions of dollars and more importantly make a real contribution to our families and to our communities.

Small, consistent changes—baby steps—in our diet and lifestyle are key to helping us achieve our optimal health goals. That is what we are encouraging at NHI's Center for Optimal Health.

We have been taking this message of healthy living around the world.

In 1997, we created the Nutrilite Experience under the leadership of Nutrilite Brand Ambassador, Bill Dombrowski. The Nutrilite Experience is an intensive three-day program for distributor leaders focusing on achieving optimal health, brand knowledge, and selling techniques. Not only do distributor leaders have the chance to meet the people behind the products—the scientists, the workers on the manufacturing lines, and other staff, but they also have the opportunity to focus on their own health and make meaningful changes in their lifestyle.

It starts with our Medical Director, Dr. Duke Johnson, sharing our Optimal Health philosophy. Then a complete fitness and blood analysis is led by exercise physiologist Sean Foy and his team of fitness experts. Participants are asked a series of questions and

Did You Know

… according to a United States nationwide survey, more Americans are saying that they are eating healthy foods and keeping fit? In a 2008 survey of more than 780 adults, who when asked about choosing a healthful diet and engaging in regular exercise, 43 percent said "I'm already doing it," versus 38 percent in 2002. Only 19 percent of those surveyed put themselves in the "don't bother me" category, not believing diet and exercise are important. This was down from 32 percent in 2002.

… the American Institute for Cancer Research and the World Cancer Research Fund published a massive tome in 1997 concluding that cancer is largely a preventable disease, with nutrition playing a major role in prevention? The report showed that between "30 percent and 40 percent of cancer incidence worldwide is preventable by the (recommended) approach to eating, weight control, and exercise," after accounting for smoking. Prevention, according to the report, saves resources as well as lives by reducing the burden of treating cancer on medical services and national economies.

… small changes to behavior, so-called baby steps, have a huge impact on our health and can inspire other healthful behaviors? For example, imagine you simply went out and got a new pair of running shoes. That small change may inspire you to get a new pair of running shorts to go with your shoes. Now you are off and walking, enjoying the smells and sights around you. In fact, you may be having so much fun that you tell a friend about it and your friend asks to join you the next day. Soon, the two of you are regularly walking. And during those sessions, you are talking about nutrition and fitness. You even decide to do a 5K event together. You tell your plan to other friends and family. They cheer you on and some eagerly want to join you. And then magic! Before you know it, you and your friends are off and running and inspiring others with good health!

THE NUTRILITE STORY

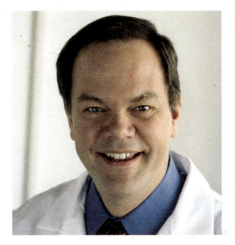 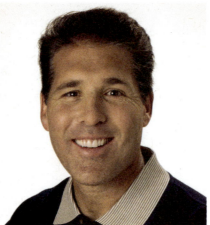 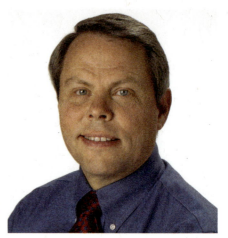

Duke Johnson, M.D., Medical Director of Nutrilite Health Institute, 2008. Dr. Johnson, author of the recently released book *Optimal Health Revolution*, has provided invaluable advice to employees and distributors since 1997.

Sean Foy, M.A., 2005. Author of *The 10-minute Total Body Breakthrough*, Sean is an instrumental guiding force in the development of fitness programs for Nutrilite employees, distributors, and the community alike.

Kip Johnson, M.D., 2004. Dr. Johnson has practiced medicine for more than 30 years, specializing in preventive medicine, and has been an advisor for us for more than a decade.

complete an assortment of tests which gauge their baseline fitness level. They also have blood work done.

After completing the fitness assessment and blood chemistry panel, participants have the opportunity to meet with Dr. Duke, Sean Foy, and Dr. Kip Johnson to design a personalized program of exercise, nutrition, and supplementation.

The program also helps our distributors share their new knowledge of the NUTRILITE™ brand in simulated sales situations at the conclusion of the program.

The impact of this program is trickling into the trenches and growing. As leaders return home from their visit, they're able to inspire their own group regarding the business opportunities surrounding the NUTRILITE brand as well as the personal benefits of following a lifestyle in alignment with optimal health.

The program was (and is) so successful that we have taken it on the road. Bill Dombrowski and his team of experts have also developed what we call the "mini-brand"

Chapter Twenty Nine: A Look at Today and Glimpse into the Future

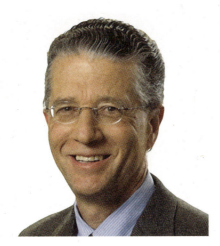

Bill Dombrowski, Manager Nutrilite Brand Experience, 2007. Since 1994, Bill has been a passionate advocate of the NUTRILITE brand and has helped my efforts to take the NUTRILITE brand message around the world.

experience tour. First launched in June 2001 in Germany and Italy, it soon was followed by the first permanent Brand Experience Center in Guangzhou, China in 2002. Subsequently others followed: Vienna, Austria in 2003, Korea in 2004. These centers offer unique face-to-face, interactive learning opportunities that have been derived from what we have learned during the Nutrilite Experience in California. The Nutrilite Experience continues to evolve each year with simpler messaging which is shared with our affiliate partners around the world to implement in their brand experience centers and programs. Today, the number of mini-brand experiences continues to grow, taking the message of optimal health to even more people.

More recently, a "bus tour" touting the value of the brand has been making its way across the United States. It's a first for the NUTRILITE brand in the United States. Along the way, festivals, expos, concerts, running events, and other activities help encourage even more people to choose optimal health and learn about the brand. It's a wonderful thing to see how the brand messaging has evolved over time.

It's hard to believe it's been more than seven decades since I first consumed my father's food supplement. Today, I'm in my 70s and continue to enjoy the health benefits of NUTRILITE products. One such benefit is helping me keep up with one of my passions: long-distance running. So far, I've participated in more than 25 marathons, and I am working toward my goal of winning one of the big ones like Boston or Honolulu—in my age bracket! Every day, I strive to reach my health goals, and the same goes for my wife and family.

In fact, it's been almost 20 years since I was able to convince my wife, Francesca, to run her first marathon. She had never done one, but figured if I could do it, she certainly could. She started with baby steps and was able to finish 26.2 miles. She was so excited about being able to achieve such an amazing goal that she was immediately hooked. Since then, she has run in more than 15 marathons. Francesca and I not only benefit from running to stay in shape, but also truly enjoy the friendly competition and camaraderie. We are not out there to beat the clock but to enjoy the moment and the benefits.

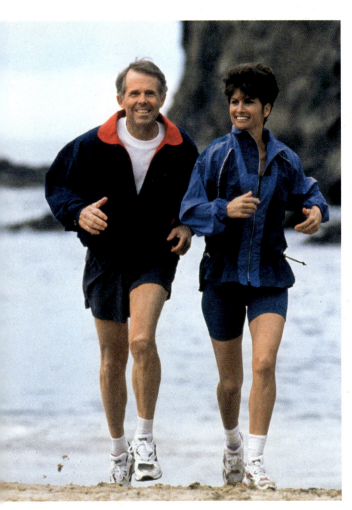

Running with my wife Francesca, 1995.

Others whom I have had the pleasure to meet, including my dear friend Leonard Kim, are also embracing a lifestyle of healthy living.

I met Leonard in the early 1990s during the downturn of the Korean business. While many distributors were complaining, Leonard approached me and said that he saw enormous potential in Amway, particularly in the NUTRILITE brand. He was determined to rebuild his business in Korea.

A few years later, Leonard visited us at the Nutrilite Health Institute in Buena Park, California, and participated in the Nutrilite Experience.

Realizing he couldn't make it through the step test of the fitness portion of the program, Leonard said he was going to take up running to get in shape so he could be a better "product of the product."

Today, Leonard is known for his running exploits and physical fitness and has encouraged many people to join him. One year, he ran the Honolulu Marathon along with many of his friends and distributors. I happened to get a phone call from my assistant, Jean Brewer. She called with concerns that it had taken Leonard 11 hours to finish the race. She needn't have worried. I told her that Leonard had been running up and down the course making sure that his entire group made it to the finish line before he did. Instead of running one marathon that day, he probably ran two!

Clement and Anita Fu—distributor leaders from Hong Kong—are also making an enormous difference in promoting an active lifestyle. Clement became an Amway distributor in 1979 and Anita in 1982. They enjoy badminton and jogging and because of the freedom of their Amway-affiliated business, are able to exercise three to four times a week for two hours. It was Leonard who encouraged and motivated them to run their first marathon. According to

Did You Know

… as I travel around the world, I often discuss the most effective way to share the benefits of food supplements? These I call the *Six Steps to Successful Selling*:

1. Use the Product – Become your first and best client! As with many things in life, experience is the best teacher.

2. Learn - Learn about the products and the role of nutrition and supplements in achieving and maintaining optimal health.

3. Be a Product of the Product - Your hearty appearance, your high energy, and your healthy outlook will tell the Nutrilite story for you!

4. Be a Friend - You will earn the trust of your potential customers and be able to make a stronger impact in helping them achieve optimal health.

5. Share the Product and the Plan - This is the most important step. Help your customer answer these key questions:

- Why do I need to supplement?
- What supplement(s) do I need?
- Why are NUTRILITE supplements the best?

By helping your potential customers answer these three questions, you will not only help them achieve optimal health, but help foster a strong business relationship as they build their own business.

6. Service, service, service!

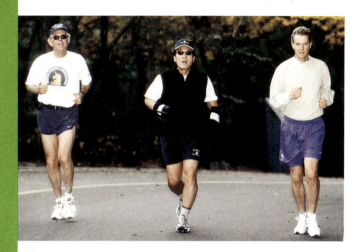

Running with Leonard Kim (center) and Jim Payne (right), March 2004. Photo taken during a training run in Seoul, Korea with Leonard's group.

Anita, "The first full marathon we ran was in 2004 at Honolulu. We finished it within 5 ½ hours. We loved it because it has the same spirit as building our Amway business, goal-setting and persistence." That first marathon led to a second in Hong Kong in 2005, a third in New York with enthusiastic spectators cheering them on, and then the AVIA Orange County marathon in early 2008 (sponsored in part by Nutrilite), where they brought more than 100 distributors from Hong Kong to run together! That's exactly what it is all about.

How many people will need to embrace the concept of optimal health before each city, country, and indeed the whole world tips toward a healthier lifestyle? No one knows for sure. But, what we do know is that small changes, one behavior at a time, one individual at a time, one program at a time, one company at a time, can make a big difference.

Years ago, my father and mother founded the Boys and Girls Club of Buena Park, California. Today, my daughter Lisa serves on the board of directors and as a company we've partnered with the Club through the Amway One by One Campaign to continue to provide safe and wholesome recreational activities for children, regardless of their economic status.

One of the projects we recently initiated, called Project Sozo, was inspired by a friendly challenge I gave Sean Foy. I challenged Sean to design a wellness and weight-loss program that could become a low-cost blueprint for schools and youth centers across Orange County—and maybe even the nation. Beginning with the Boys and Girls Club of Buena Park, the program has now been implemented in 16 youth centers in Orange County, enrolling 450 children per eight-week session. It's this kind of innovative, community-centered approach that is making a real difference.

Further from home, we've initiated the LITTLE BITS™ program, also through the Amway One by One Campaign for Children. Amway One by One Campaign rallies all resources of Amway—distributors, employees, affiliates, and customers—to make a difference in the lives of children. The LITTLE BITS program provides vitamins and minerals to undernourished children around the world. The program was first launched in Mexico in May 2009. Taken daily with regular meals, the nutrients provided by the Little Bits program are designed to help children increase energy levels, support learning abilities, achieve and maintain a healthy body weight, and generally provide nutrients necessary for children to live happy, healthy lives.

Another program that is making a real difference in the lives of people around the world is Team Nutrilite. It was created to help people lead more active lifestyles. In 2002, I met with leaders from our Nutrilite Brand Communications team to discuss how, in a simple way, we could help our consumers understand the importance of exercise in their lives. After a series of discussions around the importance of running and competing in a marathon, it was determined that the key wasn't running or competing in a marathon, but moving the body on a daily basis.

Chapter Twenty Nine: A Look at Today and Glimpse into the Future

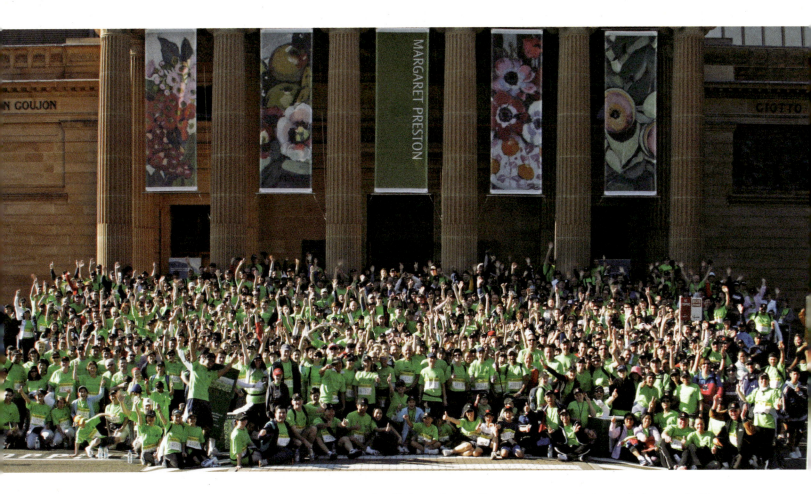

Go Team Nutrilite! City to Surf Run, Sydney, Australia, 2005.

The program was officially launched in January 2003 in India with Amway India hosting a series of 5K Walk/Jog events under the banner of Team Nutrilite. In five cities throughout India—Delhi, Mumbai, Calcutta, Kochi, and Chennai—thousands of individuals from mothers, fathers, children and seniors alike participated in the event to inaugurate Team Nutrilite into the history books of Amway and Nutrilite.

Shortly after that historic event, Australia joined Team Nutrilite by becoming one of the sponsors of the famous City to Surf 14K event. Thousands of enthusiastic runners and walkers converged upon the city of Sydney and participated under the banner of Team Nutrilite. Amway Korea soon followed by sponsoring a series of running and walking events that once again brought together distributors and customers alike, all energized to move their bodies under the Team Nutrilite flag.

Other countries around the world have also hosted health runs—countries like China and Hong Kong where thousands of people have embraced the spirit of Team Nutrilite and the concept of striving for a longer and healthier life with NUTRILITE products.

Amway Europe and other countries around the world are now looking at how distributors and Independent Business Owners (IBOs) can sponsor small local events in their communities to further embrace the spirit of Team Nutrilite while raising money for local charities under the umbrella of the Amway One by One program. Amway and Nutrilite have set the example by sponsoring small numbers of runner/walkers in the Grand Rapids Marathon Relay event, where five team members participate in a portion of the marathon and help raise awareness and money for the Helen DeVos Children's Hospital in Grand Rapids, Michigan.

Our Team Nutrilite athletes are also making a difference in the lives of people around the world as members of Team Nutrilite. For example, for every goal that soccer player Ronaldinho scores, it's another $10,000 that Amway Corporation donates to the Amway One by One campaign to benefit children.

One person at a time, one company at a time, we can all, working together, make a powerful contribution in making this a better place for all of us to live.

As my daughter Lisa reflects on her decision to work for Nutrilite more than two decades ago, she realized it was the right one for her:

> "I was so very nervous about everything and now all these years later… I can't imagine not being here at Nutrilite. I love everything about it, the employees and distributors. In addition, something I had not even considered was being a part of something so wonderful. Getting to know my grandfather even more deeply and dearly even though he is not here, I feel him with me. I am so proud to be a part of his legacy!"

There is nothing like a dream to build the future, and we at the Nutrilite Health Institute, under the wings of Amway, are positioning ourselves as the leading force in helping people all over the world embrace all aspects of optimal health. We are going to keep dreaming and building upon that dream, one day at a time, building a brighter future to help people live better lives.

Did You Know

… Team Nutrilite was launched in 2003 in India? Team Nutrilite is dedicated to helping people around the world achieve optimal health through a balance of nutrition, exercise, and NUTRILITE products. Today it consists of thousands of people around the world, as well as several world class athletes. Commitment and passion to love life and not just to live it are common threads of Team Nutrilite members.

… Canada was the first international market for NUTRILITE food supplements? Today, NUTRILITE brand products can be found in more than 55 countries.

1934	United States
1974	Canada
1976	Australia
1977	Malaysia, Hong Kong
1979	Ireland
1983	United Kingdom
1984	Germany, Taiwan, Japan
1990	Netherlands, Belgium, France
1992	Macau, New Zealand
1993	Thailand, Mexico, Panama, Guatemala, Spain, Italy, Brunei
1994	Portugal
1995	Brazil
1996	Indonesia, Hungary
1997	Poland, Honduras, El Salvador, Chile
1998	Argentina, Dominican Republic, Switzerland, South Africa, China
1999	Czech Republic, Slovak Republic, Costa Rica
2000	Philippines, Turkey, India, Venezuela
2001	Namibia, Romania, Slovenia
2002	Colombia, Singapore, Denmark, Finland, Norway, Sweden
2003	Croatia, Ukraine, Greece, Botswana
2006	Russia, Uruguay
2008	Vietnam

The Nutrilite Story

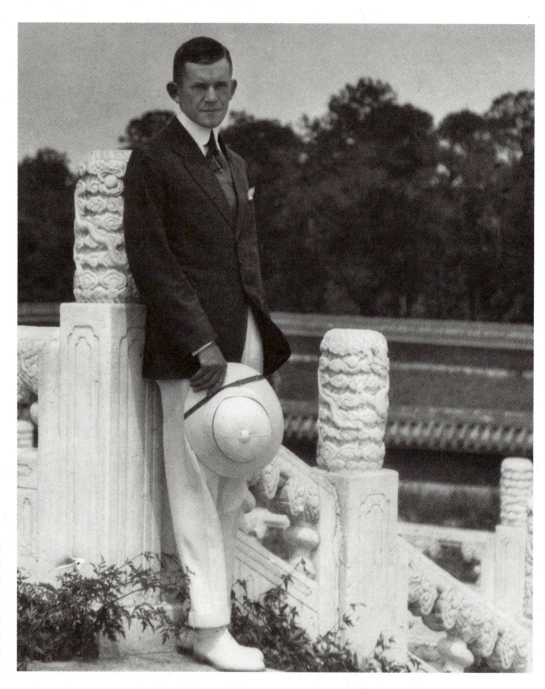

Carl F. Rehnborg in Teanen, Peking (Beijing) at the "Gate from Altar of Temples," May 30, 1917. Little did my father realize the adventure he was about to embark upon.

Chapter Twenty Nine: A Look at Today and a Glimpse into the Future

Today NUTRILITE brand products are found in more than 55 countries around the world, tens of thousands of guests visit us each year at the Nutrilite Health Institute, and annual sales in 2008 have soared past the three billion dollar mark.

"Son, one day this will be a million dollar business," my father had told me when I was a young boy. I'm sure he would be pleased to know that the supplement brand he created more than 75 years ago to help people "balance their diet" remains a top-selling brand around the world.

His message back in 1964 turned out to be more prescient than he could have ever imagined:

> *For me, who has seen our company grow, this is a grand sight. I know absolutely that even greater growth is in the immediate future, and I know equally surely that the advance will come by means of the same, simple procedures that meant your greatest advances in the past—to sell by pursuing the 'soft sell,' with truth and sincerity the guiding principles. I wish you well, and I am cheering you on.*

I look at a photo of my father taken more than nine decades ago. Pith helmet in hand, he had been happily trekking throughout China, discovering, exploring, and learning. I smile. It has been a wonderful adventure—an "adventure in the highest degree," as Dad would say. As with all good adventures, this one continues.

Acknowledgements

The idea for the Nutrilite Story has been long in the making. I've had the joy of growing up with and being part of the Nutrilite business for more than 70 years. In speeches I give around the world on Nutrilite, I'm often asked to include the Nutrilite story, but usually have only 20 to 30 minutes to do so. I'm never able to tell it completely and have been thinking for some time that I needed to sit down and put it all together for posterity.

This all came to a head back in 1998 when we launched NUTRILITE™ for the first time in mainland China. For many years, in my speeches in Asia, particularly in Hong Kong and Taiwan where we launched in 1977 and 1984, respectively, I would tell the audience that one of my big dreams was that one day we would launch NUTRILITE products in mainland China and the dream would come full circle.

So now that the dream has indeed come full circle, I realized that the time is right to tell the story in its entirety—a story that goes back more than 90 years ago when my father first set foot in China in 1915.

After a lengthy search, I found a young biographer, Chris Kelly, who had received his degree in English from Stanford University and was eager to take on the assignment. We journeyed first to Shanghai with my eldest daughter and son to find the home site of my father in Shanghai and to do a video shoot titled *The Life & Times of Carl Rehnborg*, which turned out to be a big hit with distributors and shown the world over.

Chris Kelly continued his research, which took place over the next few years. He interviewed distributors and management all over the world, and he dug through our archives, reading all of my father's early correspondence and the records that we had accumulated over the years. I told him at the outset that I wanted this book to include not only the history of my father—the complete story from his birth to his death—but also the history of China at the time of my father's stint there, the history of nutrition, the history of phytonutrients, the history and background of multilevel marketing and Nutrilite's role in its beginnings.

In 2003, he presented us with a 1,500-page manuscript complete with all the information I requested, and I quickly realized that I was probably the only one who would take the time to read such a lengthy treatise. I thought the real value of the book would be as an education and training tool for the millions of people who come into the business to share the product and who want more information about the history of Nutrilite and the role of supplementation in helping people to achieve optimal health.

I enlisted the help of a host of talented people to help me create a more simplified, condensed version that would be most relevant for our distributors and salespeople and could be easily translated for use around the world.

It is with heartfelt appreciation that I acknowledge those who graciously shared their time, talent, and tenacity to work with me on this project, both in the early stages and in this writing. They are:

Chris Kelly – For his yeoman-like job of doing the research, conducting the interviews, and pulling together most of the information that's contained in this book, as well as his review of the final manuscript.

Lorna Williams – For sharing her writing talent and expertise as a former Nutrilite trainer and nutrition scientist to help shape the final condensed version of this book to best meet the needs of distributors.

John van der Zee – For his insight and expertise in helping us to condense the original book.

Cynthia Bourgeault – For her careful read of the original book and her expert editorial comments and suggestions.

Gwen Rehnborg – For her overall guidance of the project and for her early work on pulling the book into shape, as well as her very informative and helpful changes in the final manuscript.

Gay Moritz – For her herculean effort of transforming Nutrilite's archives from overflowing boxes (containing unlabeled photos, documents, letters, marketing brochures, and artifacts) to a neatly labeled and organized collection, as well as identifying the photos that have been utilized throughout the book to bring it to life.

Shari Kline and Maritza Andrade – For their ever helpful effort in tracking down relevant images and documents for use in this book.

For their careful review of the various versions and the helpful perspective given to me on the project; Charles Savio, David King, Brad Williams, Francesca Rehnborg, Lisa Rehnborg, Rod Rehnborg, Kori Rehnborg, Jenna Rehnborg

For their careful legal review of the book: Scott Balfour, Wendy Brocker, Sherry Gunderson-Schipper, Bobbie Jones, Cary Justice, Patty Linscott, Terri Palmer, Michelle Parris, Rainey Repins, John Seurynck, Michel Terry

Jean Brewer – For her assistance at every step of the way: keeping track of all the drafts, paying the bills, helping with proofreading, etc.

Kati Boland – For her expertise in the publishing arena in helping to take the manuscript to the final print form.

Bill Dombrowski – For his careful read of the book and always thinking about the impact of the book on the distributor organization.

    It certainly takes a village to raise a child, and in this case, it takes a host of talented people to help write a book. It is with deep gratitude that I thank each of you for your efforts.

Acknowledgements

Appendix

Appendix 1. What's In a Name?

The field of nutrition is changing. It was changing very quickly during my father's time. You have probably heard of vitamins A, B, C, D, and E. But, have you ever heard of vitamins F, G, H, I, or J? Some compounds, thought to be vitamins back then, no longer have vitamin status today.

Name	Current or Obsolete Term
Vitamin A	Current Term
Vitamin B	Obsolete Term: Original anti-beriberi factor; now known to be a mixture of factors and designated as the vitamin B complex
Vitamin B1	Current Term: Synonym for thiamin
Vitamin B2	Current Term: Synonym for riboflavin
Vitamin B3	Obsolete Term: Infrequently used synonym for pantothenic acid; was also used for nicotinic acid
Vitamin B4	Obsolete Term: Unconfirmed activity preventing muscular weakness in rats and chicks; believed to be a mixture of arginine, glycine, riboflavin, and pyridoxine
Vitamin B5	Obsolete Term: Unconfirmed growth promoter for pigeons
Vitamin B6	Current Term: Synonym for pyridoxine
Vitamin B7	Obsolete Term: Unconfirmed digestive promoter for pigeons; may be a mixture; also called vitamin I
Vitamin B8	Obsolete Term: Adenylic acid; no longer classified as a vitamin

Name	Current or Obsolete Term
Vitamin B9	Obsolete Term: Unused designation
Vitamin B10	Obsolete Term: Growth promotant for chicks; likely a mixture of folic acid and vitamin B12
Vitamin B11	Obsolete Term: Apparently the same as vitamin B12
Vitamin B12	Current Term: Synonym for cyanocobalamin
Vitamin C	Current Term
Vitamin D	Current Term
Vitamin E	Current Term
Vitamin F	Obsolete term: Used to describe essential fatty acids; also an abandoned term for thiamin activity
Vitamin G	Obsolete term: Used to describe riboflavin activity; also an abandoned term for niacin
Vitamin H	Obsolete term: Used to describe biotin activity
Vitamin I	Obsolete Term: Mixture also formerly called vitamin B7
Vitamin J	Obsolete Term: Postulated anti-pneumonia factor also formerly called vitamin G2
Vitamin K	Current Term
Vitamin L1	Obsolete Term: Unconfirmed liver filtrate activity; proposed as necessary for lactation
Vitamin L2	Obsolete Term: Unconfirmed yeast filtrate activity; proposed as necessary for lactation

Name	Current or Obsolete Term
Vitamin M	Obsolete Term: Used to describe the anti-anemic factor in yeast; now known as folic acid
Vitamin N	Obsolete Term: Used to describe a mixture proposed to inhibit cancer
Vitamin O	Obsolete Term: Unused designation
Vitamin P	Obsolete Term: Activity reducing capillary fragility related to citrin, which is no longer classified as a vitamin
Vitamin Q	Obsolete Term: Unused designation (the letter was used to designate coenzyme Q)
Vitamin R	Obsolete Term: Used to describe folic acid
Vitamin S	Obsolete Term: Term applied to a bacterial growth activity probably related to biotin
Vitamin T	Obsolete Term: Unconfirmed group of activities isolated from termites, yeasts, or molds and reported to improve protein utilization in rats
Vitamin U	Obsolete Term: Unconfirmed activity from cabbage proposed to cure ulcers and promote bacterial growth; may have folic acid activity
Vitamin V	Obsolete Term: Tissue-derived activity promoting bacterial growth; probably related to NAD

Source: Modified from Combs GF. The Vitamins Fundamental Aspects in Nutrition and Health. San Diego, CA: Academic Press, Inc.; 1992.

APPENDIX

Appendix 2. Nutrition and Nutrilite Timeline

Nutrition Timeline	Year	Nutrilite Timeline
Hippocrates prescribes copper compounds for pulmonary and other diseases.	400 BC	
Clinical application of iron used to treat iron-deficient anemia.	17th century	
James Lind, M.D., a Scottish surgeon, performs the first clinical nutrition experiment to demonstrate the benefits of citrus fruits in curing scurvy.	1747	
Lind publishes results as *Treatise on Scurvy*.	1753	
British Navy requires lemon or lime juice as part of sailing provisions to prevent scurvy.	1795	
American Medical Association is founded.	1847	
Surgeon General Kanehiro Takaki introduces increased amounts of meat, barley, and fruit into the diet of Japanese sailors. This eradicates beriberi from the navy.	1884	
	1887	Carl Franklin Rehnborg is born on June 15, 1887 in St. Augustine, Florida. He is the eldest of five children born to Carl Johan Paulus ("Paul") Rehnborg and Alice Maria Upton Rehnborg. As a young boy, he lives in Savannah, Georgia.*
	1896	The Rehnborg family moves to Huntington (today known as Shelton), Connecticut.†
Christiaan Eijkman, a Dutch physician-physiologist, observes beriberi-like symptoms in chickens and pigeons fed a diet restricted to polished rice. Aspirin, a highly effective pain reliever and fever reducer, is invented in Germany.	1897	

* Presumed year as the family moved because of the historic 1887 St. Augustine, Florida fire.
† It is assumed that this is the year the family moved to Huntington, Connecticut since Paul Rehnborg's citizenship was recorded with the County Clerk in Huntington on October 24, 1896.

The Nutrilite Story

Nutrition Timeline	Year	Nutrilite Timeline
As late as 1900, diet was not believed to have much effect on health as long as it furnished adequate amounts of calories, protein, and some minerals, not yet known.	1900	The Rehnborg family also lives for part of the year in New Hampshire when Paul Rehnborg purchases a farm in Bethlehem. During Carl's formative years, he travels up and down the East Coast with his family, stopping at county fairs and resorts, to sell his father's jewelry. This exposes him to many different people and environments and sparks his lifelong interest in the histories and cultures of the people around the world.
	~1904	Carl graduates from high school in Huntington, CT (year approximate).
Cornelius Pekelharing feeds animals purified proteins, carbohydrates, fats, inorganic salts, and water and finds that they can only thrive if small amounts of milk are added to the diet.	1905	After graduation, Carl works for his father for several years—arranging catalogs and looking for a new office site.
Sir Frederick Gowland Hopkins, the father of British biochemistry, coins the term *accessory food factors* for the unrecognized essential substances in milk and vegetables.	1906	In February Carl begins a diary. Journal writing would be a habit that would remain with him for his entire life.
Two Norwegians, Axel Holst and Theodore Frölich, produce a condition in guinea pigs similar to human scurvy by feeding them a cereal-based diet free of fresh animal and vegetable foods. The addition of the restricted foods to the diet cures the surviving animals.	1907	
	1909	Carl begins work at a garter and corset manufacturer; however he's let go for failing to motivate the crew. In September, Carl enrolls at the Pratt Institute in New York studying jewelry design.

* Presumed year as the family moved because of the historic 1887 St. Augustine, Florida fire.

† It is assumed that this is the year the family moved to Huntington, Connecticut since Paul Rehnborg's citizenship was recorded with the County Clerk in Huntington on October 24, 1896.

APPENDIX

Nutrition Timeline	Year	Nutrilite Timeline
	1910	Carl leaves his studies at Pratt Institute. Around this time, he begins to research and develop a new flooring material.
Chemist Casimir Funk proposes the term *vitamine* for substances that appear to be vital for life and that contain an amine group.	1911	Carl's mother dies from pneumonia.
Funk suggests that dietary deficiency causes diseases such as beriberi, pellagra, rickets, and sprue.	1912	
Elmer McCollum and Marguerite Davis discover the first accessory food substance to be recognized as a vitamin, which they call fat-soluble A.	1913	Carl works as a streetcar conductor in Columbia, South Carolina.
[World War 1 begins]	1914	Carl enrolls at the University of South Carolina and studies chemistry and physics, but drops out after one semester. He also works as a copy editor for the *Columbia Record*.
McCollum and Davis demonstrate water-soluble factor B in wheat germ.	1915	Carl works as an accountant for Standard Oil Company of New York (Socony) in China. Before he left, he had taken a special training course and passed at the top of his class, and as a result he got the prized position, working for Socony in Tientsin, China. While in China, he studies the nutritional habits and poor health of people living in towns compared to those living in the country and makes a correlation between nutrition and health.
David Marine and Oliver Kimball conduct a study that shows endemic goiter is prevented with small amounts of iodine.	1916	Carl works as a Trader for China American Trading Company in Tientsin, China.

The Nutrilite Story

Nutrition Timeline	Year	Nutrilite Timeline
United States Department of Agriculture issues first set of dietary recommendations in a pamphlet entitled How to Select Foods. Advice based on five food groups: fruits & vegetables, meats & other protein-rich foods, cereals & starch, sweets, and fats.	1917	On April 30, 1917, Carl marries Hester Hawkes in Yokohama, Japan. They would have two children: Edward Hawks "Ned" Rehnborg (born on October 28, 1918) and Nancy Fitch Rehnborg (born on February 10, 1921).
[World War 1 ends]	1918	Carl and Hester return to the United States for a brief period. Carl is employed as Comptroller at the Lone Star Shipbuilding Corp. in Beaumont, Texas.
Jack Drummond proposes the name "water-soluble C" for the antiscorbutic factor.	1919	While in China, Carl became interested in brittle bone disease. He realized that milk was a good source of calcium and that the Chinese didn't drink it. He encouraged American Milk Products Company to launch a line of canned milk under his direction. He becomes the company's principal representative for China and he and his family settle in Shanghai.
Jack Drummond suggests that the "e" in vitamine be removed. He also proposes that the "somewhat cumbrous nomenclature" (i.e., fat-soluble A, water-soluble B, and water-soluble C) be dropped, and the substances be referred to as vitamins A, B, C, etc, until their true nature is identified.	1920	Carl launches canned milk throughout China (1920-1922).
	1921	During Carl's years launching Carnation canned milk in China, he begins to experiment with nutritional extracts from plant materials. He believes that there are probably thousands of important factors in plants that are important in human nutrition. He would come to call these unknown substances *associated food factors*. Today these are recognized as phytonutrients.

APPENDIX

Nutrition Timeline	Year	Nutrilite Timeline
Elmer McCollum and associates identify the antirachitic factor in cod liver oil that prevents rickets. Commercial introduction of iodized salt prevents goiter in large populations. Anatomy professor Herbert Evans and Katherine Bishop co-discover vitamin E, which they find in green leafy vegetables.	1922	
Tobacco mosaic virus isolated, established that viruses cause many plant diseases.	1923	The milk business wasn't growing as fast as Carl wanted (it wasn't part of the culture and many developed an upset stomach), so he decides to strike out on his own and operate his own business. He is in charge of his own agency in Shanghai as a representative for Colgate Products Company. He also becomes a member of the Shanghai Volunteers Corp.
	1924	Carl files incorporation papers for China Food Products Corporation. [On April 12, 1927, he changes the name to C.F. Rehnborg, Inc.]
The fat-soluble anti-rickets factor is named vitamin D.	1925	China erupts with political instability. Warlords and rioters are rampaging through the lands in inland China. Carl's business is affected.
The isolation and characterization of anti-beriberi factor—thiamin—from rice bran extract by P. Jansen and W.P. Donath occurs. George Minot and William Murphy successfully treat pernicious anemia with a daily diet of cooked beef liver (contains vitamin B12). Concern over health hazards of lead arsenate leads to the first pesticide regulation.	1926	Chiang Kai-shek allies with the Communist Party to form the Northern Expedition, whose goal is to eliminate the warlords and consolidate the country. The army sets out from Canton and heads north. They reach the Yangtze in the fall. Communications with Shanghai are disrupted. Foreigners are evacuated from upriver. Shanghai is flooded with refugees. Warlords seize Carl's warehouses in the inland, and in a short period of time he has lost everything.

The Nutrilite Story

Nutrition Timeline	Year	Nutrilite Timeline
	1927	Hester leaves Carl and takes the children with her. He remains. The situation continues to worsen in Shanghai. Carl puts his knowledge of Chinese food and traditional Chinese medicine to work scrounging dandelion leaves and other plants for soups, supplemented with nails and crushed chicken bones for calcium and trace elements. In November, Carl leaves China and arrives in San Pedro, California with only $24 in his pocket. In a speech he gave later, he said, "I was flat on my back and broke, but I was rich because I had a dream that I was going to pursue at all costs."
[The beginning of The Great Depression] Albert Szent-György isolates hexuronic acid. It's later called vitamin C (ascorbic acid). The word "nutrilite" is coined by Roger Williams and is used to describe vitamin-like substances other than those that are well recognized.	1928	Carl takes part-time jobs in Southern California and sets up makeshift labs in various places that he lives and begins experimenting with plant-based concentrates.
Hopkins and Eijkman share the Nobel Prize in Physiology or Medicine "for their discovery of the growth-stimulating vitamins." Henrik Dam discovers vitamin K—anti-hemorrhagic factor.	1929	From 1929 to 1932, Carl works at America Potash and Chemical Company in the desert town of Trona, California, doing statistical work. His title is Chief Clerk.
	1930	Carl marries Mildred Thompson on July 19, 1930. She tragically dies two years later while pregnant with their child.

APPENDIX

Nutrition Timeline	Year	Nutrilite Timeline
Value of iron in treating iron-deficiency anemia resolved beyond doubt. Vitamin D is isolated and its synthesis is achieved. During the 1930s, provitamin D was added to milk in the U.S. and Europe and it eradicated rickets.	1932	Carl moves to the Los Angeles area. He commits himself, heart and soul, to finding a way to supplement the diet with the necessary vitamins, minerals, and associated food factors. In order to sustain himself financially, he works at Richfield Oil Company doing statistical work. Carl marries Evelyn Berg (year approximate).
Vitamin C—antiscorbutic factor—is synthesized in the lab. It's the first synthetic vitamin. Riboflavin is isolated. The American Institute of Nutrition is formed.	1933	
Essentiality of zinc demonstrated in animals. George Whipple, George Minot, and William Murphy of the U.S. share the Nobel Prize in Physiology or Medicine for their "discoveries concerning liver therapy in cases of anaemia." By this date, all 13 vitamins have been discovered.	1934	After several years of research (and while still employed at Richfield Oil Company), Carl produces and sells what is believed to be the first multivitamin/multimineral supplement in the United States.
Riboflavin is synthesized in the laboratory.	1935	Carl registers the name of his company as Vitamin Products Company. The company's first product is called VITA-6, which received its name because of the six vitamins it contains. In July, Carl registers the name "VITAMIN" as the company's telegraph cable address. In August, Carl sets up a shop and lab in Montebello, California (at 5917 Whittier Blvd.), and leaves Richfield Oil Company to pursue his dream full-time.

The Nutrilite Story

Nutrition Timeline	Year	Nutrilite Timeline
Vitamin E (alpha-tocopherol) and vitamin B6 are isolated. Thiamin is synthesized in the laboratory. First nationwide food consumption survey is initiated by the United States Department of Agriculture. Since then such surveys are conducted at approximately 10-year intervals.	1936	Product name changes from VITA-6 to VITASOL as more vitamins are discovered. Carl Reinhold ("Sam") Rehnborg is born to Carl and Evelyn Rehnborg on February 5, 1936. California Vitamins is incorporated in California succeeding a partnership doing business under the name of Vitamin Products Company, Montebello, California.
National Cancer Institute is founded. Niacin is isolated (although its synthesis had been achieved 60 years earlier—before its vitamin activity had actually been discovered). Two biochemists share the Nobel Prize for Chemistry: Paul Karrer of Switzerland, for describing the structure of vitamin A and for his work on riboflavin, carotenoids, and flavins; and Walter Haworth of the United Kingdom, for his work on determining the chemical structure of carbohydrates as well as that of vitamin C. Albert Szent-György receives the Nobel Prize in Physiology or Medicine for his discoveries with special reference to vitamin C.	1937	On March 31, 1937, Carl moves his company's operations to Marine Avenue on Balboa Island in Southern California. In September, R. Templeton Smith inspects manufacturing aspect of Carl's company. Provides funds to turn boat shed into a real production facility. However, due to falling stock market he withdraws from the project.

APPENDIX

Nutrition Timeline	Year	Nutrilite Timeline
Richard Kuhn of Germany receives the Nobel Prize in Chemistry "for his work on carotenoids and vitamins." The synthesis of vitamin E is achieved in the laboratory. The U.S. Food, Drug, and Cosmetics Act is passed and signed into law. The new law bans any false and misleading statement when a product might be hazardous. The U.S. FDA is given the authority to seize a product, take criminal actions against manufacturers, and issue injunctions to prevent them from making or distributing a product they deem dangerous.	1938	Carl associates himself with Ferri-Min Company. Carl considers making a product called "Pick-Me-Up" (later called "Old Settler"). It's a high potency B-vitamin supplement. He eventually markets it as a hangover remedy and sells it in bars during the 1940s.
[World War 2 starts in Europe] Vitamin K, biotin, pantothenic acid, folate, as well as vitamin A are isolated. Synthesis of vitamin B6 achieved in the laboratory. A very busy year for vitamin research!	1939	California Vitamins, Inc. is renamed Nutrilite Products, Inc. and is also known as NPI. Crystalline vitamins are added to the food supplements to boost potency and make label claims. Operations move from Balboa Island to W. Slauson Avenue in Los Angeles. During this time a preliminary version of the sponsorship method of distribution is established.
Pantothenic acid and vitamin K synthesis is achieved in the laboratory.	1940	NPI's packaging and shipping operations move from Slauson Avenue to 6800 S. Hoover in Los Angeles, as more space is needed.
Food & Nutrition Board (FNB) is formed, derived from a committee of the United States National Academy of Sciences and issues the first Recommended Dietary Allowances (RDA) for calories and eight nutrients.	1941	Carl makes notes on the development of a leaf powder to add to flour to make bread dough, which would produce a balanced ration, and which could be marketed to health food stores, generally for children.

The Nutrilite Story

Nutrition Timeline	Year	Nutrilite Timeline
FDA establishes standard of identity for enriched flour, and fortification of related foods follow: 1943, cornmeal/grits; 1946, pasta; 1952, enriched bread; and 1958, rice.	1942	Carl purchases a 3.6-acre farm in California's San Fernando Valley so he can grow his alfalfa and other plant materials without using chemical pesticides and herbicides.
Henrik Dam of Denmark and Edward Doisy from the U.S. share the Nobel Prize in Physiology or Medicine for their work on vitamin K. Biotin is synthesized in the laboratory.	1943	
After World War 2, the major focus of attention in nutrition begins to shift away from acute nutrient deficiency diseases toward prevention of chronic degenerative diseases. Food and Agriculture Organization is formed by the United Nations.	1945	Mytinger & Casselberry, Inc. becomes the exclusive distributor of NUTRILITE™ Food Supplement. This is officially the beginning of the Marketing Plan.

APPENDIX

Nutrition Timeline	Year	Nutrilite Timeline
Folate is synthesized in the laboratory.	1946	Carl marries Edith Bruck, who combines her marketing ability with a belief in what Carl is doing to help grow and run the NUTRILITE business.
		NPI packaging and sales remain on Hoover Street in Los Angeles, while production facilities move to seven acres of land that had been acquired in Buena Park, California. Production takes place in a Quonset hut where Carl also lives with his family. A small farming operation also begins there.
		Dr. William Casselberry writes a 58-page booklet, *How to Get Well and Stay Well*, (formerly called *How to Cheat Death*) which while very successful, results in the FDA conducting its first factory inspections at M&C's offices and requesting copies of all sales materials.
Vitamin A is synthesized in the laboratory. Active form of pantothenic acid is demonstrated to be coenzyme A.	1947	First example of a "potentate" sponsoring a "potentate," so a two percent sponsor bonus is initiated.
		Construction begins on a large 22-acre manufacturing site in Buena Park.

The Nutrilite Story

Nutrition Timeline	Year	Nutrilite Timeline
Vitamin B12 (cobalamin)—the last of the 13 vitamins—is isolated.	1948	In April, NUTRILITE XX (DOUBLE X™) Food Supplement launches in the United States. The Roman numeral XX is chosen because the product price is $20 (U.S.). In November, the FDA seizes products and literature at potentate offices throughout the U.S., alleging improper claims. Charles Rhyne, a renowned constitutional lawyer in Washington, D.C., with lots of experience before the Supreme Court is hired to represent M&C and NPI. In November, the name potentate changes to key agent. For the first time, a key agent sponsors three separate key agent groups, so the name senior key agent originates, and a one percent bonus is added to the schedule to cover this.
	1949	Nutrilite moves to its present Buena Park location on 5600 Beach Boulevard and completes construction of a new facility. Packaging, compounding, and shipping move from Los Angeles to Buena Park so that all operations are combined. Carl and Edith Rehnborg help start the Buena Park Kids Organization, now called the Boys and Girls Club of Buena Park. Jay Van Andel and Rich DeVos become Nutrilite distributors. Nutrilite launches NUTRILITE JUNIOR Food Supplement.

APPENDIX

Nutrition Timeline	Year	Nutrilite Timeline
Role of vitamin A in vision is established. Start of fortification of commercial cereals.	1950s	The *Acania*, a 136 foot yacht, is purchased and equipped as a research vessel in connection with the feasibility of harvesting plankton as a source of protein. It makes a voyage from California into Alaskan waters with good results, but the project is discontinued due to economic reasons.
Major study documents fluoride's role in preventing dental cavities. Professor Edward Steinhaus, a pioneer in the field of insect pathology, uses bacteria to attack a caterpillar that infests alfalfa. This is the first successful use of an insect pathogen to control insects in the field.	1951	Farming operation requires expansion and moves, along with the extraction and concentration facilities, from Buena Park to Southern California's San Jacinto Valley with the purchase of a 100-acre farm at Hemet. The FDA begins a publicity campaign against NPI and M&C, which has a negative impact on sales, but NPI ultimately prevails in its court case, going all the way to the Supreme Court where the company receives a consent decree, which is the first official policy on what claims a company can make for vitamin and mineral supplements.
James Watson and Francis Crick describe double helical structure of DNA.	1953	
	1954	NPI begins its Lakeview farming operations by acquiring the Lakeview farm in San Jacinto Valley.
	1955	Under the direction of Dr. Stefan Tenkoff as vice president of production, the extraction and concentration facilities are moved from Hemet to Lakeview.

The Nutrilite Story

Nutrition Timeline	Year	Nutrilite Timeline
Denham Harman proposes the free radical theory of aging—that free oxygen radicals produced in the body cause aging.	1956	Carl became very interested in acerola as a source of natural vitamin C and establishes acerola orchards on the island of Hawaii. Acerola concentrate is used to produce the first supplement containing all-natural vitamin C. NPI gets government approval for BIOTROL—the first natural biological insect control agent in the marketplace.
Role of chromium in insulin function and normal glucose tolerance is defined in rats.	1957	The designer Raymond Loewy, famous for the design of the Studebaker Avanti car and the redesign of the Coca Cola bottle, creates a butterfly-shaped green plastic container to hold NUTRILITE DOUBLE X. Sales begin to decline due to the adverse reactions to the FDA and squabbling between M&C and NPI.
	1958	A brand new state-of-the-art research laboratory and quality control lab is built next to the old Quonset hut area. It houses quality control, some product development, and subsequently was where Dr. Thomas Jukes was going to establish and expand his world-class nutrition research laboratory—which never happened. Edith Rehnborg Cosmetics are introduced on May 19, 1958, and immediately become popular. Sam Rehnborg receives a Bachelor of Science degree in chemical engineering from Stanford University.

APPENDIX

Nutrition Timeline	Year	Nutrilite Timeline
Dietary guidelines for the prevention of coronary heart disease is published by Ancel and Margaret Keys.	1959	As a result of two separate cosmetic lines, M&C and NPI continue to feud. The feud comes to a crescendo with NPI putting an ad in the *Wall Street Journal* stating that all distributors get NUTRILITE Food Supplement from NPI. Jay Van Andel and Rich DeVos start the Amway Corporation. They develop a sales model based on the Nutrilite plan, but with significant changes to avoid Nutrilite's problems and boost individual incentives. Dr. Bill Casselberry retires and M&C, Inc. becomes the Mytinger Corporation.
Goldsmith and colleagues show that the amino acid tryptophan is used to make niacin in the body (60 milligrams tryptophan makes 1 milligram niacin)	1961	Carl and Edith are recognized for their outstanding contributions to the youth of the local community through their creation of an organization that would later become the Boys & Girls Club of Buena Park.
	1962	Dr. Stefan Tenkoff is elected president of NPI, with Carl Rehnborg continuing on as chairman of the board.
Vitamin B12 is shown to be the cofactor required for conversion of homocysteine to methionine.	1963	NPI purchases the assets of the Mytinger Corporation, reuniting production and distribution.
U.S. Surgeon General's Report on Smoking argues that smoking is a major health risk for cancer, cardiovascular disease, and emphysema.	1964	Sam Rehnborg receives a Ph.D. in biophysics from the University of California at Berkeley, and joins NPI and begins to rebuild the business based on his father's principles. Hemet farm is sold.
Discovery that vitamins E and C reduce levels of nitrosamines in fried bacon and nitrite cured products. U.S. Congress passes law requiring labels on cigarette packages: "Warning: Cigarette Smoking may be Hazardous to your Health."	1965	NPI builds a new cosmetics manufacturing facility in Buena Park.

The Nutrilite Story

Nutrition Timeline	Year	Nutrilite Timeline
The Child Nutrition Act is passed and expands food programs for children in the United States.	1966	Carl writes a series of memos describing a way to harness power using the natural pressure and temperature differences of the ocean.
First RDA recommendation is set for vitamin E. USDA researchers find tips of alfalfa are more nutrient dense than the base of the plant.	1968	
The First White House Conference on Food, Nutrition, and Health is held and with it the birth of the health and fitness movement.	1969	With publicity from the First White House Conference on Nutrition, sales of NUTRILITE Food Supplement soars.
The last vitamin—vitamin B12—is synthesized in the laboratory.	1970	
	1972	Amway acquires a controlling interest in NPI and sales of NUTRILITE products increase tremendously.
Council of Responsible Nutrition is founded. It represents mainstream dietary supplement ingredient suppliers and manufacturers.	1973	Mentally and physically active until the end, Carl Rehnborg passes away at the age of 85.
	1974	The NUTRILITE brand launches in Canada, its first international market.
Danish researchers publish initial report that high intake of fish may reduce risk of heart disease.	1975	The endowment of the C.F. Rehnborg Memorial Book Fund in Religious Studies at Stanford University Libraries is established to honor Carl's work (mid-1970s). Dr. Sam Rehnborg circumnavigates the world, studying the customs and dietary patterns of various cultures (1975-1978).
	1976	Robert Hunter is named chief executive officer of NPI. During this time, he leads the improvement and expansion of all operational facilities to meet the increased sales demand from the affiliation with Amway.

Nutrition Timeline	Year	Nutrilite Timeline
	1977	Acerola cherry orchards are purchased in Puerto Rico, insuring a continuing supply of natural vitamin C.
	1978	Dr. Sam is named senior vice president of marketing development & research at NPI.
First Dietary Guidelines introduced (updated every 5 years).	1980s	During the 1980s the Buena Park facility greatly expands; in 1981, a new food bar facility is built; in 1983, a 35,000 square foot warehouse; and in 1988, a 134,000 square foot North Complex packaging/warehouse is erected.
	1981	Dr. Sam becomes executive vice president and chief executive officer.
	1983	Dr. Sam Rehnborg is named NPI's president and CEO. A powdered nutritious drink facility is established at Lakeview.
Fish oil found to reduce mortality from coronary heart disease. Michael Brown and Joseph Goldstein receive the Nobel Prize in Physiology or Medicine for their discovery concerning "the regulation of cholesterol metabolism."	1985	*C.F. Rehnborg—A Collection of His Essays, Speeches, and Writings* is published by C.F. Rehnborg Literary Foundation. At about this time, his book *Jesus and the New Age of Faith*, which was privately circulated years earlier, is published.
Surgeon General Everett Koop releases a report on nutrition and health in which, for the first time, the federal government formally recognizes the role of diet in the etiology of certain chronic diseases and proposed labeling policies.	1988	

The Nutrilite Story

Nutrition Timeline	Year	Nutrilite Timeline
The U.S. Recommended Dietary Allowances developed by the Food and Nutrition Board have been revised nine times since 1941. In the 10th edition, published in 1989, the number of nutrients for which an RDA or safe and adequate intakes have been established has expanded from nine in 1941 to 26 in 1989.	1989	C.F. Rehnborg Professorship in Disease Prevention at Stanford University School of Medicine is established. It was funded by the Nutrilite Foundation, Amway Corporation, and the Rehnborg family. Hurricane Hugo devastates much of NPI's acerola plantations in Puerto Rico. NPI begins search for alternate supplies and growing sites.
Negotiations between the FDA and USDA lead to the enactment by Congress of the Nutrition Labeling Act. This legislation, which went into effect in 1994, makes nutrition labeling mandatory and strictly regulates nutrient content and health claims.	1990	Completion of a bridge connecting North Complex facility to main plant in Buena Park. It is the only privately owned bridge to cross the Santa Fe Railway tracks, which links tablet manufacturing with packaging and warehouse facilities.
	1991	NPI purchases about 270 acres (108 hectares) of land in Colima, Mexico for the development of an acerola plantation. The acerola plantings are moved there and the operation is successfully established. At the same time options are explored for additional land to meet the growing needs for other crops like alfalfa, which includes the purchase of 109 acres (44 hectares) in Rancho Santa Clara Maria.
A public health recommendation is issued urging all women of childbearing age to get 400 micrograms of folic acid daily, in order to prevent neural tube defects.	1992	NPI continues to develop farms in Mexico, including the purchase of about 900 acres (360 hectares) of fertile land at Rancho El Petacal in Jalisco, Mexico (in 1992 and 1993). Major expansion begins at Buena Park and Lakeview facilities, and an Agricultural Research Center is established at Lakeview.

APPENDIX

Nutrition Timeline	Year	Nutrilite Timeline
The FDA approves a health claim that states that diets high in calcium may reduce the risk of osteoporosis. Bruce Ames, Ph.D., of U.C. Berkeley, estimates that each cell of the body experiences approximately 10,000 oxidative hits daily.	1993	Amway and NPI announce a three-year promotional agreement with the National Basketball Association, with NUTRILITE becoming the official vitamins of the NBA.
Dietary Supplement Health and Education Act (DSHEA) becomes law in the U.S. DSHEA defines supplements as amino acids, herbs, botanicals, metabolites, vitamins, and minerals.	1994	Amway Corporation purchases the remaining shares of NPI from the Rehnborg family. Nutrilite becomes a division of Amway. The C.F. Rehnborg Agriculture Research Center is dedicated in Lakeview, California.
A meta-analysis of 28 studies found low levels folic acid associated with heart disease and states "policies for increasing folic acid intake could have a considerable effect on the prevention of arteriosclerotic vascular disease." Lycopene, the carotenoid in tomatoes, found to support prostate health. The National Institute of Health Office of Dietary Supplements is established.	1995	Amway Manufacturing & Distribution Center is established in Guangzhou, China, which now manufactures NUTRILITE brand products. The first Nutrilite phytochemical conference takes place.
	1996	NUTRILITE brand worldwide annual sales pass the one billion dollar (U.S.) mark and are found in over 25 countries. The Rehnborg Center for Nutrition & Wellness (later, the Nutrilite Health Institute) is established to serve as the primary source of science, education, and training for NUTRILITE brand products. Dr. Sam Rehnborg serves as its president. Nutrilite launches its first herbal line of products.

The Nutrilite Story

Nutrition Timeline	Year	Nutrilite Timeline
World Cancer Research Fund/American Institute for Cancer publishes *Food, nutrition and the prevention of cancer: a global perspective* stating that there is overwhelming evidence that fruits and vegetables reduce risk of cancer.	1997	The first Nutrilite Experience program launches with Amway IBO leaders from Germany and Italy. Today, more than 15,000 distributors from 28 countries have been part of the program. Duke Johnson, MD provides recommendations to participants involved in the Nutrilite Experience and in 2006 he becomes NHI's Medical Director.
FDA requires addition of folate to enriched grain products.	1998	Amway Corporation acquires Fazenda Planalto Grande in Brazil and a controlling interest in Trout Lake Farm in Washington State (taking full ownership in 2000). Former United States President Gerald R. Ford, Dr. Sam Rehnborg, and Amway executives dedicate the new Lakeview powder drink facility. Manufacturing facility established in Himachal Pradesh in India.
The World Health Organization produces a report that warns governments about a growing epidemic that threatens public health—obesity.	2000	
First scientific study to be published which shows that diabetes can be prevented by lifestyle.	2001	First Nutrilite "mini-brand" Experience Center launches in Germany and Italy.
An article in the *Journal of American Medical Association* states that all adults should take a multivitamin to reduce risk of chronic disease, vindicating Carl Rehnborg's theories. The American Heart Association recommends that healthy adults consume omega-3 fatty acid foods (DHA/EPA) either from fish or plant sources to protect their hearts.	2002	The first permanent Brand Experience Center launches in Guangzhou, China. [As of 2009, similar centers exist in Austria, Germany, Italy, Spain, Portugal, India, Korea, Taiwan, Indonesia, Australia, Dominican Republic, and Mexico.]

Appendix

Nutrition Timeline	Year	Nutrilite Timeline
Mapping of the human genome is complete, paving a new era for nutrition where we are beginning to understand how phytochemicals influence metabolism and gene expression.	2003	NUTRILITE brand worldwide annual sales pass the two billion dollar (U.S.) mark and are found in over 50 countries. Team NUTRILITE—Global Fitness Club is established. All Nutrilite farms are now certified organic according to the criteria established by each respective country.
Vitamin C shown to reduce C-reactive protein. CRP is a biomarker for inflammation. Lutein, a phytochemical concentrated in dark green leafy vegetables, found to support vision and eye health as reported in the Lutein Antioxidant Supplement Trial.	2004	The NHI establishes the Scientific Advisory Board, which consists of leading scientists from around the world in areas of academia, industry, medicine, and research, to provide constructive scientific evaluation, advice, and public opinion on specific topics. Acquisition of Interleukin Genetics to usher Nutrilite into a new arena of nutrition—nutrigenomics. NutriCert™ program is initiated and ensures that any plant concentrate purchased has been grown according to strict organic specifications.
Over the past 5 years, more than 10,000 scientific articles related to antioxidant nutrients have been published.[‡]	2005	NUTRILITE DOUBLE X launches in China, bringing the Nutrilite story full circle from its beginning in China in 1915. Reformulated NUTRILITE DOUBLE X launches in more than 30 markets. NIH clinical trial shows that DOUBLE X boosts blood levels of beneficial nutrients and provides functional benefits to maintain health.

[‡] Based on a MEDLINE search using the key terms "antioxidant" and "nutrient" and limiting search to the years 2000 to 2005. June 30, 2009.

The Nutrilite Story

Nutrition Timeline	Year	Nutrilite Timeline
Vitamin D is shown to support heart, immune, and bone health. Some experts believe the RDA of 400 IU is too low.	2006	Launch of GENSONA™ genetic tests and personalized nutrition. The company launches NUTRILITE™ IL-1 Heart Health Nutrigenomic Dietary Supplement—the first and only supplement formulated to address the phytonutrient needs of men and women who tested positive for variations in the IL-1 gene. NHI's Center for Optimal Health launches. Its mission is to promote the NHI's research into plant-based nutrition and to help business owners communicate the optimal health message to their family, friends, and associates. The first director is Gwen Rehnborg, wife of Rod Rehnborg who is Carl Rehnborg's grandson. She is very instrumental in getting the center organized.
Nutrilite scientists along with scientists from Interleukin Genetics publish a groundbreaking paper published in the scientific journal *Nutrition* which confirms a link between genotype and nutrition.	2007	Carl Rehnborg is honored as a pioneer in the history of nutrition in the Wellness Revolution Hall of Fame. Rod Rehnborg accepts the honor on his behalf. Manufacturing facility established in Dong Nai Province in Vietnam.

APPENDIX

Nutrition Timeline	Year	Nutrilite Timeline
Organic milk is found to contain more antioxidants and vitamins than ordinary milk.	2008	Amway Corporation signs two-time FIFA Player of the Year and soccer phenomenon Ronaldinho to a multi-year, global endorsement agreement to represent the NUTRILITE brand. The endorsement, the largest platform in the 74-year history of the NUTRILITE brand, aligns Ronaldinho with other world-class athletes who endorse the NUTRILITE brand. The NUTRILITE brand also becomes the official nutrition supplement of AC Milan—one of soccer's most renowned clubs. NUTRILITE brand worldwide annual sales pass the three billion dollar (U.S.) mark and are found in more than 55 countries. NUTRILITE is the number one brand of vitamin, mineral, and dietary supplements and is also recognized as the world's leading children's brand of vitamin and mineral dietary supplements.§
A MEDLINE search using the key words "phytochemical" or "phytonutrient" as the search criteria reported over 2,500 published scientific studies. Compare it to ~400 studies on this topic by 1999, ~300 by 1989, ~150 by 1979, 50 by 1969, 5 by 1959, and none at the time Carl Rehnborg started his work.** This excitement seems to parallel the excitement seen at the turn of the 20th century with vitamins and is confirming Carl Rehnborg's theories on the importance of plant-rich diets.	2009	The LITTLE BITS™ program, which provides vitamins and minerals to help children around the world, launches in Mexico. The Chinese version of the NUTRILITE trademark [崔 (NIU CUI LAI)] has been granted the "Famous Mark" status, giving the mark expanded trademark protection. Nutrilite celebrates its 75-year anniversary of producing quality nutritional products based on the genius of Carl Rehnborg and dedicated to his dream of improving diets of people throughout the world.

§ Based on 2008 sales, as supported by research conducted by Euromonitor International.
** Based on a MEDLINE search using the key words phytochemical or phytonutrient as the search criteria, June 30, 2009.

Appendix 3. The Nutrilite Opportunity

The Marketing Plan developed to sell NUTRILITE™ products is considered the first instance of multilevel marketing. The Mytinger & Casselberry, Inc. (M&C) Marketing Plan was developed in 1945 and blossomed from Carl Rehnborg's basic marketing ideas. Below find the concept of the M&C Marketing Plan used during the mid-1950s. Itconsisted of several levels: distributor, agent, and key agent.

Distributor: a person authorized by M&C to distribute NUTRILITE Food Supplement. Profits to distributors are based on one of two charts. The distributor chooses the chart that is most favorable to their situation

Profits Based on Number of DOUBLE X™ Yearly Savings Plans Sold	
Number of new customers each month purchasing DOUBLE X Yearly Savings Plan	Profit on total monthly volume
0-9	35%
10-14	40%
15-24	45%
	etc. up to 60%

Profits Based on Monthly Sales	
Monthly sales	Monthly profits
$0-499	35%
$500-999	40%
$1,000-2,499	45%
$2,500-3,999	50%
	etc. up to 60%

All distributors purchase NUTRILITE Food Supplement through their sponsor at a 35 percent base discount. If they sell 10 or more yearly savings plans per month (or $500 or more in monthly sales), they will receive a refund check from their sponsor for the additional earnings.

Sponsor: when a distributor has become experienced by making a given number of sales and has met the simple qualifications, he will become authorized to be a sponsor. He may then start to build a sales organization. The volume of the distributors he sponsors is added to, and becomes part of, his total purchase volume in order to determine profit bracket. For example, if a sponsor's total volume is $1,500 and the combined volume of the two distributors he sponsors is $1,700 ($850 each), the sponsor is bumped up from the 45% profit bracket ($1,500) to the 50% profit bracket ($1,500 +$1,700 =$3,200). The sponsor purchases product for his distributors and gives them a refund check based on their profit bracket ($850 x 0.05= $42.50 each).

Agent: a distributor who, through his own efforts and the efforts of his group of distributors, has attained a 17 percent refund. This puts him in the 52 percent profit bracket on his own and up to 17 percent on some of his distributor's sales. He holds regular meetings for his group, supplies them with merchandise and sales tools, and trains them in the proper presentation of NUTRILITE Food Supplement.

Key agent: a distributor who through his own efforts and those of his group has reached the maximum refund bracket of 25 percent. This means that he and his group either purchases and delivers at least $15,000 worth of NUTRILITE product each month or sells a minimum of 150 DOUBLE X Yearly Savings Programs each month. This puts the key agent in the 60 percent profit bracket on his own and up to 25 percent on some of his distributor's sales.

When a key agent directly sponsors distributors who also become key agents, M&C will pay the sponsoring key agent an additional two percent refund on the volume of the directly sponsored key agent group(s), pending certain requirements are met. When a key agent directly sponsors three or more key agents, they are eligible for an additional bonus plan.

Individuals who become key agents deal directly with M&C, Inc.

Appendix 4. Best of Science (Publications List)

By bringing together some of the world's leading experts, the Nutrilite Health Institute (NHI) has built a global scientific community – adding unprecedented focus and impact to a wide range of studies, from heart health and weight management issues, to improving our lives as we age.

The NHI draws on the expertise of over 100 internal scientists as well as outside experts for research, clinical testing, and education. Their discoveries, demonstrated in hundreds of international science and nutrition journals and presentations, have greatly expanded global understanding of nutrition science.

The list of NHI publications spans more than five decades of groundbreaking research in the areas of nutrition science, analytical chemistry, and agricultural methodology and includes the following:

1. Randolph K, Kornman K. A nutrigenetics proof-of-principle study: 12 years of molecular genetics meets 70 years of nutrition science. *Nutrition*.2009;25:258-260.
2. Corren J, Lemay M, Lin Y, Rozga L, Randolph K. Clinical and biochemical effects of a combination botanical product (CLEARGUARD™ Supplement) for allergy: a pilot randomized double-blind placebo-controlled trial. *Nutrition Journal*. 2008;7:20.
3. Herman D, Vargas M, Lin Y. Strategies for successful weight management programs: what are the options? *Nutrition in Complementary Care*.2008;10:41, 44-48.
4. Kornman K, Rogus J, Roh-Schmidt H, Krempin D, Davies A, Grann K, Randolph K. Interleukin-1 genotype-selective inhibition of inflammatory mediators by a botanical: a nutrigenetics proof of concept. *Nutrition*. 2007;23:844-852.
5. Meskin M, Bidlack W, Randolph K (eds.). Phytochemicals: *Nutrient-Gene Interactions*. CRC Press, 2006.
6. Lemay M, et al. Anti-inflammatory phytochemicals: in vitro and ex vivo evaluation. In: Phytochemicals: Nutrient-Gene Interactions, CRC Press, 2006.
7. Randolph R, et al. Proof of concept for a nutrigenomic botanical for inflammation associated with genetic overexpression of IL-1. In: *Phytochemicals: Nutrient-Gene Interactions*, CRC Press, 2006.
8. Rozga L, et al. Proof of concept bioassay and clinical evidence for a botanical anti-allergy intervention. In: *Phytochemicals: Nutrient-Gene Interactions*, CRC Press, 2006.

APPENDIX

9. Yuan Xiang-Nan, Shen Xiao-Yi, Li Ke-J i, et al. Multivitamin and mineral supplements on the quality of life of healthy persons. *China Mental Hygiene Journal*. 2006;20:506-509.
10. Brovelli E, Boucher A, Arnason J, Menon G, Johnson R. Effects of expression technology on physical parameters and phytochemical profile of Echinacea purpurea juice. *HortScience*. 2004;39:146-148.
11. Lemay M, Murray M, Davies A, Roh-Schmidt H, Randolph R. In vitro and ex vivo cyclooxygenase inhibition by a hops extract. *Asia Pacific Journal of Clinical Nutrition*. 2004;13:S110.
12. Meskin M, Bidlack W, Davies A, Lewis D, Randolph K (eds.). *Phytochemicals: Mechanisms of Action*. CRC Press, 2004.
13. Lemay M. Clinical research on dietary supplements. In: *Phytochemicals: Mechanisms of Action*, CRC Press, 2004.
14. Bone R, Landrum J, Guerra L, Ruiz C. Lutein and zeaxanthin dietary supplements raise macular pigment density and serum concentrations of these carotenoids in humans. *Journal of Nutrition*. 2003;133:992-998.
15. Botero Omary M, Brovelli E, Pusateri D, David P, Rushing J, Fonseca J. Sulforaphane potential and vitamin C concentration in developing heads and leaves of broccoli (Brassica oleracea var. italica). *Journal of Food Quality*. 2003;26:523-530.
16. Brovelli E, Li Y, Chui K. Image analysis and cichoric acid level reflect drying conditions of Echinacea purpurea. *Journal of Herbs, Spices & Medicinal Plants*. 2003;10:19-24.
17. Johnson P. Acerola (Malpighia glabra L., M. punicifolia L., M. emarginata D.C.): agriculture, production & nutrition. *World Review in Nutrition & Dietetics*. 2003;91:67-75.
18. Randolph R, Gellenbeck K, Stonebrook K, Brovelli E, Qian Y, Bankaitis-Davis D, Cheronis J. Regulation of human immune gene expression as influenced by a commercial blended Echinacea product: preliminary studies. *Experimental Biology & Medicine*. 2003;228:1051-1056.
19. Meskin M, Bidlack W, Davies A, Omaye S (eds.). *Phytochemicals in Nutrition and Health*. CRC Press, 2002.
20. Murray M. A closer look at supplement bioavailability. *American Dietetic Association Nutrition in Complementary Care Newsletter*. Summer, 2002.

21. Veltri R, Marks L, Miller M, Bales W, Fan J, Macairan M, Epstein J, Partin A. Saw Palmetto alters nuclear measurements reflecting DNA content in men with symptomatic BPH: evidence for a possible molecular mechanism. *Urology*. 2002;60:617-622.
22. Chandra A, Rana J, and Li Q. Separation, identification, quantification, and method validation of anthocyanins in botanical supplement raw materials by HPLC and HPLC-MS. *Journal of Agricultural & Food Chemistry*. 2001;49:3515-21.
23. David P. Separation of phytoestrogens in red clover by reverse phase HPLC with UV-visible and fluorescence detection. *Agilent Technologies*. March, 2001.
24. Hwang J, Hodis H, Sevanian A. Soy and alfalfa phytoestrogen extracts become potent low-density lipoprotein antioxidants in the presence of acerola cherry extract. *Journal of Agricultural & Food Chemistry*. 2001;49:308-14.
25. Jang Y, Lee J, Cho E, Chung N, Topham D, Balderston B. Differences in body fat distribution and antioxidant status in Korean men with cardiovascular disease and diabetes. *American Journal of Clinical Nutrition*. 2001;73:68-74.
26. Marks L, Hess D, Dorey F, Macairan L, Santos P, Tyler V. Tissue effects of saw palmetto and finasteride: use of biopsy cores for *in situ* quantification of prostatic androgens. *Urology*. 2001;57:999-1005.
27. Bidlack W, Meskin M, Omaye S, Topham D (eds.). *Phytochemicals as Bioactive Agents*. Technomic Publishing, 2000.
28. Bubrick P, Stonebrook K, Johnson P. Saw palmetto: critical review, chemistry and application. In: Bidlack W, Meskin M, Omaye S, Topham D (eds.). *Phytochemicals as Bioactive Agents*. Technomic Publishing, 2000.
29. Bone R, Landrum J, Dixon Z, Chen Y, and Llerena C. Lutein and zeaxanthin in the eyes, serum and diet of human subjects. *Experimental Eye Research*. 2000;71:239-45.
30. Conaway C, Getahun S, Liebes L, Pusateri D, Topham D, Botero-Omary M, Chung F. Disposition of glucosinolates and sulforaphane in humans after ingestion of steamed and fresh broccoli. *Nutrition & Cancer*. 2000;38:168-178.
31. Jang Y, Lee J, Kim O, Huh K, Topham D, Balderston B. Influence of alcohol consumption and smoking habits on cardiovascular risk factors and antioxidant status in healthy Korean men. *Nutrition Research*. 2000;20:1213-29.

32. Marks L, Partin A, Epstein J, Tyler V, Simon I, Macairan M, Chan T, Dorey F, Garris J, Veltri R, Santos P, Stonebrook K, DeKernion J. Effects of saw palmetto herbal blend in men with symptomatic benign prostatic hyperplasia. *Journal of Urology.* 2000;163:1451-56.
33. Schroder H, Navarro E, Tramullas A, Mora J, Galiano D. Nutrition antioxidant status and oxidative stress in professional basketball players: effects of a three compound antioxidative supplement. *International Journal of Sports Medicine.* 2000;21:145-50.
34. Bubrick P. Spinach alternatives for home use. The Business of Herbs. March, 1999.
35. Jang Y, Lee J, Kim O, Huh K, Topham D, Balderston B. Influence of age and obesity on visceral fat, muscle mass and cardiovascular risk factors in healthy Korean men. *Korean Journal of Lipidology.* 1999;9:393-405.
36. Jang Y, Lee J, Kim O, Huh K, Topham D, Balderston B. Relationship between plasma homocysteine levels and cardiovascular risk factors in healthy men. *Korean Circulation Journal.* 1999;92:135-145.
37. Jang Y, Lee J, Kim O, Huh K, Topham D, Balderston B. Changes in body fat distribution and antioxidant system in patients with coronary heart disease. *Korean Circulation Journal.* 1999;29:55-66.
38. Jang Y, Lee J, Kim O, Huh K, Topham D, Balderston B. Influence of alcohol consumption and smoking habits on cardiovascular risk factors and antioxidant status in healthy men. *Korean Journal of Medicine.* 1999;56(4):437-449.
39. Alcantara C. Drying rate effect on the properties of whey protein films. *Journal of Food Process Engineering.* 1998;21:387-405.
40. Bidlack W, Omaye S, Meskin M, Jahner D (eds.). *Phytochemicals: A New Paradigm.* Technomic Publishing, 1998.
41. Brovelli E, Brecht J, Cherman W, Sims C, Harrison J. Sensory and compositional attributes of melting and nonmelting flesh peaches for the fresh market. *Journal of Science in Food and Agriculture.* 1998;79:707-712.
42. Brovelli E, Cuppett S, Uhlinger R, Brecht J. Textural quality of green and white asparagus. *Journal of Food Quality.* 1998;21:497-504.
43. Bubrick P. Seed germination results. *The Business of Herbs.* November/December, 1998.

44. Calvert G, Jahner D, Stonebrook K. Research interest with botanicals. In: Nose H, Nadel ER, Morimoto T (eds.). *The 1997 Nagano Symposium on Sports Science*. Cooper Publishing Group, 1998.
45. Chiang W, Pusateri D, Leitz R. Gas chromatography/mass spectrometry method for the determination of sulforaphane and sulforaphane nitrite in broccoli. *Journal of Agricultural and Food Chemistry*. 1998;46:1018-21.
46. Gellenbeck K. Carotenoids: more than just beta-carotene. *Asia Pacific Journal of Clinical Nutrition*. 1998;7:277-81.
47. Magee, M, Jahner, D. Macronutrient fuels for sports and athletic performance. In: Nose H, Nadel ER, and Morimoto T (eds). *The 1997 Nagano Symposium on Sports Science*. Cooper Publishing Group, 1998.
48. Bubrick P. Acerola. *California Rare Fruit Growers - Fruit Facts* (www.crfg.org), 1996.
49. Buddington R, Williams C, Chen S, Witherly S. Dietary supplement of neosugar alters the fecal flora and decreases activities of some reductive enzymes in human subjects. *American Journal of Clinical Nutrition*. 1996;63:709-16.
50. Williams C, Witherly S, and Buddington R. Influence of dietary neosugar on selected bacterial groups in human faecal microbiota. *Microbial Ecology in Health and Disease*. 1994;7:91-7.
51. Lehto K, Bubrick P, Dawson WO. Time Course of TMV 30K protein accumulation in intact leaves. *Virology*. 1990;174:290-3.
52. Pusateri D, Roth W, Ross J, Shultz T. Dietary and hormonal evaluation of men at different risks for prostate cancer: plasma and fecal hormone-nutrient interrelationships. *American Journal of Clinical Nutrition*. 1990;51:371-7.
53. Ross J, Pusateri D, Schultz T. Dietary and hormonal evaluation of men at different risks for prostate cancer: fiber intake, excretion, and composition, with in vitro evidence for an association between steroid hormones and specific fiber components. *American Journal of Clinical Nutrition*. 1990;51:365-70.
54. Chapman D, Gellenbeck K. An historical perspective of algae biotechnology. *ALGOL and Cyanobacterial Biotechnology*. 1989;1:1-27.
55. Edwards D, Beegle B. No till liming effects on soil pH, corn grain yield and earleaf nutrient content. *Communications in Soil Science and Plant Analysis*. 1988;19:543-562.

56. Gellenbeck K, Kraemer G, McMurtry L, Chapman D. An experimental culture system for macroalgae and other aquatic life. *Aquaculture*. 1988;74:385-91.

57. Gellenbeck K, Chapman D. Feasibility of mariculture of the brown seaweed, *Sargassium muticum* (phaeophyta): growth and culture conditions, alginic acid content and conversion to methane. *Beihefte Zur Nova Hedwigia*. 1986;1:107-15.

58. Gellenbeck K, Chapman D. Seaweed uses: the outlook for mariculture. *Endeavour*. 1983;7:31-7.

59. Hall I, Dulmage H, Arakawa K. The susceptibility of the eye gnat *Hippelates collusor* to entomogenous bacteria and fungi. *Journal of Invertebrate Pathology*. 1972;19:28-31.

60. Chauthani A, Rehnborg C. Dosage mortality data on the nuclear polyhedrosis viruses of *Spodoptera exigua*, *Trichoplusia ni*, and *Prodenia ornithogalli*. *Journal of Invertebrate Pathology*. 1972;17:234-7.

61. Chauthani A, Snideman M, Rehnborg C. Comparison of commercially produced *Bacillus thuringiensis* var. *thuringiensis* with two bioassay techniques based on toxicity units. *Journal of Economic Entomology*.1971;64:1291-3.

62. Dulmage H, Boening O, Rehnborg C, Hansen G. A proposed standardized bioassay for formulations of Bacillus thuringiensis based on the International Unit. *Journal of Invertebrate Pathology*. 1971;18:240-5.

63. Miller R, Pickens L, Gordon C. Effect of *Bacillus thuringiensis* in cattle manure on house fly larvae. *Journal of Economic Entomology*. 1971;64:902-3.

64. Ikeshoji T, Mulla M. Overcrowding factors of mosquito larvae. 2. Growth-retarding and bacteriostatic effects of the overcrowding factors of mosquito larvae. *Journal of Economic Entomology*. 1970;63:1737-43.

65. Chauthani A, Claussen D, Rehnborg C. Dosage-mortality data on a nuclear-polyhedrosis virus of the bollworm, *Heliothis zea*. *Journal of Invertebrate Pathology*. 1968;12:335-8.

66. Chauthani A, Claussen D. Rearing Douglas-fir tussock moth larvae on synthetic media for the production of nuclear-polyhedrosis virus. *Journal of Economic Entomology*. 1968;61:101-3.

67. Chauthani A, Murphy D, Claussen D, Rehnborg C. The effect of human gastric juice on the pathogenicity of Heliothis zea nuclear-polyhedrosis virus. *Journal of Invertebrate Pathology*. 1968;12:145-7.
68. Chauthani AR. Bioassay technique for insect viruses. *Journal of Invertebrate Pathology*. 1968;11:242-5.
69. Chauthani A, Hamm J. Biology of the exotic parasite Drino munda (Diptera: Tachinidae). *Annals of the Entomological Society of America*. 1967;60:373-6.
70. Weaver N, Chauthani A. An all-liquid pollen substitute for honey bee colonies *American Bee Journal*. 1967;107:134-5.
71. Dunn P, Hall I, Snideman M. Bioassay of *Bacillus thuringiensis*-based microbial insecticides. III - continuous propagation of the salt-marsh caterpillar, *Estigmene acrea*. *Journal of Economic Entomology*. 1964;57:374-7.
72. Mechalas B, Anderson N. Bioassay of *Bacillus thuringiensis* Berliner-based microbial insecticides II. Standardization. *Journal of Insect Pathology*. 1964;6:218-24.
73. Mechalas BJ, Dunn PH. Bioassay of *Bacillus thuringiensis* Berliner-based microbial insecticides I. Bioassay procedures. *Journal of Insect Pathology*. 1964;6:214-7.
74. Rehnborg C, Nichols A. The fate of cholesterol esters in human serum incubated in vitro at 38°. *Biochimica et Biophysica Acta*. 1964;84:596-603.
75. Dunn P, Mechalas B. An easily constructed vacuum duster. *Journal of Economic Entomology*. 1963;56:899.
76. Dunn P, Mechalas BJ. The potential of *Beauveria bassiana* (Balsamo) Vuillemin as a microbial insecticide. *Journal of Insect Pathology*. 1963;5:451-9.
77. Mechalas B, Beyer O. Production and assay of extracellular toxins by *Bacillus thuringiensis*. *Developments in Industrial Microbiology*. 1963;4:142-7.
78. Nichols A, Rehnborg C, Lindgren F, Wills R. Effects of oil ingestion on lipoprotein fatty acids in man. *Journal of Lipid Research*. 1962;3:320-6.
79. Mechalas B. Microbiological insecticides. *Agrichemical West*. 1961;4:9-10.
80. Nichols A, Rehnborg C, Lindgren F. Gas chromatographic analysis of fatty acids from dialyzed lipoproteins. *Journal of Lipid Research*. 1961;2:203-7.
81. Westall E. Progress report on microbial insecticides. *Food Processing*. June, 1961.

82. Ershoff B, Hernandez H. An unidentified water-soluble factor in alfalfa which improves utilization of vitamin A. *Journal of Nutrition*. 1960;70:313-20.
83. Mechalas B, Rittenberg S. Energy coupling in *Desulfovibrio desulfuricans*. *Department of Bacteriology*. 1960;80:501-7.
84. Liles J, Dunn P. Preliminary laboratory results on the susceptibility of *Aedes aegypti* (Linnaeus) to *Bacillus thuringiensis*. *Journal of Insect Pathology*. 1959;1:309-10.
85. Maciasr F. Acetate stimulation of Lactobacillus delbrueckii and its replacement by nucleosides. *Journal of Bacteriology*. 1959;77:497-501.
86. Maciasr F. Effect of oleic acid on the response of *Lactobacillus fermenti* to thiamin and its moieties. *Journal of Bacteriology*. 1958;75:561-6.
87. McWilliams H. Vitamin-mineral deficiencies in the American diet. *Experimental Medicine & Surgery*. 1958;16:265-75.
88. Maciasr F. Improved medium for assay of thiamin with *Lactobacillus fermenti*. *Applied Microbiology*. 1957;5:249-52.
89. Novak A, Gama J, Liuzzo J, Rubloff E. Factors affecting the microbiological assay of pyridoxine in multivitamin products. *Journal of the American Pharmaceutical Association*. 1953;42:581-3.

For additional information on the science behind the brand, please visit www.nutrilite.com.

Reference Materials

Much of the information found within this book was culled from my father's personal and business correspondence—most of which is found in the archives at the Nutrilite Health Institute. This includes, but is not limited to, an extensive collection of handwritten journals, letters, speeches, essays, memos, photos, videos, slides, brochures, books, and artifacts. Additional information, such as that pertaining to family history, births, deaths, marriages, residences, and various jobs my father had was also gathered by Genealogy Research Associates—all of which has been confirmed by such documents as Census records, Vital Statistics, death records, Registries, and Parish records.

Additional information was gathered from individuals who graciously shared their time and knowledge regarding Nutrilite, my father, and or other aspects associated with this book. These interviewed individuals include: Dr. Viopapa Annandale-Atherton, Barney Bailey, Neal Brophy, Dewane Bunting, Helen Bruck, Katie Berry Cortright, Matt Cox, Audra Davies, Rich Devos, Dug Duggan, Basil Fuller, Sara Frances Harkness, Sally Rehnborg Hayes, Atea Hintze, Bob Hunter, Ken Jacobsen, Nancy Rehnborg Kahalewai, Clair Knox, Lester Lev, Marty Loos, Dan Montgomery, Gay Moritz, Leverne Parker, Kay Rehnborg, Joan Rehnborg, Lisa Rehnborg, Meridith Rehnborg, Ned Rehnborg, Charlie Rhyne, Archie and Lu Richardson, Ed Richardson, Rick and Jean Rickenbrode, Ned Ross, Charlie Savio, Adam Schawula, Russ Smith, Esther Spangenberg, Stefan Tenkoff, Jay Van Andel, Fuzzy Vaughn, and Sara Rehnborg Vaughn.

Chapter 2

1. Crow C. *Foreign Devils in the Flowery Kingdom*. New York: Harper & Bro; 1940.
2. Hobart A. *Oil for the Lamps of China*. Indianapolis: The Bobbs-Merrill Co; 1933.
3. Denby J. *Letters of a Shanghai Griffin*. Shanghai: Kelly&Walsh; 1923.
4. Directory and Chronicle for Japan, China, Korea, etc. 1918.
5. Rosenfeld L. Vitamine-vitamin. The early years of discovery. *Clin Chem*. 1997;43:680-685.

6. *The Voyages of Jacques Cartier*, translated by Henry Percival Biggar. Toronto: University of Toronto Press; 1993.
7. Carpenter KJ. A short history of nutritional science: part 3 (1912-1944). *J Nutr.* 2003;133:3023-3032.
8. Wardlaw G. *Perspectives in Nutrition*. 4th edition. The McGraw-Hill Companies, Inc.; 1996.

Chapter 3

1. Collier EC. Instances of Use of United States Forces Abroad, 1798 - 1993. Washington DC: Congressional Research Service — Library of Congress — October 7, 1993. Available at: www.history.navy.mil/wars/foabroad.htm. Accessed July 17, 2009.
2. Hobart A. *Oil for the Lamps of China*. Indianapolis: The Bobbs-Merrill Co; 1933.

Chapter 4

1. Marshall J. *Elbridge A. Stuart: Founder of Carnation Company*. New York:Stratford Press Inc.; 1949.
2. Rosenfeld L. Vitamine-vitamin. The early years of discovery. *Clin Chem.* 1997;43:680-685.
3. Simoni RD, Hill RL, Vaughan M. The nutritional biochemistry and the discovery of vitamins: the work of Elmer Verner McCollum. *J Biological Chem.* 2002;277:16-18. Available at: www.jbc.org. Accessed April 30, 2008.
4. Hopkins FG. Feeding experiments illustrating the importance of accessory factors in normal dietaries. *J Physiol.* 1912;44:425-60.
5. Semba RD. Vitamin A as "anti-infective" therapy, 1920-1940. *J Nutr.* 1999;129:783-791.
6. Carpenter KJ. A short history of nutritional science: Part 2 (1885-1912). *J. Nutr.* 2003;133:975-984.

7. Funk C. The etiology of the deficiency diseases. *J State Med.* 1912;20:341-368 [Taken from Carpenter KJ. A short history of nutritional science: Part 3 (1912-1944). *J. Nutr.* 2003;133:3023-3032.]
8. Ensminger AH, Konlande JE. *Food and Nutrition Encyclopedia.* 2nd ed. CPC-Press; 1993.
9. Alfalfa Production Guide for the Southern Great Plains. Plant & Soil Sciences Department, Oklahoma State University, 368 Ag Hall, Stillwater, OK 74078, p 50. Available at: lubbock.tamu.edu/othercrops/pdf/alfalfa/Okla%20St%20Alfalfa%20Production%20Guide.pdf. Accessed August 3, 2009.
10. Nestlé corporate website. Available at: verybestbaking.com/brands/carnation_history.asp.
11. Butler G, Nielsen J, Slot T, et al. Fatty acid and fat-soluble antioxidant concentrations in milk from high- and low-input conventional and organic systems: seasonal variation. *J Sci Food Agri.* 2008;88:1431-41.

Chapter 5

1. Gaan M. *Last Moments of a World.* New York: Norton; 1978.
2. Crow C. *Foreign Devils in the Flowery Kingdom.* New York: Harper & Bro; 1940.
3. Tse-tung C. *The May Fourth Movement.* Cambridge, MA: Harvard University Press; 1960.
4. Ling P. *In Search of Old Shanghai.* Hong Kong: Joint Publishing Company; 1982.
5. Hoyt EP. *The Rise of the Chinese Republic: From the Last Emperor to Deng Xiaoping.* New York: McGraw-Hill; 1989.
6. Chen J, Weng W. Medicinal food: the Chinese perspective. *J Med Food.* 1998;1:117-122.
7. Beinfield H. Cracking the code of Chinese medicine. *Natural Health.* 1996; November-December:100.
8. Deering MC. Ho for the Soochow Ho. *National Geographics.* Washington, DC:National Geographic Society; June 1927.
9. Hobart A. *Oil for the Lamps of China.* Indianapolis: The Bobbs-Merrill Co.; 1933.
10. Wilson EH. The Kingdom of Flowers: an account of the wealth of trees and shrubs of China and of what the Arnold Arboretum, with China's help, is doing to enrich America. *National Geographics.* November 1911.
11. Burrows T, ed., *Visual History of the Twentieth Century.* London: Carlton; 1999.
12. Collier EC. *Instances of Use of United States Forces Abroad, 1798-1993.* Washington DC: Congressional Research Service — Library of Congress — October 7, 1993. Available at: www.history.navy.mil/wars/foabroad.htm. Accessed July 17, 2009.
13. *Oscar R. Ewing, Federal Security Administrator, et al., Appellants vs. Mytinger & Casselberry, A California Corporation,* Supreme Court of the United States, October Term, 1949, No. 568, filed January 30, 1950.

Chapter 6

1. Lactose intolerance in the Chinese population. Website for European Centre for Allergy Research Foundation. Available at: www.ecarf.org. Accessed August 3, 2009.
2. Colgate website. Accessed October 2005.
3. Ling P. *In Search of Old Shanghai*. Hong Kong: Joint Publishing Company; 1982.
4. Sergeant H. *Shanghai: Collision Point of Cultures 1918-1939*. New York: Crown; 1991.
5. Ensiminger AH, Konlande J. *Food and Nutrition Encyclopedia*. 2nd ed. CPC-Press; 1993.
6. Young JH. *The Medical Messiahs: A Social History of Health Quackery in Twentieth-Century America*. Princeton, NJ: Princeton University Press; 1992.

Chapter 7

1. Roberts J. *A Concise History of China*. Cambridge, MA: Harvard University Press; 1999.
2. Lazzerini EJ. *The Chinese Revolution*. Westport, CT: Greenwood Press; 1999.
3. Gamer R. *Understanding Contemporary China*. 2nd ed. Boulder, CO: Lynne Rienner Publishing; 2003.
4. China timeline. Available at: http://www.worldvitalrecords.com/chinatimeline.html. Accessed on July 11, 2009.
5. Hoyt EP. *The Rise of the Chinese Republic: From the Last Emperor to Den Xiaoping*. New York: McGraw-Hill; 1989.
6. Moss R. The Fourth Marines in China, 1927-1941; May 21, 1996. Available at: history.sandiego.edu/ GEN/projects/moss/chinamarines1.html. Accessed July 17, 2009.
7. Abbey PR. United States Navy Yangtze Patrol & South China Patrol: A Brief Historical Chronology. Available at: http://www.geocities.com/Vienna/5047/yangpathistory.html. Accessed July 17, 2009.
8. *All About Shanghai and Environs: A Standard Guide*. Shanghai: The University Press; 1934.
9. Collier EC. *Instances of Use of United States Forces Abroad*, 1798 - 1993. Washington DC: Congressional Research Service — Library of Congress — October 7, 1993. Available at: www.history.navy.mil/wars/foabroad.htm. Accessed July 17, 2009.
10. *National Geographics*. Washington, DC: National Geographc Society; June 1927.
11. Gaan M. *Last Moments of a World*. New York: Norton; 1978.
12. *North China Daily News*. April 4, 1927.
13. *New York Times*. May 27, 1929 [Taken from: Isaacs H. *The Tragedy of the Chinese Revolution*. Stanford: Stanford University Press; 1962.]

Chapter 8

1. Starr K. *Material Dreams: Southern California through the 1920s (Americans & the California Dream)*. USA: Oxford University Press; 1991.
2. Trona on the Web: Trona Money. Available at: http://www.trona-ca.com/trona-money.htm. Accessed June 13, 2009.
3. *The Trona pot-ash*. Trona, CA:H.D. Graessle. November 30, 1929.
4. *The Trona pot-ash*. Trona, CA:H.D. Graessle. March 5, 1932.
5. Merck Manual. Available at: http://www.merck.com. Accessed June 2, 2002.
6. Rehnborg C. Reflections on Living and Dying; February 19, 1964. In: *C.F. Rehnborg—A Collection of His Essays, Speeches, and Writings*. Buena Park, CA:C.F. Rehnborg Literary Foundation; 1985:300-304.
7. *The Trona pot-ash*. Trona, CA:H.D. Graessle. March 19, 1932.
8. Civil Action #5208-48. Ewing v. Mytinger & Casselberry.

Chapter 9

1. Rosenfeld L. Vitamine-vitamin. The early years of discovery. *Clin Chem*. 1997;43:680-685.
2. Combs GF. *The Vitamins Fundamental Aspects in Nutrition and Health*. San Diego, CA:Academy Press, Inc.; 1992.
3. *Scientific American*. December 1932: pp 360-362.
4. Szent-Györgyi A. Observations on the function of the peroxidase systems. *Biochemical Journal*. 1928; 22:1387-1409. [Taken from: The Cambridge World History of Food. Available at: http://www.cambridge.org/us/books/kiple/vitaminc.htm. Accessed May 16, 2009.]
5. Carpenter KJ, Harper AE, Olson RE. Experiments that changed nutritional thinking. *J Nutr*. 1997;127:1017S-1053S.
6. The Noble Prize in Physiology or Medicine 1934. Available at: http://nobelprize.org. Accessed May 15, 2009.
7. Pizzi RA. The Roaring Twenties and the Great Depression: This era of vitamins and hormones also witnessed the development of new drugs and vaccines. [Taken from: The Pharmaceutical Century (American Chemical Society) ACS Publications website. Accessed Dec. 24, 2000.]
8. Ogden RL, Kehr WR. Field management or dehydration and hay production. *In* Proc. 10th Tech. Alfalfa Conf, USDA-ARS; 1968.
9. Without Medicine Chests. *Orange County Business*. 1st Quarter; 1969: p 59.
10. Great Depression in the United States. MSN Encarta website. Available at: http://encarta.msn.com. Accessed July 25, 2009.

Chapter 10

1. Richard Kuhn and the Chemical Institute: Double Bonds and Biological Mechanisms. Available at: nobelprize.org. Accessed July 30, 2009.
2. Yahoo Financial. Available at: http://table.fianance.yahoo.com. Accessed July 11, 2002.

Chapter 11

1. BenVenue Laboratories website. Accessed June 14, 2002.
2. Folic acid fortification. U.S. Food and Drug Administration, Office of Public Affairs Fact Sheet; February 29, 1996.
3. FDA History Part II: The 1938 Food, Drug, and Cosmetic Act. U.S. Food and Drug Administration website. Available at: http://www.fda.gov/AboutFDA/WhatWeDo/History/Origin/ucm054826.htm. Accessed August 11, 2009.
4. Swanson B. I just found out about Orange County—Vitamins. *Santa Ana Journal*. October 28, 1938.

Chapter 12

1. Combs GF. *The Vitamins Fundamental Aspects in Nutrition and Health*. San Diego, CA: Academic Press, Inc.; 1992.
2. Larrick G. Testimony in Ewing vs. Mytinger and Casselberry, October Term, 1949, pp. 385-387.
3. The vitamin content of foods. Chart from *Live: the Helpful Guide to Healthful Living*; December 1940 (found in Carl Rehnborg's scrapbook).
4. Beamon AR, as told to Terhune E. This vitamin age. *Los Angeles Sunday Times*. June 26, 1940:, p 11.
5. Vita-Diet brochure, date unknown.
6. Escrow and Safe Deposit Company (Reseda farm escrow paper. Escrow No. 4203); February 28, 1942.
7. Description of Whizzer from Doug Clark. Rare old whizzers delight pedal pushers born to be wild. *Spokane Spokesman-Review*. July 7, 1998:, p B1.
8. Brittanica Online. Nobel prizes: medicine, timeline of achievements. Available at: search.eb.com/nobel/medtime.html. Accessed June 16, 2002.
9. Vitamin History, from Lasker Awards website.
10. Williams R. Nutrilites. *Science*. 1928; Vol. LXVII: pp607-608.

Chapter 13

1. Without Medicine Chests. *Orange County Business.* 1st Quarter 1969: p 58.
2. The Organization Behind the Product You Sell; Volume 1. Mytinger & Casselberry, Inc.; 1952.
3. *Oscar R. Ewing, Federal Security Administrator, et al., Appellants vs. Mytinger & Casselberry, A California Corporation,* Supreme Court of the United States, October Term, 1949, No. 568, filed January 30, 1950.
4. Stanford-Binet Intelligence Scale. Available at: www.Britannica.com. Accessed September 3, 2009.
5. Mahoney T. *The Great Merchants.* New York: Harper; 1955.
6. How to Cheat Death, first sales manual prepared by Mytinger & Casselberry for Nutrilite, September 1945.

Chapter 14

1. Barrett S, Herber V. *The Vitamin Pushers.* Amherst, NY:Prometheus Books; 1994, p 2.

Chapter 15

1. *Oscar R. Ewing, Federal Security Administrator, et al., Appellants vs. Mytinger & Casselberry, A California Corporation,* Supreme Court of the United States, October Term, 1949, No. 568, filed January 30, 1950.
2. The mess called multi-level marketing. *Money Magazine*; June 1987:, p 144. Available at money.cnn.com/magazines/moneymag /moneymag_archive/1987/06/01/83883/index.htm.
3. Poe R. *Wave 3: The New Era in Network Marketing.* Roseville, CA: Prima; 1994.
4. The Organization Behind the Product You Sell. Mytinger & Casselberry, Inc.; 1956 revision.
5. Fuller B. Basil Fuller Tells How to Make Your Fortune As Big As You Want It! *Salesman's Opportunity*; November 1953.

Chapter 16

1. *Oscar R. Ewing, Federal Security Administrator, et al., Appellants vs. Mytinger & Casselberry, A California Corporation,* Supreme Court of the United States, October Term, 1949, No. 568, filed January 30, 1950.
2. Know Where You're Going. Mytinger & Casselberry, Inc.; 1952. Contains the Final

Consent Decree (civil action no. 10344-BH) and provides information in order that all agents and distributors, M&C officers, employees, and representatives will have a complete understanding of the Decree.
3. Address given by George P. Larrick, U.S. Commissioner of Food and Drugs at the American Medical Association's National Congress on Medical Quackery, Washington, DC, October, 1961 [Taken from Levenstein H. *Paradox of Plenty*. Berkeley: University of California Press; 2003, p 167.]
4. Dunbar PB, Administrator, Food and Drug Administration *Food Drug Cosmetic Law Journal*. January 1952, p 51 (Text of speech given to Food Law Institute on his retirement from FDA, November 14, 1951).
5. Fletcher RH, Fairfield KM. Vitamins for chronic disease prevention in adults: Clinical Applications. *JAMA*. 2002; 287:3127-129.
6. Fletcher RH, Fairfield KM. Vitamins for chronic disease prevention in adults: Scientific Review. JAMA.2002; 287:3116-126.

Chapter 17
1. Van Andel J. *An Enterprising Life: An Autobiography*. New York: Harper Collins Publishers, Inc.; 1998.
2. Collin J, Porras JI. *Built to Last*. New York:HarperCollins Publishers Inc.; 1994.
3. *Time Magazine*. August 18, 1952. Available at: www.time.com. Accessed September 3, 2009.

Chapter 18
1. Rehnborg C. The Purpose of the Boys Club; August 3, 1960. In: *C.F. Rehnborg— A Collection of His Essays, Speeches, and Writings*. Buena Park, CA:C.F. Rehnborg Literary Foundation; 1985:183-187.
2. Pennington J. *Food Values of Portions Commonly Used*. 15th ed. Philadelphia, PN: JB Lippincott Co.; 1989.

Chapter 19
1. Rehnborg C. Excerpt from Tahiti—An Island Paradise; 1958. In: *C.F. Rehnborg— A Collection of His Essays, Speeches, and Writings*. Buena Park, CA:C.F. Rehnborg Literary Foundation; 1985:262-279.

Chapter 20
1. Rhyne CS. Penalty Through Publicity: FDA's Restitution Gambit. *Food Drug Cosmetic Law Journal*; October 1952, p 67.

Chapter 22

1. Carpenter KJ. Thomas Hughes Jukes (1906-1999). *J Nutr.* 2000;130:1521-1523.
2. Williams R. Nutrilites. *Science.* 1928; Vol. LXVIII, pp 607-608.
3. Rosenfeld L. Vitamine-vitamin. The early years of discovery. *Clin Chem.* 1997;43:680-685.
4. Nelson H. New insecticides to aid race for food supply. *Los Angeles Times*, June 19, 1959.
5. Chevalier L. They sell your patients...'Good Health at $19.50 a Box.' *Medical Economics.* August 3, 1959, pp 115-128.
6. Williams WL. History of the Start of the Biochemistry Department, memo to Professor David Puett, University of Georgia Department of Biochemistry, March 2, 1993. Available at: bmbiris.bmb.uga.edu/history/williams1.htm. Accessed March 24, 2003.

Chapter 23

1. Rehnborg C. Distributor speech at Fiesta de Oro Convention, Los Angeles; June 20, 1964. In: *C.F. Rehnborg—A Collection of His Essays, Speeches, and Writings.* Buena Park, CA:C.F. Rehnborg Literary Foundation; 1985:1-5.

Chapter 25

1. Rehnborg C. Reflections on Living and Dying; February 19, 1964. In: *C.F. Rehnborg—A Collection of His Essays, Speeches, and Writings.* Buena Park, CA:C.F. Rehnborg Literary Foundation; 1985:300-304.

Chapter 28

1. White RE. Natural born killers: ladybugs, wasps, and worms replace toxic pesticides as gardeners go organic. *Wall Street Journal.* August 13, 1999.
2. One by One. Rancho El Petacal Health Clinic, Jalisco. Amway website. Available at: www.amwayonebyone.com. Accessed June 2, 2009.
3. Nutrilite Health Institute Fact Sheet. Available at: www.nutrilite.com. Accessed August 2, 2009.
4. Ornish D, Magbanua MJ, Weidner G, et al. Changes in prostate gene expression in men undergoing an intensive nutrition and lifestyle intervention. *Proc Natl Acad Sci USA.* 2008;105:8369-74.
5. Kornman K, Rogus J, Haeri Roh-Schmidt H, et al. Interleukin-1 genotype-selective inhibition of inflammatory mediators by a botanical: nutrigenetics proof of concept. *Nutrition.* 2007;23:844-852.

Chapter 29

1. Nutrition and You: Trends 2008. Paper presented at: Annual Meeting of the American Dietetic Association; October 25-28, 2008; Chicago, IL.
2. World Cancer research Fund/American Institute for Cancer Research. Food, Nutrition and the Prevention of Cancer: A Global Perspective. Washington, DC: AICR; 1997.
3. Social Responsibility Corner. *Leaflet*. Issue 3; 2008.
4. Rehnborg C. Reflections on Living and Dying; February 19, 1964. In: *C.F. Rehnborg—A Collection of His Essays, Speeches, and Writings*. Buena Park, CA:C.F. Rehnborg Literary Foundation; 1985:300-304.

Appendix

1. Srilakshmi B. *Nutrition Science*. 2nd ed. New Delhi, India: New Age International; 2006.
2. Guggenheim KY. Chlorosis: the rise and disappearance of a nutritional disease. *J Nutr*. 1995;125:1822-1825.
3. New World Encyclopedia. Lind, James. Available at: http://www.newworldencyclopedia.org/entry/James_Lind. Accessed May 4, 2009.
4. Rosenfeld L. Vitamine-vitamin. The early years of discovery. *Clin Chem*. 1997;43:680-685.
5. Combs GF. Celebration of the past: nutrition at USDA. *J Nutr*. 1994;124:1728S-1732S.
6. Hopkins FG. Feeding experiments illustrating the importance of accessory factors in normal dietaries. *J Physiol*. 1912;44:425-60.
7. Carpenter KJ. History of nutrition. *J. Nutrition*. 2003;133:975-984.
8. Vandamme EJ. *Biotechnology of Vitamins, Pigments and Growth Factors*. London, England: Springer; 1989.
9. Oliver Perry Kimball Papers. Dittrick Medical History Center. Case Western Reserve University. Available at: http://www.cwru.edu/artsci/dittrick/site2/archives/perry.html. Accessed May 13, 2009.
10. C. F. Rehnborg—A Collection of his Essays, Speeches, and Writings. Buena Park, CA: C.F. Rehnborg Literary Foundation; 1985.
11. Drummond JC. The nomenclature of the so-called accessory food factors (vitamins). *Biochem J*. 1920;14:660. [Taken from Rosenfeld L. Vitamine-vitamin. The early years of discovery. Clin Chem. 1997;43:680-685.]
12. Timeline: Discoveries and contributions by UC Berkeley scholars. History of U.C. Berkeley. Available at: http://berkeley.edu/about/hist/timeline.shtml. Accessed May 11, 2009.

13. Agriculture Research Service. Available at: www.ars.usda.gov. Accessed June 24, 2009.
14. Szent-Györgyi A. Observations on the function of the peroxidase systems. *Biochemical Journal*. 1928; 22:1387-1409. [Taken from: The Cambridge World History of Food. Available at: http://www.cambridge.org/us/books/kiple/vitaminc.htm. Accessed May 16, 2009.]
15. Williams R. Nutrilites. *Science*. 1928; Vol. LXVII:607-8.
16. The Noble Prize in Physiology or Medicine 1934. Available at: http://nobelprize.org. Accessed May 15, 2009.
17. Why Nutrilite. Available at: http://www.nutrilite.com. Accessed May 18, 2009.
18. Bronner F. *Nutrition and Health: Topics and Controversies*. Farmington, CT: CRC Press; 1995.
19. The Nobel Prize in Chemistry. Available at: http://nobelprize.org. Accessed May 15, 2009.
20. The Nobel Prize in Physiology or Medicine. Available at: http://nobelprize.org. Accessed May 15, 2009.
21. Escrow and Safe Deposit Company (Reseda farm escrow paper. Escrow No. 4203); February 28, 1942.
22. Nutrition and health. Available at: http://profiles.nlm.nih.gov/NN/B/C/Q/K/_/nnbcqk.ocr. Accessed May 15, 2009.
23. Food and Agriculture Organization of the United Nations. Available at: http://www.fao.org. Accessed June 26, 2009.
24. ARS Research Timeline. Available at: www.ars.usda.gov. Accessed June 26, 2009.
25. Harman D. Aging: a theory based on free radical and radiation chemistry. *J Gerontol*. 1956;11: 298–300.
26. Kuhn D. *A World of Opportunity*. Amway. Amway Corporation: Ada, MI; 2009.
27. United States Department of Agriculture. Food and Nutrition Services. Available at: http://www.fns.usda.gov/cnd/Governance/nslp-legislation.htm. Accessed June 29, 2009.
28. Ogden RL, Kehr WR. Field management or dehydration and hay production. In *Proc. 10th Tech*. Alfalfa Conf, USDA-ARS; 1968.
29. About CRN. Council of Responsible Nutrition. Available at: http://www.crnusa.org/who_about.html. Accessed May 18, 2009.
30. Vollset SE, Heuch I, Bjelke E. Fish consumption and mortality from coronary heart disease. *N Engl J Med*. 1985;26;313:820-4.
31. *Jesus and the New Age of Faith*. Buena Park, CA: C.F. Rehnborg Literary Foundation; 1955.

32. The Surgeon General's Report on Nutrition and Health. U.S. Department of Health and Human Services, 1988. Available at: http://profiles.nlm.nih.gov/NN/B/C/Q/G/_/nnbcqg.ocr. Accessed June 26, 2009.
26. Kiple K, Ornelas KC. *The Cambridge World History of Food. Vol 2*. Cambridge, UK: Cambridge University Press; 2000.
27. CDC (Centers for Disease Control). Recommendations for the use of folic acid to reduce the number of cases of spina bifida and other neural tube defects. *MMWR*. 1992; 41 (No. RR-14).
28. Ames BN, Shigenaga MK, Hagen TM. Oxidants, antioxidants, and the degenerative diseases of aging. *Proc Natl Acad Sci*. 1993;90:7915-7922.
29. Dr. Duke's Phytochemical and Ethnobotanical Database. Available at: http://www.ars-grin.gov/duke/. Accessed June 28, 2009.
30. Boushey CJ, Beresford SA, Omenn GS, et al. A quantitative assessment of plasma homocysteine as a risk factor for vascular disease. Probable benefits of increasing folic acid intakes. *JAMA*. 1995;274:1049-57.
31. Giovannucci E, Ascherio A, Rimm E, et al. Intake of carotenoids and retinol in relation to risk of prostate cancer. *J Nat'l CA Inst*. 1995;87:1767-76.
32. National Institutes of Health: Office of Dietary Supplements. Available at: http://ods.od.nih.gov. Accessed June 28, 2009.
33. WHO Technical Report Series 894. Obesity: preventing and managing the global epidemic. WHO, Geneva; 2000.
34. Tuomilehto J, Lindström J, Eriksson JG, et al. Prevention of type 2 diabetes mellitus by changes in lifestyle among subjects with impaired glucose tolerance. *N Engl J Med*. 2001;344:1343-50.
35. Fletcher RH, Fairfield KM. Vitamins for chronic disease prevention in adults: Clinical Applications. *JAMA*. 2002; 287:3127-129.
36. Fletcher RH, Fairfield KM. Vitamins for chronic disease prevention in adults: Scientific Review. *JAMA*.2002; 287:3116-126.
37. Kris-Etherton PM, Harris WS, Appel LJ, et al. Fish consumption, fish oil, omega-3 fatty acids, and cardiovascular disease. *Circulation*. 2002;106:2747.
38. Human Genome Project Information. Available at: http://genomics.energy.gov/. Accessed May 19, 2009.
39. Juurlink B. The beginning of the nutr-geno-proteo-metabolo-mics era of nutritional studies. *PBI Bulletin* (Plant Biotechnology Institute, NCR, Saskatoon); 2003,1 pp 9-13.

40. Block G, Jensen C, Dietrich M, et al. Plasma C-reactive protein concentration in active and passive smokers: influence of antioxidant supplementation. *J Am Coll Nutr*. 2004;23:141-7.
41. Richer S, Stiles W, Statkute L, et al. Double-masked, placebo-controlled, randomized trial of lutein and antioxidant supplementation of atrophic age-related macular degeneration: the Veterans LAST study (Lutein Antioxidant Supplementation Trial). *Optometry*. 2004; 75:216-30.
42. Sligh T, Sall K. Clinical research update Double X: Effects of daily multi-supplementation on nutrient status and risk factors in healthy adults. Undated. Available at: www.nutrilite.com. Accessed June 2, 2009.
43. Stampfer MJ. Vitamin D in the spotlight. *Newsweek*. December 4, 2006.
44. Kornman K, Rogus J, Haeri Roh-Schmidt H, et al. Interleukin-1 genotype-selective inhibition of inflammatory mediators by a botanical: nutrigenetics proof of concept. *Nutrition*. 2007;23:844-852.
45. The Wellness Revolution. Available at: http://thewellnessrevolution.paulzanepilzer.com/carlrehnborg.php. Accessed May 19, 2009.
46. Butler G, Nielsen J, Slot T, et al. Fatty acid and fat-soluble antioxidant concentrations in milk from high- and low-input conventional and organic systems: seasonal variation. *J Sci Food Agri*. 2008;88:1431-41.
47. Quixtar (2008). International soccer superstar Ronaldinho signs with Nutrilite. Available at: http://www.nutrilite.com. Accessed May 19, 2009.
48. The NUTRILITE™ brand partners with football's most successful club—AC Milan—in global marketing and training pact. Available at: www.nutrilite.com. Accessed August 13, 2009.
49. Nutrilite Leading Children's Vitamin Mineral and Dietary Supplement Claim, Euromonitor International, July 7, 2008.
50. The Nutrilite Opportunity. Mytinger & Casselberry, Inc., circa 1956.

Reference Materials

Index

Acania, 232–233
Accessory food factors, 60
Acerola, 237-238, 274, 338-339
Addison, Dick, 155
Alfalfa, 58, 63, 116-119
American Milk Products Company, 59
Amway Corporation, 261-264, 299-300
    acquisition of Nutrilite Products, Inc., 306-310
Armstrong, Gay. *See* Rehnborg, Gay
ARTISTRY, 316
Associated food factors, 77
Bacillus thuringiensis, 270
Bailey, Barney, 192, 276, 285, 287, 307, 327
Balling, Joan. *See* Rehnborg, Joan (Joni)
Beach, Donn, 243
Berg, Esther, 158
Berg, Evelyn. *See* Rehnborg, Evelyn
Beriberi, 47, 61, 89, 184, 214
Berry, Katie, 292, 298, 311
Best of nature, best of science, 340-347
Big-Eared Du, 86
BIOTROL, biological pest control. *See* Early products
Blades, Les, 235
Bossie the cow, 23
Boys and Girls Club of Buena Park, 226, 233-234, 356, 380
Brockman, John, 285
Brophy, Neal, 339-341
Bruck, Edith. *See* Rehnborg, Edith
Bucklin, 131, 135-137
Buena Park Kids. *See* Boys and Girls Club of Buena Park
Bunting, Dewane, 182, 223, 238
Burlingame, Ray, 137, 145
Business locations
    Balboa Island (Marine Street), 128-130
    Buena Park (Beach Boulevard), 184
    Buena Park (Grand Boulevard), 177
    Long Beach (Hartwell Building), 136
    Los Angeles (Hoover Street), 177
    Los Angeles (Slauson Avenue), 152
    Montebello (Whittier Boulevard), 116
Butz, Robert, 192, 197
C.F. Rehnborg Professorship in Disease Prevention, 340
Calcote, Lela, 135–137, 151–152, 154
    See Rehnborg, Lela (Cal)

California State Polytechnic University, 340, 344
California Vitamin Sales Company, 137
California Vitamins, Inc., 128
Calvert, George, 341-342
Carl F. Rehnborg Museum, 336
Carnation's Experimental Farms, Washington, USA, 66
Carter, Roy, 287
Cartier, Jacques, 48
Casselberry, Bill, 156, 164, 167–174, 203–213, 253-275
Center for Genetics, Nutrition and Health, Washington, D.C., 340
C.F. Rehnborg—A Collection of His Essays and Writings, 295
Charity, Richard, 339
Chen, Junshi, 345
Chiang Kai-shek, 89, 92–96
China
    era of warlords, 53, 69, 93-96
    NUTRILITE products enter Chinese market, 329-331
    map, from 1927, 34
    politics, mid-1920s, 93–98
China Food Products Corporation, 85

Chou En-lai, 92-93, 96–98
Citizens' Magazine Society, 68
Claus, Cliff, 276, 287
Colgate Company, 85
Colgate, Harry, 85
Consent decree, 212
Cox, Matt, 140
Crawford, Charles, 319
Cresci, Francesca, 293, *See* Rehnborg, Francesca
Crown Prince Tungi, 244
Dam, Henrik, 116
Davies, Audra, 341-342
Davis, Marguerite, 60
Dead Sea Scrolls, 235
DeBusk, Ruth, 345
Dennis Day Show, 218
DeVos, Rich, 216-218, 224-225, 258, 260-264, 305-308, 380
Doisy, Edward, 145, 161
Dombrowski, Bill, 350, 352-353
DOUBLE X™ Food Supplement, 203, 250-251, 316
Duggan, Dug, 219, 254, 275
Dye, Ruth, 276, 287
Dykhouse, Robin, 341-342

Early products
- BIOTROL, biological pest control, 270
- ECO-LITE home care products, 286
- Edith Rehnborg Cosmetics, 252–257, 316
- HI-B, 146
- JUNIOR Food Supplement, 166
- K-9 capsules, 161
- MAINTENANCE, 146
- NUTRILITE 100, 316
- NUTRILITE Capsules, No. 5, No. 7, No. 10, and No. 15, 189
- NUTRILITE XX Food Supplement, 202-203
- OLD SETTLER, 158
- One-a-day vitamin capsules, 157
- SPECIAL, 147
- STANDARD, 146
- VITA-6, 120
- Vitamin E Concentrate (with B&G Proportions), 126
- Vitamin-fortified candy, 144
- VITAPHYLL, 126
- VITAPOTENT, 134
- VITASOL, 120, 126-127

Edith Rehnborg Cosmetics. *See* Early products

Efficacy substantiation continuum, 346

Egyptian earthworms, 223

Eijkman, Christiaan, 47

Ewing, Oscar, 212

Facts Folder, 218-219

Farming operations
- Buena Park, California, USA, 179
- El Petacal, Jalisco, Mexico, 336, 338
- Fazenda Nutriorganica, Ceará, Brazil, 338–340
- Hawaii, USA, 237-238
- Hemet, California, USA, 221
- Lakeview, California, USA, 237-238, 334-336
- San Fernando, California, USA, 160
- Trout Lake Farm, Washington, USA, 337-338

Ferri-Min, 135–137

Fields, Bob, 195

Fiesta de Oro convention
- 1958, 256-257
- 1964, 279

Finding of Fact, 207

Firebird, 314, 317-318

Food and Drug Administration (and M&C, Inc.), 204-213

Food and Your Family, 255

Food, Drug, and Cosmetics Act, 1938, 137

Ford, Gerald, 336

Foreign concessions, 41

Fortmann, Stephen, 345

Foundation for American Resource Management (FARM), 236-237

Foy, Sean, 350, 352, 356

Franklin, Walter Scott, 117-118

Frisk, 262

Frölich, Theodore, 63

Fu, Anita, 354-355

Fu, Clement, 354-355

Index

Fuller, Basil, 187-192, 211, 217-218, 223, 253, 262-264
Fuller, Lena, 190-192
Fuller, Warren, 188-191
Funk, Casimir, 61
General Assembly of Nutrilite Distributors, 186, 191-192
Germ theory, 76
Gofman, John, 280
Goldberger, Joseph, 88
Griffin, 41
Guthrie, Bernie, 287
Halverson, Spence, 113, 151
Harvey, Jack, 147-153
Harvey, John, 209
Hauser, Selman, 199
Hawkes, Hester, 28-29
    See Rehnborg, Hester
Haworth, Norman, 128-129
Hazell, Pete, 254
Helen DeVos Children's Hospital, Grand Rapids, Michigan, 358
Hester, Luther, 249, 256, 267, 272
Ho, Z.C., 345
Hoard, Ralph, 137
Holst, Axel, 62
Hopkins, Fredrick, 60-61
Horizontal integration, 336
Hosking, Kay, 135
How to Cheat Death, 172-173
How to Get Well and Stay Well, 203, 205-208
Hua, 41–42
Hunter, Bob, 305-306, 316, 318-319, 323-326
Hydroponics, 223

Interleukin Genetics, 343, 345
Ja-Ri Corporation, 261
Jesus and the New Age of Faith, 235
Johnson, Duke, 350, 352
Johnson, Kip, 352
Johnson, Lee, 287
Jukes, Thomas, 232, 267-269, 272, 280
Kahn, Lloyd, 281
Kaizen, 325
Karrer, Paul, 117, 128
Kemp, Tom, 281
Kettle, Fletcher, 249, 256, 267, 272
Kim, Leonard, 354-355
Kline, Dick, 276
Knox, Clair, 255, 264
Kornman, Kenneth, 345
Kuhn, Richard, 127
Kyoto Prefectural University of Medicine, Kyoto, Japan, 340
L.O.C.™, 262
Ladder for Salesmen, 138
Lakeview's Agricultural Research Farm, 334-336
Larrick, George, 147, 156, 204
Lernoux, Maurice, 254, 287
Les Tropiques, Tahiti, 242-243
Lev, Lester, 151-152, 159, 176, 183, 204, 209-210, 221-222
Liersch, Al, 179
Lind, James, 48
Lindseth, John, 341
Loewy, Raymond, 250-251, 254
Lone Star Shipbuilding Company, 56
Loos, Dottie, 192-194
Loos, Marty, 192-194, 211, 263, 286, 307-308

Maaskant, Neil, 191, 217
Madame Chiang, 250
Magicare, 254
Manufacturing
    early days, 119-120, 125–131, 178-182
Mao Tse-tung, 75, 92-93
May Fourth Movement, 95
McCollum, Elmer, 61, 77
Merck, George, 220, 232
Minot, George, 117
Moss, Faraon Jay, 154, 156
Murphy, William, 117
Myers, Lee, 204-206, 208-209
Mytinger & Casselberry, Inc., 171, 239, 261, 284
    marketing plan, circa 1956, 392-393
    staff and facility, 1954, 225
Mytinger Corporation, 275
Mytinger, Bob, 176, 189-191, 219
Mytinger, Lee, 164, 168-173, 188-190, 207, 225, 253-275
Nelson, Walt, 287
New Tide Society, 68
Nichols, Alex, 280
Nishino, Hoyoku, 345
Nixon, Richard, 210, 286, 293
Nord, Otis, 182
Northern Expedition, 94
NutriCert™ program, 336-337
Nutrigenomics, 344-345
NUTRILITE brand, markets (today), 359
Nutrilite Farming Practices, 222-223, 334-340
Nutrilite Foundation, 233

Nutrilite Health Institute, 341-347
    Center for Optimal Health, 348-349
    Mini brand experience, 352-353
    publications, 394-401
    Scientific Advisory Board, 344-345
Nutrilite Products, Inc.
    acquisition of Mytinger Corporation, 275-276
    acquisition by Amway Corporation, 306-310
    creation of a nutrition laboratory, 1950s, 267-269
    early logo, 161
    early sales and promotion, 154, 167, 175, 218, 239, 304
    early sales kit, 175
    facility expansion, 1970s and 1980s, 324
    management, circa 1966, 287
    origin of name, 149-151
    sales, 1945 to 1947, 185
    sales, 1948 to 1954, 219
    sales, 1955 to 1959, 259
    sales, 1960 to 1963, 277
    sales, 1964 to 1971, 289
    the marketing plan, 169
Nutrilite timeline, 369-391
Nutrimana, 298-299
Nutrition timeline, 369-391
Oceanographic Research at Woods Hole, 232
Oconomowoc Condensory, Wisconsin, USA, 62-63
One by One Campaign for Children, 356
    Little Bits program, 356
    Project Sozo, 356

Index

Optimal health, definition, 349
Paraminobenzoic acid (PABA), 161
Parker, Leverne, 130-131, 143
Payne, Jim, 355
Pepper tree talks, 223-224
Performance Teams, 324, 326
Permacultural practices, 334-338
Pet Milk Company, 59
Plankton project, 231-233
    vitamin A and D extraction, 133
Potentate salesmen, 186-201
Pow Wows. *See* General Assembly of Nutrilite Distributors
President's Team, 325
Profit sharing, 325
Quonset hut, 179, 336
Rankin, Lee, 249
Redwood house, 179-180
Rehnborg Center for Nutrition & Wellness. *See* Nutrilite Health Institute
Rehnborg, Alice, 18-21, 23, 29
Rehnborg, Carl, 10, 16, 20, 22-23, 26, 31, 56, 60, 66, 69-70, 87, 91, 121, 124, 132, 174, 177, 218, 220, 223-224, 226, 238-239, 245, 257, 271-273, 278, 282-283, 287, 291, 313, 360
    astronomy, 292
    becoming a *keeper of custom*, 43-44
    building the milk business, 69-83
    childhood, 20-24
    confined to International Settlement, 97-100
    developing flooring material, 29
    essays, 30-31, 294
    hosts American Bar Association dinner, 1957, 249-250
    impressions (South Pacific), 241-246
    in Tsinanfu, China, 17
    infected with influenza, 56
    jobs as a youth, 24, 27-31
    jobs as an adult, 35, 51, 55, 57, 59, 115
    journaling as a youth, 24-25
    letters, 100, 123, 135, 147-149, 178, 181, 183, 227-230, 245-248
    life in Beaumont, Texas, 56
    life in Pinehurst, North Carolina, 25-26
    life in Savannah, Georgia, 20-22
    life in Shanghai, China, 67-99
    life in Tientsin, China, 40-56
    negotiating in China, 73-74
    nutrition experiments, 80, 98, 106, 114–115, 148
    observations in China, 42, 46-49, 57, 62, 73, 77, 83
    passes away, 310
    peace of nothingness, 110
    recounts story of a friend's experience in a prison camp, 184
    reflections, 65
    religion, 47-48, 233-234
    report for Richard Nixon, 293
    schooling, 23-24, 28-34
    Shanghai Volunteer Corps, 89
    speech, 1958, 257
    speech, 1964, 279
    teen years, 24-27
    thoughts (importance of soil), 69, 77
    travel to China, 35-41
    travel to Chinese Interior, 75
    world tour, 1953, 227-230

Rehnborg, Carl Gustaf, 20
Rehnborg, Carl Reinhold.
  See Rehnborg, Sam
Rehnborg, Edith, 174, 177-180, 218, 221,
  223-224, 226-230, 236, 245,
  252-253, 282, 287, 297, 308, 311
Rehnborg, Edward (Ned), 60, 65-67, 69-70,
  79-80, 90, 183, 221
Rehnborg, Emanuel (Manny), 18
Rehnborg, Evelyn, 114-115, 119-120, 125, 131,
  139-140, 144, 158-159
Rehnborg, Francesca, 319-320, 353-354
Rehnborg, Franklin, 22
Rehnborg, Gay, 241, 273
Rehnborg, Gweneth, 328-329
Rehnborg, Hester, 51-56, 66-67, 79, 90,
  99-101, 106
Rehnborg, Jenna, 320
Rehnborg, Joan (Joni), 280-282, 300, 311
Rehnborg, Kay, 21-22, 227
Rehnborg, Kori, 320
Rehnborg, Lela (Cal), 160, 162
Rehnborg, Lillian, 30
Rehnborg, Lisa, 273, 317, 326-327, 330,
  356, 358
Rehnborg, Lydia (Lillie), 18
Rehnborg, Mildred, 108-110
Rehnborg, Nancy, 79, 90
Rehnborg, Paul, 17-30, 84-85, 109
Rehnborg, Pauline (Pump), 20
Rehnborg, Roderick (Rod), 298, 317,
  327-330
Rehnborg, Sam, 124, 282-283, 285, 287,
  298, 317, 324, 327, 336, 345,
  354-355
  aboard the *Acania*, 232
  begins work at NPI, 282
  childhood, 124-125, 159-161, 179-182
  circumnavigates the world,
    1975-1978, 317-319
  graduate studies, 280
  message of optimal health, 348-358
  Six Steps to Successful Selling, 355
Rehnborg, Sara (Sallie), 22, 84, 90, 96,
  See Vaughn, Sallie
Rehnborg, Tucker, 300
Rhyne, Charles, 209-213, 243, 249-250,
  293, 313
Richardson, Ed, 131, 185
Rickenbrode, Jean, 195-199
Rickenbrode, Rick, 194-199, 262-263, 285
Rogers, Danny, 285
Romo, Sandra, 338
Ross, Ned, 199-201, 308
Rowing Club, Shanghai, China, 89
Santa Ana Journal, 1938, 138-139
Savio, Charlie, 282
Science Magazine, 1928, 150
Scientific Advisory Board, 344-345
Scurvy, 46
Senior Key Conference, 1957, 253
Senior Key Study Group, 1959, 262-264
Serra, Tony, 247, 281
Shanghai Volunteer Corps, 89, 91
Shawula, Adam, 287
Silly Billy, 44
Simopoulos, Artemis, 345
Slaga, Thomas, 345
Smith, R. Templeton, 129-134
Societe Hoteliere de Tahiti, 243

Index

Somodi, Joe, 287
South Seas Enterprises, Ltd., 244-245
St. Augustine, Florida 1887 fire, 19-20
Standard Oil Company of New York (SOCONY), 35
Stanford University, California, USA, 340
Stay Well!, 154-155
Stephens, Henry, 113-114, 117-118, 148
Sterling, Penny, 287, 327
Stevens, CS, 59
Stewart, Alma, 120-121
Strategic Planning, 324-326
Strawberry Wall, 180, 223
Stuart, Elbridge, 63-65
Sun Yat-sen, 92-93, 94
Sun Yat-sen University, Guangzhou, China, 340
Surh, Young-Joon, 341
Sustainable Farming, 334-338
Swanson, Bob, 138
Szent-Györgyi, Albert, 117
Takaki, Kanehiro, 47
Telescope house, Idyllwild, California, 290
Tenkoff, Stefan, 220-221, 232, 237, 247, 273-276, 282-284, 287, 298, 310-311, 318-319
Thompson, Mildred. *See* Rehnborg, Mildred
Trona Pot-Ash, 107, 110
Trona, California, 106-107
Umpleby, Merle, 287
Umsted, Ed, 192
Upton, Alice. *See* Rehnborg, Alice
Upton, Benjamin, 19, 29
Van Andel, Dave, 336
Van Andel, Jay, 217-218, 224-225, 258-264, 305-306, 324-325
Vaughn, Fuzzy, 53, 89-90, 133, 161, 221
Vaughn, Sallie, 133, 160-161, 211
Vaughn, Sara, 133
Vertical integration, 336
Vitamin Products Company, 118-119, 127-128
Vitamins
    adding to product, 140
    current and obsolete terms, 366–368
    synthetic, 148
VITASOL. *See* Early products
Wales, Sam, 123, 127
Wall Street Journal ad, 1959, 259
Warren, Frank, 147, 151, 153
Westall, Ed, 287
Whipple, George, 117
White House Conference on Food, Nutrition, and Health, 1969, 286, 288-289
Williams, Roger, 150-151
Yearly savings program, 197, 392
Yin and yang, 73
Yonsei University, Seoul, Korea, 340